# Copyright

Note:

Paul Cathcart is not a Doctor or Medical Professional of any kind. All content is based solely on personal experience and opinion. This book is a memoir only.

This book is not intended as a substitute for the medical advice of physicians. The reader should regularly consult a physician in matters relating to his/her health and particularly with respect to any symptoms that may require diagnosis or medical attention.

# Persona non grata with

# diabetes

# Simply, Natasha

"To my family, for dragging me out from hell. Victor, I want to be just like you when I grow up. Nolan, you hold me up when you don't even know you are doing it. I have been waiting a long time to say those words. //And '*Little*' Jo Day and Natasha for catching the man whores and genital harpies (sub-editing)."

"I tell you how messed up diabetes is: the medical community actually looks at you funny when your blood sugar is level. – He must be cheating, they think to themselves."

Paul Cathcart

# Preface

Thank you for giving me this opportunity to speak with clear voice as an everyday diabetic.

My bet is that through diabetes we are all going through roughly the same. We live together-though-worlds-apart in some variation of the same highly stressed society, set within an ever more-anxious day and age; we share in the same (often-broken) *ideal* fundamental social grouping of family, standing surrounded by the same choices. So chances are you have either been through, are at present going through or may encounter the same diabetic screams as I have.

Life's everyday factors of broken hearts and social influence; becoming lost and swallowed in a loved one's emotional turmoil; pulled down by an inner depression, that stuff you keep at the back of your mind or career fatigue. Chances are at some point you are going to be left buckling under pressure with diabetes giving way under your feet, desperately trying to find a way out. Waiting for someone to convince you that you're okay, that what you are going through is perfectly normal and that it's not your fault. – And it's not, you are, so please relax and everything will be fine. And just for your thoughts, what you are going through is very, very real.

As diabetics we must factor in the stresses and strains of everyday life with the fluctuations they cause to our condition. My core belief is that the *Diabetes Industry* has yet to fully come to terms with this (us), continuing to treat lightly the impact day-to-day living has on our health, and health has on our quality of life; overlooking the diabetic in the treatment of diabetes.

I've been mixing bottled insulin with life now for just over seventeen years, implementing a system of trial and error toward errant sugar (read: emotion) along the way. Such an approach has given me freedom to pursue the potential of my career; to often surpass the limits of sense, entering into excess in my private life, and perhaps most importantly, it has allowed me to body swerve reluctance, entertaining myself with the quality of life that I want.

However, for all the varying levels of success returned, trial and error has only ever dragged me through: failing to prepare for the life confounding constant drama this condition would conspire, negating to reveal the severe underbelly of true ill health or the spiralling self-doubt and distress caused by simply imperfect blood sugar. In the absence of any real world insight as to what we're struggling with (comfort blanket); or rejuvenated health care system; what would really have been useful is some sort of heads up, an indication to the tough times that lay ahead, a pocket guidebook for living a *real life* with diabetes – or a compendium for that matter. Ideally though, a *'Big Brother'* diabetic buddy system and confidence of shared experience with someone to say,

> *"Hey, that same thing happened to me and look out for this or don't feel bad about that. I've been through this already and it got me too but look on it like this and it's not so bad plus you can avoid it happening again in the future by..."*

Taken from *'A book I wish someone had written'*

In essence, someone who understands my on-going needs; my potential and future difficulties, someone who has been around the block a few times who can advise or at least reminisce on the profound professional, social and personal challenges to be overcome should I wish to continue with any resemblance of normal life – more than that, an idyllic life. A friend who can talk me through getting over the worst of it – or at least getting on top of it, even if it may already be too late for them.

And with that (and you) in mind I have written '*Persona non grata with diabetes*,' a lowbrow walkthrough of real life with diabetes, hoping that from within these shared pages we are able to draw parallels and exchange in lifetime experience, exemplified throughout in life defining moments. None of which stray too far, if at all, from a life with diabetes but all of which touch on this condition in one way or another; offering comfort in the knowledge that what we are going through both physically and emotionally is shared by us all.

Paul Cathcart · Diabetic, class of 1993

# Heads, diabetes

So what's the point to this open memoir? Contemporary outlook and well designed as it is. There are countless books already stacking shelves on the subject of *diabetes*, covering everything from introductions to, diets for (essentially fast food brochures), how to spot and even miracles to cure. – Although if *Dr. Young* with his '*pH Miracle*' looked deep enough into my blood cells all he would find is confusion and guilt.

We have courses for sufferers with long, supportive and understanding names such as *S.A.D.I.E (Skills for Adjusting Diet and Insulin in East Sussex)*, *D.A.F.N.E (Dose Adjustment for Normal Eating)* and *D.E.S.M.O.N.D.S (Diabetes Education and Self-Management for Ongoing and Newly Diagnosed)* enabling us with new coping mechanisms for a *modern, life balanced* approach to *diabetes*. – Unfortunate then that my Diabetes Specialist Nurses refused to share any answers till *week four*.

As for experts, we have unprecedented access to *Diabetes Experts* in every major hospital both private and state; sharing with them a wealth of tens of thousands of years combined medical knowledge. The benefits of which are then distilled and filtered throughout proven chains of communication, via Consultants to Doctors, Dieticians and Nurses, right down to Pharmacists and the

Optometrists. – My Doctor does not know his arse from his elbow.

Supporting these are the multi trillion dollar *Global Pharmaceutical Industries*, where the white coats of the scientific and medical professions break down *diabetes* even further, on a molecular biological and genetic level: additional insight gained only through the diligent and meticulous cross referencing of clinical trial outcomes in a million other research fields. – Before piecing and packaging it all back together again with the latest product developments (plastic pens), marketing trials data and foresight from Public Relations *Ribena Executives.*

Not to mention, *Diabetes Aware* Human Resource Departments offering assurance to every major corporate entity, complementary medicine – Herbal Therapy Stores on every high street corner and *Diabetes Proficient* Personal Trainers at every gym. We even have *diabetes iPhone* apps and websites offering to sell·on our unused equipment. – HR departments in their insufferable role to placate the diabetic employee, whilst assessing the company's legal standpoint prior to sacking. – David Cameron, I will get to you later.

As for registered Diabetes Charities and advocacy, advocating what exactly? Smiling faces, corporate sponsorship, helium balloons and tax avoidance for the benefit of whom? And all of this just for us to be instilled with an understanding of our condition and given the support necessary to cope with and conquer our life as a *person with diabetes.*

Heads or tails?

# Tails, diabetic

Health Sectors refuse to even acknowledge our real physical and day-to-day burden; failing entirely to address a diabetic's tireless aftermath of symptoms and complications. They practice instead a rudimentary knowledge of mock diabetes, the simple to conceptualise though difficult to maintain principle of *normalising* (not even a real word) blood sugar levels between numerals four and eight: instigated by administering more and more insulin on instruction of the *Pharmaceutical Industry* (*moo*) under the false impression that this *harmless hormone* has side effects overcome simply by having more sugar. Pushing all responsibility back into the hands of the hapless diabetic to avoid the consequence of having a *dry mouth* or feeling a *touch tired* (bore) etc., before delving effortlessly into the black revelation, 'Your kidneys will fail, your feet will go black and complete loss of sight awaits... if you are not a good boy.'

As for our state of mind and emotional wellbeing, complications, relationships and long-term future: less obvious to the outside world of course but of equal importance for us, forget it! Don't even bother, the *Diabetes Industry* does not wish to contemplate (*our pish*) an obligatory responsibility for even one moment, 'Buy a *Diet-Coke*, read a diet book and just get on with it,' don't go rocking the *cash cow* business model by mixing up real world expectation for expensive scientific observation with financial models stretching out higher and higher into years ahead. They don't want resulting mental anguish (*more of our pish*) hurting business, interrupting a main stream of income, when sticking to the easy to theorise assumptions of, 'Tired and grouchy but nothing too serious,' proves so efficient. Until that is, the day you fall angrily down a manhole like a mad Pirate, and then they say, 'Oh, it must have been the high sugars not *normalising* really getting him down.'

*Out of sight out of mind;* altogether it's the equivalent of everyone you so desperately need to know putting their fingers in their ears and shouting, 'I CAN'T HEAR YOU, I CAN'T HEAR YOU.'

The problem is that *they* see diabetes only as a disease, not as the *state-of-being* it has become for the diabetic. *They* study a life with diabetes, but it's not my life. *They* don't cover panic attacks as my blood sugar spirals out of control for reasons unknown; or the frustration, upset and pointlessness I feel when I can't figure out why, taking my confidence levels from that of a thirty-two year old man and reducing them to those of a frail seventy year old in a matter of minutes. *They* don't relate to my inability to concentrate at points throughout the day as blood sugar levels fluctuate and no one wants to know about the, 'FUCK. FOR FUCK SAKE, FUCK,' like anger I feel when my sugar is high. This leaves me feeling like a complete bastard when it all comes crashing back down.

*Nor do they acknowledge the disparity that pregnant women are expected to go positively nuts due to hormonal imbalance, to the point where in England they are unlikely even to be arrested for shoplifting and they have the right to urinate anywhere; including some say the inside of a Policeman's helmet! – Yet we who are injecting ourselves with synthetic-foreign hormones all day everyday, whilst sharing similar food craving, are supposed to hold it together – and not even have an ugly day.*

I ask myself, how are we to cut past poor decision; let down and left off balance as the ones we depend upon have given way to ignorance: accepting their role of *Sales Team* for an industry as our suitable health-care solution? Therein lies the state of the *Diabetes Industry*, shackled to the state of our condition and the purpose of this book.

This book is not about diabetes the disease of medical definition; this book is about diabetics. The flip side of the coin; an open memoir, a written sketchpad of my life without faceless diagrams or conditions, serving to honestly assess this *state-of-being* we all share in its highs and lows: the soul of this disease, the textures leading up to the cause of, and living. Offering you on the way a chance to say, 'I know just what you mean. I know exactly how that feels, and Oh Jesus I won't be drinking that!' whilst I recap to find and learn how to fix myself.

As much as this world thinks it knows about diabetes, I find it can often be a very difficult and lonely place, and to my comprehension the only way we're ever going to get through this is with a *rightful understanding* based upon shared experience. Only then can we accept a *just responsibility* toward our health. We should not be willing participants in any *Diabetes Industry* settling for second best. That's not the diabetic I am willing to be. I've waited around for seventeen years already, a lifetime when you consider it was all entirely avoidable in the first place.

Before I go, I know we have access to a thousand more websites and forums offering up group support and enabling us to share our thoughts, but who wants to bicker about how much sugar is really in a banana or start a bun fight to determine which blood sugar test monitor is the best? Don't we all just want to have a healthy, uncomplicated and great life with plenty of room for big nights out and not having to stop half way through a shag for a *Mars Bar*!


Tails.

# Persona non grata with

# diabetes

Well my passport describes me as, "Cathcart, Paul, Stuart, British Citizen, Date de naissance 04 Feb 77, Sexe M, Lieu de naissance Glasgow," and displays me in an out of date photo, a couple of stone overweight and badly needing a shave.

Supporting this is a letter from my Doctor – which he charged me twenty pounds for the privilege of, informing the thick people of *easyJet, "The above mentioned has Type 1 Diabetes Mellitus confirmed at the age of sixteen and is insulin dependent requiring that he carry insulin and the necessary equipment with him."* Approval sought proving just enough to scupper reservations of bright orange persons behind a bright orange check-in desk and wipe away contrary expression as I *\*highly nasally accented,* 'GO THROUGH,' my bag of sharps intact. – Is that a fake tan or are easyTracy and easySharon sporting all out nicotine stains? '\*THEY MIGHT ASK YOU TO PROVE IT AGAIN AT THE GATE... SO KEEP IT, YOUR LETTER, WITH YOU,' it screams like a banshee, obviously not wanting to let things pass quite so lightly, but one up for the *everyday diabetic* I tell myself as I skip on through the rest of my trip uninterrupted. A completely different state of affairs from that afforded when I fly *BA*, who being far more compos mentis, preside, 'Welcome aboard Sir, diabetes, yes that's fine and if there is anything that we can do to help?' before further reassuring, 'We have plenty of *Diet-Coke* on board sir, for all that complimentary vody soon to be in your body Sir.' – A gentleman's understanding I feel.

I've never been a diary person, not one of those people who write everything down into a secret notebook hidden under their bed, but I do like those people. Nor am I one of those who *tweet* and blog thoughts not belonging to them; though I do follow one-thousand live feeds of *persons with diabetes*, screaming out and falling down; and I'm certainly not one to force-feed the world status reports. – Posting pretty pictures, collecting compliments and as many friends as possible; never speaking directly mind, just talking down *en masse* and confusing high numbers for self-confidence. I'll stop this French thing in a minute, it just makes me chuckle.

I see diaries and autobiographies as fascination, the epitome of human being, not the ghost written dwindling of a hard faced tart breaking up with her boyfriend in time for Christmas publication. Anne Frank – no, she's not a hard faced tart – now that's a diary, although it bored me silly at school. Malcolm X, now that's an autobiography, I just need to get around to reading the second half. I rarely write anything down at all, except ideas for my comic book, which I scribble down and sketch into a secret notebook then I hide it under my bed.

I've never actually read a memoir; to be honest I got into this completely oblivious as to how hard it would be. I hadn't realised till half way through, how much writing this book meant to me; though this open approach feels poised to the ethos of this communication, plus it's nice to write down ones musings in not such rigid a structure as a formal diary would dictate. Whereas autobiographies, those seem at their best when on the subject of the deceased ...three, two, one ... no still here.

It's become very fashionable of late to write a letter back to ones sixteen year old self, with the age old adage, 'If I knew then what I know now.' And If you happen to be around sixteen and reading this, *you lucky bastard!* As hard as it may be at times, life is great and diabetes won't slow you down, frankly there is no reason for you to become any more ill.

Maybe this is a little bit like that, a letter to my childhood self, expressing comfort that I'm going to be okay. But more so it's about reliving and unwinding, with pendulous levels of laughter and deep breaths, the circumstance, cause and affect which place me where I am. A time-out chance to think through every key moment, summoning memories long since buried. Head-in-my-hands-realisations of love and life in startling clarity: staring into open hands remorseful and peering into nothingness, owing, thankful and letting go. I hate even admitting to myself I have a disease.

My life as a red balloon if you will, unclasped and rising, let go by a child's hand: taken form around the questions a sick diabetic asks themselves on any given day. Why did I become diabetic? I never felt this ill before, so when did I become a sick person? When did I become a weak person? Worse still, when did I become a meek person and how am I ever going to make myself better? And, am I still worthwhile?

My current situation is that I am lost, my character as thin as my skin pale, confidence gone, expectation extinguished; soaked through with doubt, nurtured in worry, close to giving up entirely. I used to be better than this. I used to look the world dead in the eye and swore I could stare down the sun, now the world's gotten the better of me. Responsibility for everything and it's all too hard I fear I am letting everyone down. But I'm making myself better. Maybe it's the time I find on my hands, or my current health status, this book just seems right.

*It's just turned a minute past midnight on the 24/Dec/2009, so I'm popping over to give Natasha a kiss on her head. We're getting married a year from today.

Note // Please excuse coarse and colourful language throughout: all natural reactions to real life recollections and I would be a liar if I were to be all, polite and flowery, about everything that has happened; especially those bastards who should have known better. On top of that, I'm typing away on a half broken *Dell* laptop with a screen consistently flickering before going blank on receiving the slightest nudge.

# Dating, late twenties

An orchestra of tits and bums: two au pairs in my one very small bed, caressing and touching, stroking and oohing. I'm standing there a useless prick testing my sugar for the sixth time; reduced to an onlooker at the world's most interactive show. The only thing stopping me from cumming is the shock of all the excitement that this is happening to me, and adrenalin mixing with sugar making me shake.

Walking down West End Lane, returning from *Sainsbury's* and a severe hypo in their customer car park, she sputters from prolonged silence, 'I know you're diabetic and everything and when that happens it's important you have sugar and everything – then the Australian tan lined face of fucked off – but I've had a bad headache all day and I haven't gone on about it.' Then she dumps me.

*Bradleys' Spanish Bar*, just off Oxford St, Sunday afternoon, boozy conversation with an out of hours client, discussing what colleagues she has fucked and my sugars fallen in the background to two point eight. I'm munching through a *Snickers* bar; head still halfway into my bag. I turn back to her, she leaps backward three feet, 'Stay away from me, I'm allergic to peanuts.' I'm glad she never wanted to see me again. I'd give up sex before I'd give up on *Snickers* bars.

I met her on *Myspace*, tall, blonde, size zero; she drinks as much as I do, and not only gets her round in but returns with a packet of cigarettes from the bar; returning to find me having my night-time insulin when her face falls. Her ex-boyfriend was diabetic, he went out of control when his sugar was out of control, then slapped her around. Didn't help his name is also Paul.

'In my country, where I was a Nurse, so many men they have this. And then their toes go black and feet need to be cut off.' One step at a time; whatever it takes to get away from this Czech Princess.

Saw her sitting on a bench reading her book in Paddington Station; long blonde hair as in her description, pretty face as in the photo. Shoulders on down getting wider and rounder to seemingly no end, certainly not in her profile; no way am I dating this heifer. So I slip on by, facing the opposite direction, hand in my jackets right pocket turning down the volume rocker. Out of the station, heading back toward trusty Abbey Road and a quick text message to say, "*Sorry I can't make it my diabetes is playing up.*"

My mobile phone goes and it's the Art Student; she had only just started driving home twenty minutes ago, 'Tears, crying, upset, you treated me like you never wanted me there all weekend. You made me feel completely in your way.' I certainly didn't mean to, I really quite liked the Brightonian girl, and she looked great wearing nothing but a red cowboy hat.

# Today

*Today* I opened a letter from the Diabetes Eye-Screening Clinic. I'm going to go blind.

The only thing holding in hysteria is fear. It's over isn't it? Please tell me it isn't over. I can't be over before I've even gotten anywhere, before I've even given up on myself. Everything once so promising has been taken, like a vicious knife attack but slow, far slower, couldn't really twist it in more. "The first stages of Background Retinopathy." black print on white paper, an accompanying leaflet listing all the ways it can go wrong from here. I can't feel anything. I'm less than numb and unbalanced from the knees up. I guess this is the shock. I fold it back into the pile of faceless letters from the bank and hold onto Natasha for dear life, 'It's not even highlighted in red. It doesn't even say urgent on the envelope.' It's been laying there for months now amongst a pile of loose bank letters. We stand together frozen, a nightmare where the scream does not come out. White letter and black text.

But how can this happen? I was there at the test; the woman was short and Spanish, she was apologising for the machine having being broken previously and this being a return visit. She put me at ease, told me I'd be fine when I told her how I was scared of eye tests, of how my mum now had glaucoma in the family history and that I was

3

terrified of losing my sight; as my hands trembled.

She said from the first looks of photographs she had taken of the backs of my eyes, that there was nothing obviously wrong, no apparent damage; a couple of marks to be expected following near seventeen years of diabetes. Though nothing of obvious concern and some much needed reassurance these were yearly tests set directly to pick up any *early warning* signs of decay; so as to give the experts to whom these photographs would be sent much advanced notice. 'Were they to find anything serious, they can treat a patient in advance with all the wonders of modern medicine and laser eye care therapy. Being able to eradicate it there and then,' she said. Words taken and held onto like a comfort blanket.

But this letter doesn't mention any of that; black text on white paper with no personal signature it reads I have the first stages of Background Retinopathy and the accompanying tissue-thin colour brochure states that *one direction* this *may go* in can be treated *in some instances* with laser eye care surgery: that this can work for a *small percentage of some people with diabetes.* Presenting next on profoundly colourful print another half dozen or so untreatable ways it'll no doubt accelerate.

Back to the letter, they want to see me again in a year to track what route of deterioration my eyes have taken. A YEARS TIME before looking into possible treatments, if any and in the meantime I am to sit tight and it is most important I should keep my blood sugar(s) level. I can't deal with today's letter, it is again sealed, folded then stacked and shelved amongst the bottom end, two-thirds down a stack of white paper envelopes that I'll never open.

...

I'm sitting at the kitchen table, exquisite finish stone floor and back to a wood burning stove; Natasha clasping both hands in hers, forcing me to make eye contact and promising me I'll be fine, that everything is going to be okay. I know I won't be. 'The *NHS* is wrong, these people are always wrong. So poorly fucking trained half of them could not get a job anywhere else. We will have a professional evaluation done, a private second opinion. How can they say something like this then tell you to wait a year? It must be wrong.' Our heads say it's wrong, our hearts say it's wrong, all fairness says it's wrong. 'My life is over.' Her diamond engagement ring sparkles; life together forever and already I know I can't put her through it. I can't and it will hurt her but in the long run she will be better off.

I'm only forty percent in the room, the rest of me burrowing down into the spot of the mind which copes with grief as we move upstairs to be more comfortable in some strange continuation. Sat on the edge of the couch staring blankly at the television, the screen's a familiar bright blue media hub. Staring at walls in the bathroom; a green hue clearly defined by *Farrow & Ball*, a room full of keen designers who mulled it over for months. Vinyl recordings passing over me in the bath as river clear water licks at my form in tiny waves making equal-delicate splashing sounds. Green flash of light in my right eye when I blink, how much of this is real concern, how much of it obsessing? Days pass days with no real sleep in between; I'm saying goodbye in my head to the kittens as I stroke them on the curve of pale yellow beech wood flooring, framed against a chocolate box window, clasped shut and leading out to the courtyard. And I'm welling up on answering the front door; it's all I can think about. It's my own fault for not being more careful. It's too late and it's my own fault. I am to blame. I am the one who pissed it all away. I'm saying goodbye to people in my head. I'm too scared to even hold my eyes closed just for one moment to imagine forever blindness.

How will I come to terms with this? How can I tell Nathan and the people I care about? Tell them I want to see them face-to-face one more time because eventually I'll never see them again, and I want them to see me and remember me strong? – Though I could use the hug. How can I tell Nolan? He was shit enough already when I told him my dad was dying, "I, how do you feel about that then?" how is he going to cope with this? I can't tell my mum or Angela it will kill them. That blind girl in *Nice n Sleazy*, she held her head with such dignity, she was poised and beautiful. I can't even touch on being able to begin to imagine how she deals with this. How will Natasha look after me; how will I ever manage to be a Dad, how will I manage not to ruin her life? What if my eyes go all white and I have the shame of wearing dark sunglasses so as not to make people around me feel uncomfortable. Can I expect her life to become that of a full time Care Worker? I won't do it. I won't make her poor; I won't drag her life down with mine. I won't put her through this. The shame in that. – Kind of a null point, but if I get a Guide Dog then I want a blonde one; somewhere in my mind I do fancy getting a dog. Blue would have made an excellent Guide Dog.

When we were kids we used to talk about, 'What would you prefer if you had to choose between going deaf or going blind?' Deaf of course always being the answer, no more having to listen to stupid questions. When I'm walking down the road I not-often see these old men pushing ahead so slowly and the pity that falls on them as they find footing on bobbled red stone as indicator to the vicinity of traffic lights and the road in front on which they might stumble. Guide Dogs, those Labradors give them nothing but patience and love. Mum and Gran knew of a blind man local to them, he was led half way across the Shettleston Road then left to fend for himself. This plays on my mind. What I would give to be heartbroken right now, heartbreak is easy. Or sacked for being shit and ill, I miss that. – I'd never complain about that again: it never closed down my world like this. It all seems so pointless now, so nonchalant, and so bloody mediocre; reality has changed so much, and I want it to go back to how it was and for this to be simply wrong.

I remember being in the lifts of fancy hotels, in run down flats; numeric metal pads with arrows for ups and downs, the ding of a bell if you were lucky and perhaps a green light of indication on arrival but last on any list was some braille centred within an inch squared barely embossed button within enormous bustling-chandelier foyers or glumly lit green on blue mosaic tiles drenched in bleach. In either case how the fuck was a blind person supposed to find that button? When Mum first told me she had glaucoma I naively tried to comfort her by saying, 'But Mum, the Doctor said that it's really slow. That you might not get bad till you're in your seventies.' And she explained to me that's no better, that it's worse, that this is when she is old and she is frail, fragile and scared: a defenceless old lady without even her sight. I haven't felt so close to her in such a long time and I can't tell her why. Why did I not spend more time with her when she found out, why did I not hold her more, why was I not more there for her?

This reminds me of being on the plane to Philly one day and asking a Nun to pray for my mum's eyes as I knew her prayers would be more powerful than my own. Then I went onto sin; as if asking someone to do better work for me would help her, while I went on being horrible and getting worse.

Now there is the thought of my early conversations with my very first Diabetes Specialist Nurse, Sister Shepherd, of how I would need to sit my driving test every four years due to, "Potential quick eye deterioration caused by poor diabetes control." This would never happen to me. Then there is the joke about Jake the blind man; he turns up at a Nun's door and on knocking she calls out, 'I'm in the shower, who is it?' and he replies, 'It's Jake the blind man.' So she thinks to herself, no harm there, I'll pop out and see everything is okay. Jake just smiles and says, 'Nice tits love, and there's your blinds.'

# Burn out

Hollow bag of nerves; I can't be the only person going through this. If this is happening to me then it has to be happening to a thousand others every day. The constant not knowing where you stand; the bullshit reassurance whilst being pushed into obsolescence; being led down the path with the same fucking lies, by the same fucking people in their same fucking stations peddling their same bullshit un-illuminated knowledge to us damn idiots who hold out our hands hoping things will get better. 'FUCK, FUCK, FUCK, FOR FUCK SAKE FUCK.' Natasha watches me kick the wall and cries into her hands. 'Fucking cunts have killed me.' I'm in tears, 'Fuck I'm only thirty-two.'

When I close my eyes it stings. The sting details what I can lose. Maybe the tears will well to wash my nerves. Remedy my blindness. At least before I was only on the shelf, now I'm a corpse. I thought I had this all figured out in time.

And I'm so sorry it's my own entire fault. I've dropped myself through the cracks. That's what I've always been so afraid of: dropping through the cracks, left rotting. But I bet I can make them take notice; sit up and take notice, fucking stand to attention, maybe help others avoid making the same mistakes I have in the first place or at least make sense of it. A book would be my answer, justify some kind of self-belief. Give me some point, but can I honestly risk the time and money it will cost to take such a leap? Am I actually well enough to return to normal work anyway? I don't think so.

More than that, I'm too scared to re-join the real world. I've been hiding. My blood is again acid and my heart heavy and still. Everything is difficult and working against me; it's worth getting angry about, and God I am angry. And the fear and the panic then the calm: I'm not scared of the diabetic pain; I'm in no real fear of dying. I'm afraid of being afraid. Sleepless nights, pools of sweat, bouts of confidence; my own blood is a traitor dissolving me from the inside; like a son going against the will his father; I feel it burning through my arteries and taste it in my spit. Anxiety trickled down raw nerves, my heart palpitates, thoughts again turn negative; always waiting in the background for panic and worry to set in and it's all just high sugar; deep down all I need is a couple, maybe a few months of good blood sugar and I know I'll be fine.

The thought of travelling into work seems exhausting enough and memories of waiting to become ill are not helping any. The problem is that so many no longer want me around; I'll be honest with you, I'm not the easiest person to be around. Quivering; struggling to get in the front door in the first place, and my blood sugar being so rancid that I had to turn around and go home with my tail between my legs to everyone's bemusement; feeling like the elephant leaving the room; made worse when they choose not to believe me, laying blame rather than accept. What is the difference between weak and meek? It's the inability to deal with life. When did diabetes become my full time occupation? Isn't it now irrelevant?

At least here I can have a stab at this in my own time, in my own hours, see how things pan out and concentrate on my recovery with some sense of purpose. A book will give me good enough reason to make some sense of myself and soul searching seems the proper place to start.

# Blind

And diamonds shine as they always have, on an engagement ring displaying to me all the colours of the world. How do you be blind? I mean, how will I tell what I like anymore? Doesn't it all become a single endless black space, me a worthless void? Won't I miss the noise and bustle of people surrounding me when I'm standing on the platform, when meandering the streets of Marylebone?

Blind, London plays out her wares before me; easier to remember Baker St, July through September's evenings than it is anything else; amber lights merging, alternating between greens and reds, dusk fading through deeper warm blue; high stools around barrels, smiles and the chink of wine glasses. Gloss black taxis streaming by fast food monopoly neon signs, cheap iconic glow reaching farther than the sweet stench of their contents. Cigarette ends balanced on bin lids, the numbers of a thousand lost girls in telephone booths, countless repetitive office blocks and air so polluted as to damage your lungs the equivalent of ten cigarettes per day, yet still heralding triumphant the air Queen Victoria.

Black kids being pushy in *KFC*, white guys feigning superiority but lacking confidence stand at the bar of the *Sherlock Holmes Hotel*. Chinese people doing whatever it is a Chinese person does, hacking on us smelling of butter maybe. Polish girls looking grumpy working

12

in *Tesco*; 'Eastoes,' as I had heard some drunken Australian girl referring to them; as I picked her an orange from a crab apple tree; and their love of nineteen eighties bleached hair with stonewash fashion. Far side of the world superiority to rubbish our gainfully employed Czech, Slovak and Polish population; two year return Visas on which to travel Europe, along with the rest of their classmates; resulting in some long vacation spent in Kilburn or some South London dive where three tenant a shared two-bed accommodation and ten bed-down for the customary, late, five pounds a night. Working in bars; rejecting Scottish currency, working in call centres and banging on about the great beaches back home. A single trip to Italy and the rest spent on the Heathrow Injection: getting fat and high reminiscing on the Bush. 'Aww Yeahh, I know *Fosters* tastes *heaps* better over here and you can't drink it back home. It's simply not made by the same company as *Fosters* in Australia; try reading the back of the tinny while you get blotto on a Sunday morning throwing fruit at each other will you?' Kiwi's pretending to be Australians but can't keep pace, laughing in the face of the TV license, God forbid you even entertain the idea of paying Council Tax. Surprised they won't let you extend your Visa? Really? 'Honestly, you believe cider is made by mixing beer with wine?' Now on with the classic Indians, all bold and swearing out of earshot from their parents, and Iranians calling themselves Persians as they chain-smoke outside the *Globe Bar* on the corner; seriously intelligent, peaceful and kind people.

An undercover Bomb Squad Officer with a seventies style moustache in tight blue denim passes trained eye over our bags and fellow passengers on the upper deck of the one three nine to Waterloo Road as we pass *London-Tokyo Property Services,* coming to a soft stall at the entrance to Baker Street Station just south of *two-two-one B*. Looking down over the flower salesmen standing in the rain, but just happy to

13

be out; collective hearts in our mouths; can't he just stay on till our stop? We'd feel much safer with him on here with us, - even half expecting him to dive through a window into some empty cardboard boxes.

Accelerating past a *Ferrari* from the bus lane, noticing the spiralling weight gain and loss of the woman who only ever acknowledges me when I'm wearing a suit and then she can't stop looking; pulling a left at the pink neon *"Salt Beef"* sign, now crawling past the world-class displays of *Selfridges* as I step off with a jolt at Oxford Circus, cutting right down Little Argyle St – Fuck me *'Chitty Chitty Bang Bang'* is still on and I grab a couple of bags of *Chilli McCoy's* and a twenty deck from the Turkish body builder attending the crate over from *Liberty*. Puffing on a couple of cigarettes down Great Marlborough Street makes me smile, skipping on by puddles and the woman with the worst frizzy hair who never says hello, then on into work at *Megalopolis-Transmission*, Great Chapel St, Soho for seven years. Think I'll walk home tonight if it brightens up, to capture the last part of summer.

Taxi Driver deciding spur of the moment whether or not he likes the young woman as she exits, 'Snotty cow,' he thinks to himself as he *struggles* deliberately foraging for change; pilfering suited flocks descending down for that quick drink after work the English do oh so well. Well maybe a bottle but not four in the morning, well not tonight. A surprising lack of Scottish and Irish tramps on the streets this evening, we must have been forced along Edgware Road so as not to offend the tourists.

People down here have the wrong perception of us as a nation of tramps; we do not have a preoccupation with urine, nor are we a race of drunken train spotters. My brethren stuck here could just never fully fathom the overly complicated Underground Rail Network with its double pronged Northern Line or shape of the Circle Line; unable to justify the value of a ticket so they missed that vital job interview and languish incarcerated here, backs to station walls instead. Having a few cans, baking in the sun, tops off, practicing for public speaking engagements: just getting ready and figuring a few things out. And it's not the packed location from which to beg spare change they gravitate toward; it's the close proximity to a good chip shop whilst pissed. Since London has so few, these vagrants are instead getting by sipping on *rose* wine and dining out on *Halal Fried Chicken*. Occasionally walking face first into automated doors at *Tesco Metro* past closing time and scaring shitless the Polish girl, stacking shelves. – 'It just shows ye how clean they can get they windies, din't it?' instructing with quivering arm, all bearded and wet against glass. Oh look, five Nigerian Traffic Wardens and a blonde transsexual one.

*The girl nearly trips out of her cab, left foot sticking then twisting in the curb. He is staring on through the wing mirror hoping to chance a glance of something; leg or cleavage anything will do so long as he can tell his mates about the sort he had in the back earlier. Pondering, should he give her the duff fiver? She narrowly avoids a puddle, talk about exhausted, 'Thank god I got my hair blow dried at lunch time, I looked like a French Poodle by the time I got into work this morning. Twenty-five pounds in a taxi for two tube stops and it's worth it to see an old friend I haven't seen in ages,' she tells herself. 'Wonder how he is getting on? Seems to be doing really well!' pulling back on the steel arm of heavy glass, the Door Man nowhere to be seen, 'I hope he is here,' as her hair turns again to frizz and a group of rich Arabic men watch her struggle as though she were filth. 'I need three drinks already, one just to settle down from my day, one to wake up and maybe another two to have a good laugh at my hair,' – Still talking to herself.*

15

*He is at the bar all pissed up and getting lairy with himself, no one else will pay him any attention. Kisses on the cheek and a hug, he does not want to let her go. Wanking off about her all last night and again twice this morning: met her in a hotel bar for a reason, she must know it; must be into him. He knows that she fancied him when he was with his ex.*

'Christ, what time have you been here since?' – *Polite question, his hand still on her hip.*

*'I went out with the boys from work. Boozy lunch, well you know. We kept the plonk going and did shots till three.' – Oi Oi Jack the lad.*

*Bullshit, he has been in here since five-past-six, arrived sober as a Judge and knocking back Russian Standard to calm his nerve; plans of taking the lead and just booking a room in advance ending faster than an email trail to bored colleagues about his spoils for this evening.*

'Do you want to get a table? My feet are killing me. It's so good to see you.'

*Sitting together, secluded table at the back of the room: fashionable lighting and no room for elbows.*

'So how are you? What have you been doing? Are you still living in Clapham with Kirsten?'

'No I moved out; I'm staying at a mates, things got too heavy. I thought you never liked Kirsten anyway?'

'What? Why? No, I thought she was lovely. Why would you think that?' – 'She was way out of your league as far as I can remember. Oh shit, now I'm starting to remember, he was a bit of a sleaze while he was drunk,' – Inner voice.

*Waitress comes over, 'Hi, Are you ready to order? What can I get you?'*

'Oh could I see the wine list please?'

16

*'Same again?' – The waitress smiling too much: clearly he has been tipping hard.*

*'What is it that you're having?' – Already not fancying the idea.*

*'Two double Vodka Red Bulls?' he garbles.*

*'Oh, I thought I could smell Red Bull. No. I'll just have a glass of Sauvignon Blanc,' she interrupts.*

*'So what about you? You are still single?' lurching forward peeking down her top.*

*'No, I met someone special; really special, I was going to say that I wanted to introduce you...'*

*'What, I thought you were here to see me!' – All goes quiet. The Ohhh did I just say that / Oh did he just say that staining the air. Some movement of cutlery and menus before the waitress leans over with more drinks. Neither having to look to notice he is staring at her tits.*

*Quick change of subject, 'So how is your work, are you still trading?'*

*'Fucking nightmare,' as he pours in more Red Bull than the glass will possibly allow. Any attempt at pretending to be sober now over the table with the ice cubes.*

*'Oh, what's happened, are you not enjoying it?' – Concern? – All but indifference and clearly searching out an entertaining story.*

*'I love the money but I lost a boat?'*

*'WHAT?'*

*'I've lost a boat filled with LNG, Liquid Natural Gas.'*

*'WHAT? Are you joking? How can you lose a boat?' – As she giggles: not even*

*trying to hold it in, 'Patronising turd, I know what LNG is,' – Inner voice.*

*'Don't laugh, it's not funny.' – All stern like a crap Dad.*

*'You have lost a boat, who loses a boat, how can you even lose a boat?'*

*'The radio is broke and it has a leak, the Coast Guard cannot raise them.' Bla bla bla he stammers on for a furthermore polite drink and excuses are made before he tries to grasp her wrist as she stands to leave. Letting go before she even tries to pull away.*

*Now in KFC and made eye contact with a boy with a patois, 'Tsss, look at you babes, you can go before me, your boyfriend must be one lucky guy. WHICKED, you get me?' – Finally someone has been nice to her today and she smiles coyly.*

*Taxi to Abbey Road.*

*My door chaps, an impish Natasha popping her head around when I answer. Six foot one and a half inch stands giggling, clutching her powder blue cardigan pocket to the left of her smile, her right paw holding out a paper bag and a plastic carrier of KFC.*

*'He lost his boat!' Kisses and smiles.*

*'What?'*

*'He is a complete fucking idiot. What a sleazy, eeeyyyhhhh,' noise from the back of her throat, Jewish descendancy in full flow, 'He lost his boat!' – Grinning like a loon.*

*'Laughs, Who? What? What are you talking about? Get in, you're soaked.'*

*'Look at my hair? I look like an Afghan Hound.' – Pleased to be home.*

*'You look lovely, you're mental, what are you talking about, how can you lose a boat?'*

*'He was a total nightmare; mmmm Rolo Ice Cream I forgot I got that, get spoons please.' – Grin. 'He has lost a tanker containing liquid gas, the communications are down and it's got a leak, HA.'*

This is my London and I'm not willing to let it go. This is where I made my world. It is where I met this beautiful woman who would take me as her husband.

How she will describe the world to me? How can she spend her life trying to make up to me all that I miss? Would I do it for her? Yes in an instant, but will I put her through it? I do not have a choice, neither of us have. We couldn't live without each other, well we wouldn't want to no matter how bad it gets.

To see someone happy, will I be able to tell that only by her voice? Maybe you're reading this and you know me; maybe you're thinking, 'I know him, he can get through this, he finds joy in hopelessness, he finds the good in life and he will smell her beauty, touch her breast and the light of her life will bring joy to his heart; being blind is far from being dead.' Maybe you're thinking, 'He can't do this. Better him than me,' and it's perfectly natural.

# State-of-being

And there was me, sitting on the pavement for hours in the sun; picking my nose and eating it; built like a little tank, dressed in a tightly fitting rainbow coloured t-shirt, and navy blue shorts all covered in dust; clutching luminous green and aquamarine thick cordial ice poles, watching formations of birds gather and glide together in the sky, rising and tumbling then looping back over, a handful falling out only to be swept back in then dive again.

How I love the smell when moisture from raindrops falls upon the summer's dust.

He would make my sister hold onto his lit cigarette while he beat our mother. She could handle herself when it came to the violence, but even as the strongest woman in the world, she could no longer endure the psychological torture so we ran.

...

Yells fell silent, as the sky dimmed its summer blues and yellow for an autumnal orange gone thick blood red. Shadows cast of chimneys falling over buildings as birds flocked back to nest; flustered, chirping and panicked, caught off guard by this venerable relapse of nature. Deep chills ran thick down through us all, paused and vulnerable in this sudden stillness of night. A heartbeat would last a second and this moment would last forever? Nature had shown us the true meaning of nurture. Pupils dilated and thoughts stammered; we stand here a series of silhouettes barely acknowledging one another, staring uniformly up at the sun. Heavens rewind as quickly as they had played out before us, the sky lifting into its rightful place. Child's hands dropped aghast in mutterings expressed of relief, mild clapping uplifting to euphoria. The sun shone clear once more with no obtrusion. I'm left standing there, an awkward expression on my face, totally lost in thought and as confused as the sparrows.

How I love the smell when moisture from raindrops falls upon the summer's dust.

...

Drunk with a cut in his hand from breaking glass, forced entry through the front door; pitch-dark bathroom and Mum in tears, clutching onto a towel: he has disconnected the electricity. Slamming the living room door against her to scold with hot plates she is carrying, and the time he had made a huge drama of going out with a large kitchen knife to get the, "Black man," who had pushed him out of a phone box; well these were only a handful of incidents I had witnessed first-hand, reducing this place to only almost a home.

...

At the age of around eight, sitting on my big sister's bed, in her tiny box room with its sloped ceiling she loved so much; the summer's sun kissed evening spellbinding in through a small clasped open window. Chocolate box and full of femininity, the kind of things a boy would never show interest in, other than my big sister Angela was here. Angela and our best friend James Duffy from across the street, whom both took this opportunity to tell me, 'In the morning, instead of

21

going to school, Mum is going to take us, and we're going to run away to live with our gran up in Scotland, because Dad keeps on hitting her.'

They told me this as a secret, there was an element of having to have me prepared in their sentiment, as the sun falls down lower, glistening onto their, not so much older than mine, children's faces. A secret I agreed, and tiptoed up to peer down over my back garden. The sky had gone pink, yellow clouds with purple edges; I had a secret now. I could hear their voices below, him and Mum pretending to get on but the tension was there. A secret from Dad, I would only have to hold onto till tomorrow, which wasn't so far away as soon we would be going to bed. I very much disliked being sent to bed when it was still sunny outside, still bright and the birds chirping.

So sure enough, the following morning with my father safely away at work, we never went to school. The magic three of us instead began making our way to Gloucester Coach Station, having said goodbye in words and with a stroke to our Labrador Blue, and waving goodbye to James's house. A fond memory for every cobble passed, bats and ball games played out along our row of perfectly ill-fitting properties grouped tightly on either side: a single ball's throw road, and bouncing back from the curb to form Widden St, Gloucester. Carrying with us only a leather holdall, some plastic bags and a suitcase full of essential items; leaving behind our childhood pets, and near middle class family home.

...

Now on a bus heading for Cranhill, Glasgow, noted in 'The Paper' as being the seventh worst Council housing estate in Europe, and here we will, all of us cram into our grandparent's home. All of us sharing a two-bedroom accommodation on the fourteenth floor of the seventeen story cement grey Longstone high flats, framed within an even more dreich battle ship grey sky. Sleeping bags and plates of chips for dinner: always missing Blue.

...

Orange street lamps polluting any view of the stars, to gaze upon; this place is so alien to me, it's so cold. No houses on cobbled streets or traditional corner shops, no friends to run around with or adventures to be had; only three sets of identical towering seventeen story boxed high flats meeting the crest of a motorway, and an odd shaped water tower on the horizon. Fences gating in fences leading to pathways and small areas of grass, further fenced off but from what?

Identical buildings containing identical flats, running four floors high and two doors wide for streets on end; foreboding communal entrances lead to communal verandas, but no one sits out on them, people barely nod to one another, other than when taking it in turn to clean urine from the stairwells. Everyone is white and depressed and looks the same; shrunken jaws with wiry hair gelled down over pale foreheads, and fierce expressions. Everyone is angry about something all of the time, murderous angry. Kids play hide and seek in *midgie* bins, and flat school roofs used as climbing frames. God forbid anyone lucky enough to actually have a front or back garden, is to make any effort to maintain flower beds or neat hedgerows, as these will simply become hurdles upon which to bound over in games of *Grand National*, with crowds of us stampeding through *the backs* from the top of Milford St to the bottom. – Oh, grassed myself up there.

Here I stand; now a complimentary English bastard, with an accent like '*Worzel Gummidge,*' *and* no Father for support, surrounded by the vilest of little shits on the planet.

23

...

We keep in communication with Victor through an intercom system, at the foot of my gran's high flats. Pressing fourteen/six, then a call button; half shout, half talking through muffled speakerphone, 'He's, still isn't here yet, and we're freezing,' we call out over the wind together, hours of this, yet unwilling to return fourteen floors to wait within strange adult tension.

A car pulls around from the only road leading in, one way to go, though still driven without purpose; we almost don't want it to be him. Instinctively it's wrong. I sense in Angela, she feels the same as I do, that this is not what we were expecting. Something is wrong, not even the car is the same. We make him out clear enough through the downpour, his silhouette frame between lashing rain and illuminating city orange, distanced by bluish light surrounding headlamps.

He is looking around the interior cabin, in no rush to get out. Narrower eyes than before, straining back, was he sure it was us? He gets out and approaches, gesticulating and playful that it's windy; we begin to walk forwards, and I don't know if we feel more uncomfortable than before, or was he always funny to be around and we had just gotten used to it? Paler skin, chafe, more deadened complexion than before; red broken vessels feigning a flush of rose, raising unevenly to cover his cheeks; sharper purple veins curtailing onto pattern his nose. Lips shrunken thin are cracked. He smells unclean, before he is even close enough to touch, stale alcohol and tobacco: Dad has not been looking after himself, since we have been gone, and I think he wants us to know.

Whites of his eyes contrasting blood red deliberately neglected to wanting pupils; shivering as if in trauma, 'I miss you, I love you,

Angie, I love your mum. I need to speak with your mum, Angela, are you okay? Paul son, are you alright?' I don't know if I believe him. I don't think he really believes it in himself. How hard must he have tried to convince himself? And it is occurring to me, it strikes me; that at age eight this is a terrible way to think of my father, but he shouldn't have done the things he has, and I'm all too aware of them now. I listen to everything around me, what everyone says about him; they hate him. 'It's going to be all fine son, I miss you too, I miss the both of *yees*, and I miss your mum.' Big lump in his dry throat under grazed skin sounds like it hurts to swallow, then weeping all over the place, wiping snot and drool from his nostrils and the guttering of his mouth.

Diminished and alone, my father, and I don't even know if we have missed him at all, it's occurring to me that we're here primarily to get Blue back. 'But where is Blue? Where is Blue, Dad? You said you were bringing Blue. Where is he?' *'Lies, spite, excuses and blame...'* pat on the head, and he hands us over from the back seat my stuffed *'ET'* teddy and some plastic bags of belongings, 'Everything else I had to sell, because your mammy took you away, and I lost the house. Couldn't stay in the house without your mum.' He tells it sincere, we should blame her, and that will never happen.

Behind him the hum of wave after wave of cars, my gran's flat facing the other direction, leaves us standing worlds apart in the light of this stranger's car; all I can see in front of me are crashing raindrops, and Angela; empty is our only emotion, sick with upset, cold rain falling down our backs following sharp vertical lines, reminding us just how far out of reach the sky now was, how far rain had fallen. And we are trembling, completely inconsolable before stepping back into the hollow corrugated metal shell, in its stench of faint piss through bleach. I am glad she is here with me and not him. By the

25

time doors open on the fourteenth floor, any chance of returning *home* was gone.

...

Mum, distraught he has not returned our photo albums, 'Out of spite he has destroyed them.' Out of spite all of our childhood memories are gone, save a few she managed to tuck away as we were leaving, and the handful already at my gran's.

School pictures mostly, of Angela in brown uniforms and me all chubby cheeks and freckles, perfectly presented in a blue shirt and tie that would be coming off the instant the photographer called, 'Next!' or the flash bulb dimmed. Some of us all in the house prior to Gloucester, back in Livingston with my grandparents; a sunny day in the garden, everyone's standing around my buggy; bleached in sunlight, soft around the edges, only the over exposed reds and greens still shining through, and now all with his face sharply cut out, a silhouette remaining where half my life should be.

My first memory was around this time, around the time in Livingston, of me hurtling down a hill in my buggy, backwards momentum bumping in time with the ground, looking up at the sky. We were in the park that sunny day, on the verge of a concrete paved hill with a tunnel at the bottom. My grandparents had let the buggy slip from their grasp, no doubt distracted by conversation of, 'What a bastard that Stuart is,' and I went drifting off. No harm done, the buggy having come to a soft halt at the bottom. Though it had not tipped over, they fell silent, too afraid to tell Mum. When it finally comes to light, over a late drunken evening, plenty of time spent to heal, and a laugh expected, my mother goes berserk; absolutely berserk, "YOU DON'T JUST KEEP A THING LIKE THAT TO YOURSELF. YOU HAVE TO TELL ME. HE COULD HAVE BEEN

HURT. YOU SHOULD HAVE TAKEN HIM TO THE HOSPITAL. YOU HAVE TO TELL ME, I'M HIS MOTHER. YOU HAD TO TAKE HIM TO THE HOSPITAL TO BE CHECKED. YOU HAD TO TELL ME." Rage that continues on long throughout the night, bass lined echoes and murmurs travelling as I try to sleep, tension and the gentle calming of Victor's voice, 'That's it Irene, I know, I know hen. It won't happen again, and he's fine, he is fine. Irene come own, you are all fine now hen.'

...

We quickly harden to my father's tears and cries; the end of weekend visits, goodbyes always ending in him crouched down in pathetic whimpering by the traffic lights to the far gates of Cranhill Park, over on the Edinburgh Road side, over from the off license and the chip shop, next to *The Dalriada 'The Dal'* Motel where he is staying. Embarrassed by it, it is so uncomfortable to watch this grown man feign suffering, and we stand powerless to do anything about it, we can't just walk away. Instead having to watch and wait, listening to him tell us how he loves our *mammy,* how we were to tell her how he loves her, that his life is so bad without hers and he wants us all back. We can tell he wants us to press her, to tell her how she was wrong.

Ritual humiliation of watching a man who had once been our strength, broken, worn and stubbled; those diseased red eyes staying with me all week; he can wear all the poor gardening clothes in the world, we know it is all his fault. Angie and I speak together, of how we wished he would stop behaving in this way, on our confused walk back home through the park. Finding Victor asleep on the grass, all sunburnt and surprised to see us, 'Oh, ah must ave nodded aff there in the sun, are youse twos ohright?'

27

We want Blue back, and in my own way I still want them back together, while the message delivered back to Mum, 'Dad was crying again. We wish he would stop doing that.' Mum is more upset that he is keeping his promise never to give her a penny in Child Maintenance, and to never give her a divorce. – The only two promises he ever keeps in his life. By now he will be busily stealing towels from *The Dal*, and driving back in his new car to his new home, the one his brother has purchased for him in Ayrshire. By now everything we had ever owned has been sold for a sad song. While he tells himself that it is all her fault, tells anyone who will listen that it is all her doing. The worst kind of lie, the kind you convince yourself is true.

...

Two months in and we're moved to *emergency housing*; accommodation comprising a draughty yet spacious three-bedroom maisonette, with features including; low stucco ceilings with damp patches, stairs that move when you climb them, wall after wall of stuck-shut-forever windows and paper thin doors split by ill-tempered foot holes. A small blessing lies inherent, in the previous tenants '*Batman*' wallpaper (my room); we notice this when looking up at our *soon to be* new residence, weeks before from the road below, 'Careful not to tread in that broken glass, and dog mess,' Angela says. The rest is coated in layer upon layer of yellowed gloss enamel and damaged plaster, while nicotine stains every surface. Washes thick of *minging* blue poured down white doors; lashes on skirting's, frames with drips enveloping handles encrusted into fittings, making stiff access to a burnt out gas central heating unit. Vents in walls, surely designed to keep us cold. The smell of something, not damp but not belonging, lingering in our sinuses, a heavy air filling our lungs over prolonged exposure. Pigeon feathers fall from taps, taking days to run them clear, while the, *Yale*

*Lock* (one key), means we can come and go without having to chap on the door, but best to leave it locked for now.

We spend weeks scrubbing filth-covered floorboards, 'What manner of hair is this?' Chipping back broken tiles, peeling away mottled vinyl; finding as many green toy soldiers as two pence pieces before bleaching, paint stripping, and bleaching again these now fluorescent magnolia base coated rooms. Laughing together, as a family, at the instruction on Victor's *Black and Decker* Paint Stripping Gun, *"Do not use as a hair dryer."* Gran greets us every time with plastic containers filled with smaller plastic containers, plastic bags filled with poly bags, coat hangers, and countless bars of *Imperial Leather* soap. The only place to put them is in with the last weeks' plastic containers containing sachets of salt and pepper and tomato sauce she has taken from the canteen in *BHS*.

Our presence in Cranhill has become known; a light box illuminating the Bellrock Court, beaming out high voltage bulbs; a birdcage for public humiliation, those English who don't belong here. Only I am excited to be able to watch my family, while sitting in the park, everyone else is tired of ignoring the people who are, 'Always fucking looking in the window.' My dear Mum always awaiting the next benefits payment from which to furnish with light shades and something other than just a patchwork of net curtain, we live a public existence. Only outshone by the bright orange social climbers sparkling in the night sky, their *as soon as it gets dark and everyone can see* ultraviolet sun bed lights on full pelt for the evenings roasting. 'Is that you just back from Spain again? Because you never leave that hoose.'

An old orange couch arrives from somewhere, new for us; courtesy of a charity donation given into John Care at the *Credit Union*; perfectly fitting with my cast-me-down jumpers and out-grown *Farah* trousers, whilst playing with Altar Boy Gerard *'GT'* Taggart's old *'Star Wars'* toys and reading his hand-out *'Dandy'* comic book annuals. The magic three of us cuddling up for the evenings together, covered up in quilt, and munching on our new favourite delicacy of toast and melted nuclear orange cheese with garlic powder sprinkled over on top; Mum holds onto our hands and says, 'It's alright, we will be on our feet soon.' By eleven in the p.m. Angela and she are having an argument; Mum is crying into her hands and running out of the house. I am crying and banging on the window as she passes below; terrified she is not coming back. She is the only thing keeping us alive. She is only going to get some air and cigarettes from the garage; she says she will not sleep tonight.

...

'It's *no* the man in the lift way the slash marks doon his face you are to be frightened aye, it's the man who did it tay him,' Victor explains to us, following our first finding of syringes in the stairwell and resulting questions on our new environment. 'Who was the boy who had the concrete slab dropped onto his head?' Long afternoon walks to the *Huggy* and Victor walks comforting and softly behind me; his little ritual of rolling Shag Tobacco from the pouch and shaking sometimes unsuccessfully the match before dropping it on the ground, 'You're an arsonist,' I call back. 'What did you call me there?' 'An arsonist, for dropping flames.' 'Oh. Ha. I thought you called me an arsehole there,' pats my head. 'Can we go fishing tomorrow?'

Angela arrives home in tears: chalk white, her left eye blood shot with pain: scratched face, nail marks down her cheeks and neck, arms covering her head. Child's hands trying to hold long ribbon blonde hair back in place, clumps falling from between her fingers, she is picking them up from the floor and trying to pass them to my mum. Two girls her own age she befriended had turned on her, beaten her and torn at her. No one else tried to stop them; no one offered to help this child as she staggered home from street to street.

...

Sat up on the unit at the kitchen window near every second Friday after school; four o'clock he would be here this time, he will make it this weekend, 'That's half past seven, come on son. Your dad's not coming.' I wait another hour, then a bit more.

All of this, residing within a stack of maisonettes, in a slum where the sewage system overflows drains with tampons, soiled nappies, toilet paper and excrement during stormy days. A place where I get kicked and they scream abuse every time I set foot outside, where two Doberman Pinschers jump for my throat on the landing directly above ours as their owner struggles for control, a place where no human being should be left to fend. It is becoming clear to us that we have arrived into hell, and escalating to the point where I am too afraid even to go outside and play anymore. At least my gran and Victor live just up the hill, a flashing light bulb to communicate that I have made it there safe, a flash back to acknowledge that I can stay overnight anytime I like; Victor's blue-fishing-sleeping-bag will always be here for me on the tanned leather sofa with the comforting drone of cars passing by on the motorway below.

We get to pick a kitten, a little orange ball of fluff. I select him because he is the smallest of the litter; Angela gets to pick his name, 'Dempsey,' after her favourite television show. All sharp clingy claws, he brings us warmth missing from our hearts.

...

31

As a child christened in the kitchen sink, by a mother too ashamed of my father's behaviour to risk him ruining such an important day; it was the obvious choice to send me to the Protestant, Lamlash Primary School; a no questions asked institution, where all but three of my class mate's had parents separated.

*Adam Ant* and *Bananarama* were no more, not when it seemed you could fuck a Fenian bastard, whatever that was,

"HELLO. HELLO. We are the Billy Boys. HELLO. HELLO. You'll know us by our noise. WE'RE up to our knees in Fenian blood. Surrender or ye die. Cos we are the Brigton Derry Boys."

They sang this in the playground whilst whipping the fuck out of each other with skipping ropes; one kid was always pulling down the skirts of *Barbie Dolls* and leering at their smooth parts. Everyone else ranked on how good at fighting, they were: Best Fighter, Second Best, Best Fighter in the Class, Best in the School, I was categorised as, '*No into fighting.*' I was known now only as Cathcart, and only ever referred to as Cathcart, 'Cathcart ya prick, here you ya prick. Fuck up. Fuck you ya prick. Fuck you ya wank. Ya skinny dyin bastard. I'll boot you in the haw maws. I right Cathcart ya prick. Fuckin dobber.'

I just wanted to run around the playground pretending to be on a motorbike, but eventually giving in, I started saying sorry for everything all of the time as a nervous twitch. Colds were lasting longer, Mum thought I was playing up, the ten minutes past nine bug; our GP concurred. I guess this was the beginning of me running away from the world, on antibiotics waiting on this odd feeling of weak, sickness and flu, of just not right to disappear.

I would get really upset in class; I used to fall apart now and again thinking about what had gone wrong, but I couldn't get out the words, so they left me be, by the sinks so as not to disturb the rest of class. Here is where I would drink from makeshift plastic beaker tumblers; also used for cleaning primary watercolours from brushes, rubbed hard into solid circles of pigment; here is where I would gulp down cup after cup of tap water trying to quench a first that would not abate: till my tummy felt hard and full, it hurt with fluid.

I drew a picture of a gnome reading a book, and on the cover of his book was a picture of himself reading the book and so on and infinity. It made a nice change from being furious inside, at my classmate's lack of symmetry.

I remember being jealous because some of these kids had special, *Social Workers*, and got to spend a full day out each week being taken on *day trips* with these adult *friends*. And I remember a loose fence giving way to the bushes, leading to a grass verge separating us from motorway traffic; here Rab Crowlin and I found at arms-reach a little brown sparrow's nest. Eggs tiny, of turquoise and brown speckled with yellow, so fragile and full of purpose they made us gasp. These we held out in open palms, absolutely tenderly and delicately for closer inspection. A moment before I dropped one, the moment before it broke over the grass, that same moment my conscious fell into despair. We panicked, I dropped another. I had never hated myself before.

One of the boys with a Social Worker is off today, his mum is embarrassed because last night his Uncle pointed a shotgun at my sister and her friends when they were playing hide and seek in the *bottom* set of high flats. All the police were shouting at everyone to get in their houses and pointing guns at him.

...

33

'Dinghy man! Pure rubber dinghy, he pure dinghied you,' this boy's face scrunched up and flapping his left ear forward, laughing, 'He dinghied you a cracker!' Three minutes of intense *dinghied* debacle, from a child dressed in dirty, torn school trousers on a Saturday and all because the ice cream van pulled away just as I got to the closing sliding door. – *Cairnsey.*

I did make one friend, a best friend in Steven *'Cairnsey'* Cairns. A proper latch key kid from the *middle* flats, his father had recently died from flu. Cairnsey got kicked out early every morning with a few pence in his hand, forbidden to return home till dark. It's not that his mother never loved him; the parents round here just seemed to want their children out playing all of the time. Cairnsey stole milk from people's front doors, while streets lay vacant, their inhabitants tucked up nicely in bed on a procession of Council mattresses. Picking cigarette ends from the ground, he called them doubts; never lifting one with fewer than four draws remaining. He would puff on them as we hung around playing with matches in empty swing parks, and me signed off from school again, this time with a cold sore on the side of my mouth, smeared thick in pineapple cream. Shielded from the wind together by broken wooden stumps and monkey bars with the words, *"Fuck, shag and Sharon,"* carved into them; seemed everyone had been here.

By the entrance to my gran's high flats: the *top* high flats, gales would foster and amplify to forces on which we set sail. Hitching inverted quilt jackets over our heads, arms held tightly into sleeves; with t-shirts tucked firmly into scuffed jeans, we would jump up to be caught in gusts and drift if only for a fraction of a second. But those repeated flights of inches measured in square concrete slabs, generated so much excitement and laughter, they made us yearn for life.

Cairnsey told me of how these plots of land surrounding the top and middle high flats used to be the *Sugarolly Mountains*; of how all the streets in Cranhill were named after lighthouses, and the space between Cranhill and Ruchazie where the motorway droned and echoed, used to be a fresh river running. We dreamed of those days, the idea of having a place to swim during hot summers and wondered whether their demise was partly to blame for Old Nelly and Tommy the Tulip going mad. Local faces whose ranting and raves were so muddled we could never tell if they were being supportive or angry, 'I that's it son, that's the gem, come own the young team, I ya we bastards, tell yer ma ah know her, you're in for it now, you're gonna get it noo, away and play, enjoy yourself, I son, I, that's the gem.'

Another month passes, another week spent absent from school with flu virus; coughing, sneezing, bit dizzy, sore stomach, more antibiotics, whatever it was this time. Contagious maybe, but after some days I felt just fine and rain would not be enough to deter me from playing outside in the peace and quiet, while the animals were trapped inside. More time spent with the truant Cairnsey; talking to him about my dad, looking for some kind of understanding, but he seemed lost in a different way. Pretending instead to be a robot, with *Tennent's Lager* cans crushed then folded around my feet to clank along with. Crossing grit-covered paths and clambering over fences, running down dirt tracks and kicking off the cans to scale the big tunnel to avoid packs of stray dogs roaming the area. They would either want to bite us or shag us. Standing within the concrete tunnel to avoid getting soaked, watching floods of rain plaiting and stream beneath, Cairnsey's fingers curled around damp doubts trying to find a dry one. It occurs to me, he is in complete shock.

...

Christmas day and the Police are at my gran's door. 'Is your mother home, could we speak with your mum?' 'Yes. Happy Christmas!' Angela and I say, 'MUM,' we shout down the hallway, and Victor sticks his head around the door, 'Whit is it? Oh Jesus, haud own, Irene, Katie, haud own a minute, be quiet, the Police are it the door.' He ushers through two very solemn Officers, we follow up the hall. 'Could we speak with you alone Mrs Cathcart? Without children present.' We are walked back down into the bedroom by Victor, 'I don't know. I'll come get yees in a minute, stiy there.' All goes quiet, back listening to the few cars that pass on the motorway this special day, till we hear screams. 'YA DANCER!' Mum's voice. 'That's the gem son,' Victor's voice. 'Sit doon, sit doon, have a drink, come own,' we see my gran encourage shocked Officers, already making their excuses as we look in through semi opaque glass partitioning the hall running to the living room door. 'Your arsehole father has tried to overdose on Christmas Day. Christmas Day! And he canny even get that right.' 'I, who needs the attention noo?' they all take it in turns, everyone saying it, every repeat emphasising it more. I picked up my juice from the table, looking to Angela.

...

My gran and Victor drank a lot of *Irn-Bru*, which they referred to only ever as, 'Ginger,' ginger also being their term for everything else fizzy; be that *Irn-Bru*, *Coca-Cola* or *Schweppes Lemonade*. Yet instinctively they knew of which the other was referring. It seems this should have been instinctive in me also, bubbling away at some level between my strong English accent and predication for the term, 'Fizzy-pop,' which had me laughed out of most Cranhill newsagents. Washing out the *Bacardi* bottle with *Cola*, as I boxed into Victor's hands, Abba's '*Chiquitita,*' playing in the background. – I can't believe it has only just now occurred to me that they were able to do this only as mixers to alcohol, and as such each knew what the other had in their *Bacardi, Bells* or *Smirnoff Vodka.* Unbelievable.

Summer's afternoon, I arrive at my gran's soaked through from playing in jets of ice-cold water, fresh from the numerous fire hydrants set off all over Cranhill; quickly nominated by everyone because I'm flooding the house, to, 'Go and get us some Ginger.' In the lift, musing over what to bring back, having gotten it wrong on so many occasions and disappointed everybody. Body lurches forward in time with the hint of oiled mechanics, slowly and sickeningly, down then up, jarring to a complete standstill. Leaving me in a corrugated makeshift urinal for what seems a very long time. Pressing buttons one through seventeen, rubbing my thumb against braille dots to see if it will make them work better. Open, close, concierge button, nothing, 'HELP!' and no response is the answer.

Attention soon passes from my current dilemma, and onto reading graffiti, just who is Sharon? Why was she here? Going through my pockets now for a bit, some interesting fluff, not sure if that was chewing gum or toffee, then the lightning rod of realisation; that these empty bottles I hold in my arms as I tip-toe over puddles of piss brought fresh to life from my cold soaking shorts and t-shirt are worth ten pence each. That's ten pence in my Paulie pocket for every bottle I redeem, and my gran has heaps of them by the fridge. I'm doing the sums now, that's at least two pounds and there are some more at my house. This is going to be as big as Christmas.

The lift shakes back into action with a bump and some g-force, lifting my stomach to my neck, and taking the rest of me to the ground floor, where I am greeted by irate neighbours presuming I have been playing and pissing in the lift. Further arms raised in fury of buttons one to seventeen being alight, allowing them plenty more time to ignore each other as the lift stops at each and every floor.

By now Angela had been sent to find me, and she hunts me down on the return leg of my triumphant journey, 'Where have you been?' 'I got stuck in the lift.' 'You've been out playing and everyone is waiting on you.' 'No, I've no,' carrying with me two bottles of Limeade and some American Cream Soda. Twenty pence change left in my pocket; I was not going to risk getting it wrong this time. 'Aww Paul son, whit's that? You've goat the rang Ginger.' – Thanks, Victor.

In my gran's kitchen now, filling bag after doubled bag with *empties* and instructed down to the sixth floor where her friend Iza will have loads more for me, 'Aaaannnny Gingies?' then I notice this lady is pissing herself laughing to the point of hysteria; it becomes clear that in Glasgow, it's a *red-neck* to return more than two bottles at any time, and they are all cheering me on; loving the thought of the look on Kitty's face when I fill up her wee van with ginger bottles and she has to hand me over money.

'Am no takin thame, all gee you seven pence each?' Kitty's husband croaks at me through his half frog half robot voice box, over the heads of the queue. And I'm left waiting with my heaving bags of *empties*, stuck behind people ordering, and listening to scum drivel for the following fifteen minutes.

'Eh, alllll hiv eh, a double nugget, an oyster, no-no, two cones two *Flakes* in thame, two bottles aye *Irn-Bru*, twinty *Bensons*, twinty *Club*, a *Double Decker*, a *Marathon* for him, a *Fruit and Nut* for him, allll iv a *Toffee Crisp* fir me, two bags aye *Skips*, a bag ah pickled *Monster Munch*; a better take some matches case ave ran oot, an eh, I, I'll hiv two bags oh five p crisps for the waines, there getting fuck ahh else,' says the woman in her housecoat and one slipper.

'Am pure no shagging him. Ah don't care,' she says to her friends, the girl not that much older than me. 'It might be wee, but it's gem,' he calls over. 'I au right then, get us a *Twix* then, and a single and two matches, and some *Polo Mints* so ma mah doesney smell ma breath.'

'Don't know about that man, fffftt,' sound made blowing air between the teeth, over the bottom lip, tongue impacting on the back of the teeth, 'Don't know. Am no sure. Am pure no sure. Whit is it?'

'Quality man, that's pure quality. Look it this man,' gesturing for friends to come over. 'Pure quality in it? Whit is it?'

'Ah like that. Ma daahs goat wan. Ma uncle collects thame. Hivney seen wan like that fir ages. Am gonna get wan for Christmas. Whit is it?'

'Ye would just piy the extra win't ye? If ye wir piying that fir a *Porsche*, ye wid just piy the extra and get a *Ferrari*? Here, is someone goat a loan a nine pence so a can get an ice cream coan?' says the man in his thirties, brand new sixty-pound trainers on, while his wife living on the balcony upstairs from us scrapes together dole money, and money borrowed from anywhere to buy food for their three kids.

'Here wee man, they are pure shit hot,' he points to my trainers. I think he is saying I have shit on my shoe, I'm checking the back of them and the sole on them, till it's finally my turn at the counter. More *Refreshers* than I can chew on and near three pounds cash, a short-lived result; every kid in the area has gotten over the *red-neck* to copy my scam and Kitty's offering less and less in return: now charging a penny for the now nine pence mixture paper bag; the jig is up. Although I do have one new idea, to start delivering bread rolls alongside milk in the morning. But the only person offering cash to fund my operation is my father, and bearing in mind he still owes me back the six pounds I'd collected for *Bob-a-Job* week, it seemed a touch foolish to go into partnership with him.

...

GT tries getting drunk and we see the Police take him away because he keeps falling over; he comes back and they have broken two of his fingers in the back of their car to make him say, 'Sorry.' Cairnsey falls out with me because he has nothing, and his mum has bought him a pair of *Nicks* when he'd asked and told everyone he was getting a pair of *Nike*. 'That's not a cat, that's a kitten. Is that you shagging your cat? Are you scared of the baird?' he calls up to my landing, and I was alone again, surrounded only by people even I knew to be scum.

There is this great respite in Glaswegian culture my mum taught me, which is when a person becomes a parent, all past sins are forgiven. It does not matter whether they have *dinghied* you three times, or even if your families have hated each other for generations; as soon as that person has a child, all is forgotten. I wondered if this was the true basis of religion. Maybe it's what the adults were playing at once a year, when wishing each and every one a Happy New Year.

...

As if things weren't bad enough, some *hot shot* goes and makes a movie glamorising the *Kray Twins*, wrapped in Hollywood gloss, protected by an eighteen certificate, and connecting with embittered youth.

Where I was living, ignorance could not differentiate piss poor folklore with its essence in London's East End working class roots, a clip around the ear and the fabled respect, from real life. We had never seen Barbara Windsor as one of our own and those times of

40

questionable morality, as myths and legend of post WWII, where family stuck together, so many could barely tell the difference between that and every day.

And now every kid my age and above is walking around saying, 'Crocodile,' and, 'Say thank you,' in reference to one man having a sword pushed down through his hand, into the pocket of a billiards table. Of another held petrified while a long knife is inflicted between his mouth: slicing through meat and flesh of his cheeks, leaving flaps of skin open to black-deadened-shocked-eyes to the admiration of onlookers and inhale of sickening power by the violator. Brutally, convincingly re-enacted by the *Kemp Twins* of former *Spandau Ballet* fame; two guys who sang along to *'True'* and *'Gold,'* before the New Romantics Scene ran out on them. One of them now selling sofas for a living, having played joint inspiration for a thousand brutally slashed faces up and down the city of Glasgow in a legacy that continues today. *Right then,* I'm off home for a cup of tea with my mum.

Angela goes head first off a friend's bike down the steep hill in the park. The left hand side of her face removed; she screams like a banshee, her soul as light projecting through a shattered mirror all her pain. She screams in hysteria for my mum, she screams at the Police as they try to take her to hospital. I am the only one she will be kind to.

A boy sneaks up behind me and bangs my head off paving. The guy selling t-shirts left slow and disfigured, we recognise him as the boy who had the concrete slab dropped onto his skull over by the motorway bridge. Kids stamping each other's heads during simple playground fights; even our local ice cream van drivers are in turf wars resulting in the firebombing and murder of a family of six and

41

now GT has started selling his stuff to buy hash.

On a recurring visit to a loose relative, a cousin of my mum's and her kids, 'Last time you were here Irene, did you hear anything?' 'No. How?' 'Because there was a guy o'er there in the junkies close getting his haunds chapped aff.' – I'm eleven; I really didn't need to hear this.

We stand near enough to signposts that the bus will stop but as far back as possible from the bus shelter, still drenched in blood and bound in ripped yellow tape from last Friday's murder. Jogging quickly, heads down past pubs we know to be filled with violent offenders, we peer from bus windows at a rainy *Lea Rig* on Alexandra Parade, and drinking dens along Duke St, recently featured in the *'Daily Record'* for shootings; always-careful not to make eye contact with the regulars.

Waiting on a bus at Bellrock St, and some reasonable enough in appearance woman approaching my gran's age turns around to my mum and says, 'An new they've goat they coloured people stiyin in the high flats. Gee them the special treatment and we get nothin.' Mum interjects, 'Those young men and women are training to be Doctors within the *NHS*. They are a great resource to our city.' 'I, ma son, he never goat tay be a Doactor.' – To be fair love, you can't even pronounce the word Doctor, and your son tore a man's ear off in a fight the other month. People in the *top* high flats are still trying to clean his ingrained blood from the stairs. I don't know if he would have the human touch to be a Doctor. I think to myself, with my mum giggling to me.

Budgie McCulloch has become the new interpretation of Devil; skin taut around his skull he looks like fear itself, he looks right through you and cries of, 'JUNKIE!' raise the alarm as his black greasy hair and sheepskin waistcoat come into view; everyone scrambling for safety, even Kitty's Ice Cream van closing for business and driving off. No one sticking around long enough to take a closer look at the red pot marks over his greasy olive arms, except for Willie Copper, who too petrified to move is approached and then taken up a stairwell. His yoyo borrowed; its string wrapped tightly around Budgie's arm as he taps for a vein, releasing the contents of his orange-capped syringe. It was more a zombie who handed Willie back his yoyo. Willie had a little accident in his pants.

A suffering pigeon lands at my feet. Its face and eye have been shot multiple times by an air rifle. I had to finish it off with a stick but it wouldn't die. I had never felt such blind panic, and so wrong before.

...

I could smell the cold from late night snow coming in through the single pane window. It was beautiful. Bright as daylight reflecting into my bedroom, there were no creases in the world. Cranhill was white and pure and innocent. The stars had fallen on us. Someone had forgiven us. Everyone was deeply asleep, except for me. I had been swept up to enjoy this night all alone; the true value of being alone, and no one could touch me, no one would want to. God has taken away all the bad parts and replaced them with good. The stars fell upon us. I slept.

...

Moved onto a Catholic School; Mary blue highlights to interior decoration and a glass wall two extremely tall floors high containing the canteen and assembly hall; catching reflections from a paler blue sky on days where the moon shone full amongst faint white cloud. A sky upon which airplanes streaked on way to someplace different; someplace that existed even within reach of us regular Glasgow people. Abstract reflections form, where the sun and sky have been broken apart and pieced back together, now forced in confinement into meeting with the shapes of windowpanes. But they were still alive.

Returning to inaugurate primary six, following on from a *sixteen-degrees* summer heat wave adorned by fourteen year olds getting drunk and pregnant in the park. I blame '*Three men and a baby*' for this (no, not really). And the girls in our very own class have started wearing bras. We're bra pinging, bra staring, having bra conversations every day; we have excited smiles on our faces extending well into autumn as the efforts of prayer standing up are taking their toll on my legs, which feel heavy and tired and I want to sit down and recharge. Especially when Mr Gallagher takes the reins and has us doing the Rosary Beads at the beginning, during and end of lessons; how many times must you repeat prayer over and over before God will take you seriously? I can't get my head around that at all. Class milk comes to a sudden halt and kids start dropping like flies, fainting all over the place. I see them coming in late like broken clockwork; collapsing face first at the teacher's desk. The same teachers have begun hammering on about having more rest and us going to bed at a more reasonable hour. My third generation, shrunken jawed; pale skinned and round foreheaded Irish Catholic immigrant friends couldn't manage any more rest. 'You have just taken away their meal of the day,' say some of the parents. 'But there is nothing we can do,' teachers reply. I stumble through red gravel on the football pitch on my way home for lunch, dizzy, hungry, shaking, weak, confused and unknown to anyone.

Time spent in the playground with white shirt untucked, loose tie's a scruff and my feet still aren't big enough for trainers with Air Bubbles in them. There is a kid in the year below nick named Riddles

44

with a mottled scalp and tufts of black curly hair, they often de scant him (pull down his tracksuit bottoms), and we laugh because he wears the same Union Jack boxers on every day. The curved metal fountain tap that jets cold water into my mouth has become my resting place with my mouth firmly attached to it through most breaks.

Freddie brings in porn mags and we can't stop staring at women with scaffolding poles; Peter, Lachie, Scott and I hiding out of sight round the sides of the bike sheds; meanwhile Ben Longstone has popped back into class to steal my green skull rubber. He digs pothole marks into it with his pencil, pretending graphite marks were left by him weeks ago; denial continues even as Mrs Hunter tears him a new arsehole for stealing, and leaves him standing outside her private side entrance in the cold all afternoon in near dark beside human faeces. Calling me up to her office at half past three to collect my belonging, she informs Ben, 'Do not to be surprised should Paul give you a well-deserved smack once outside.' I take my rubber and take one look in his dark watery eyes, and wished I had never said anything. If I had understood for a second what was going on in that boys life I would have given him my rubber, my blue, my green and my red pencils plus the first six inches off my transparent shatterproof rule. I leave him to it, turn towards home on the frost coated red gravel pitch. I become all shaken, and get real hungry real fast. I panic a little, and walk all dizzy for a few moments, the floor rising up to meet me before pulling myself together as I unclasp the *Yale* and enter my front door.

Primary seven and we are shaping up for big school; I have a couple of eye tests because I keep having problems seeing the board, but each time I go they say my eyes are fine but I may need glasses in the future. I overhear Mrs Shields mention me on her list of pupils

45

she thinks could make it to University. This means the world to me. Though often she uses me as a prime example to castrate some of the other not so pressured to perform kids, 'For God's sake Fred, Paul is a PROTESTANT and he knows more about this Communion than you do!' A Holy Communion, for which I receive mixed blessing.

Freddie Skerryvore was some kid, he certainly had problems of his own and the wild eyes and energy that went with them, but he was a deeply good kid who needed that constrained and supportive environment to hold his world together. Carrying a knife into class gave him a whole new edge, and us an insight into where his life was going; left to cry a deep hurt cry on the final day, that boy knew he was heading for despair. As Catholic school children we were taught how to pray and seek forgiveness for everything. Pray standing up and everything was forgivable. Pray sitting down and you don't need to feel guilty all the time; it's a fifty/fifty.

...

Weekend visits to my father's homes in the towns of Ayr, Kilwinning and Kilmarnock, where coastal skies bleed like ink from grey, through silver linings, yellow and dark blue; we make camp in sand dunes and watch waves crash, alighting sheets of cardboard and sticks of driftwood, flames blowing turbulently in all directions. It looks so warm from inside but you get out here and the wind bites at your lips. Venturing into the sea, it's not so cold and you soon adjust. Mouthfuls of salt water as waves crush against, but they are more silky than rough and I'm left buoying myself up, arms open, hopping up and down with the tide, gradually pushed forward then back. A step too far and I've lost footing, having to push with my arms now to keep tiptoes on the sand and gain momentum on which to escape; one more wave and my head knocked forward: it's all over, salt water

46

goes down my throat, pushed in my eyes and up my nose. I'm straining to see anyone on a horizon of silver-soft waves, voices are barely audible and I'm being pulled back. I'm gone, I'm going to be gone, but I keep flapping my arms and the next wave pushes me. Feet firmly planted in the sand now; with everything I've got I'm treading forward, walking ahead, film of water in my eyes I can see their forms, hear them, a couple of smooth pebbles and a few more to go. I had never felt ashamed before.

Sand grated off layers of my skin, drinking *Cola* till my teeth itch and eating *Rolos* till I get sick and overly tired; looking at this man in the kitchen cooking lunch, spaghetti bolognese for us, ham haugh for him, repeating his mantra, 'I'm not proud. I'm not proud.' This guy has not eaten an apple in years, he dry boaks when trying to drink tea, and he can't hold down anything but pig's trotters, tramps in red lace garter belts, cheap cider and *Guinness*. So yeah, something kept him full, but mostly *B&H* smokes, 'Hooers,' and liquor kept him going. Anything else made him gag up a mouth full of vomit, and his nose run down his Christmas blue jumper. It's not even the right colour for a Christmas jumper. What a fucking man, thank fuck for *Brut* aftershave. I'm off now, to grow up big and strong.

...

Cycling past the water tower atop of Bellrock St, on which Glasgow City Council has spent one million pounds on décor for the passing motorist; whilst local housing rots in condensation, freezing to sheet ice over stripped window frames, their tenants hacking bronchitis. Turning down past the *Phoenix Bar*, head down and quickly then left past the statue of an onion, representing the different layers in society. – I mean fucking seriously. Jacques René Chirac, Prime Minister of France would be visiting in the next few years. The purpose of his trip: to gain inspiration from visionary ideas on the development of city planning in poorer areas. I bet he went home thinking, 'Well that's that sorted then? Are they taking la pisse?' Or did he go home thinking, 'I never understood a single word any of them said, and who is Sharon?'

My mum brought home from work a copy of '*The Story of Art,*' by *EH. Gombrich* she had found in the drawer of an abandoned desk, inscription still intact, and a gift to someone with its photographs of '*The Dying Slave*' by *Michelangelo*; it blazed a light of the world onto me.

A trip to Pitlochry, organised by John Care, paid for by *Children in Need.* This tremendous hushed blue for which the birds sing and never disappoint; I could for once feel the trees and their autumnal leaves forming moist covering to pathways, leading to a tree house; crisp yellow light, brightest and sharp; shallow low-lying sun clenching on every matt stone, and horizons ending over conifer clad mountains. Ice-cold streams impossibly clear, lochs deep and black, still managing to reflect the sky. The temperature fluctuates around me; I shiver to inhale fresh air. I try to stick twigs up another kid's nose.

Sitting on my mum's bed, Saturday afternoons as always, chatting and listening to the window cleaners clatter up the sides of buildings, ours and over the road. 'I wish he would fall off his ladder,' says my mum, about a particularly noisy one, Angela and I laugh and Mum begins opening the mail, one letter in particular grabbing her attention. Hand scribbled, black handwriting on white envelope, Mum knew what it was before she even began to read out loud, 'I miss yees, I love yees, I need yees back, bla bla, blas,' followed by, 'You may have noticed this is not my handwriting, I was in a car accident with a train at a crossing and have broken both of my arms.'

We burst out laughing together, the magic three of us falling about giggling, then we hear like something from a cartoon, 'Whaaaaaa-metallic-crash,' as the window cleaner over the road has fallen a considerable height from his ladder. Then we all get up and start bouncing about on the bed together.

'You two come here,' Mum wakes us both on a Saturday morning earlier than usual; it's usually we who awaken her, 'Your gran in Ireland has died. Are you two okay?' We didn't even know her, well other than a handful of forced phone calls when we used to visit Dad. An old lady with a Belfast accent so thick I could barely understand a word, other than that she would always ask for my little sister, which made no sense at all. ... Six hundred pounds! We were millionaires, no more second hand clothes for me.

...

For my other gran, we would sing, 'No ye canny throw yer granny aff the bus. No ye canny through yer granny aff the bus. No you canny throw yer granny, because she's your mammy's mammy. No, ye canny through yer granny aff the bus.'

Catherine was her Sunday name. Friends and family called her Kate, Katie or Cathy, depending on when they met: followed by Munley, McEnroe, McGarvie, Lindsay or Waugh. Her proudest moment, receiving a personal letter, *signed* from the *Pope* himself; instructing her she was forgiven; not for marrying an evil man who tore out her hair, not for divorcing to escape or even given permission to marry again, but forgiving her for marrying a Protestant in the first place. Before she went onto re-marry, to my Protestant, grandad, Victor, the best move she ever made.

Hearing what my father has done to a girl in Ayrshire, I felt something break inside of me. – He left you without so much as a look of recognition. He never taught you anything, never encouraged you, never made you happy when you were down and never blinked an eye when he could do without you. He never wanted you back, and you never wanted for anything more; he forgot and you remembered. It's like being killed over and over again; this wound that never heals.

'Paul son, you're a natural worrier like me,' she said. And that was it; anxiety had a home, stress and upset defined our default state of mind. Our trusted *state-of-being* to fall back upon; no matter what happens the comfort of anxiety will be there, waiting. Better the devil you know.

I'd open the fridge as a very proud child, watching the light come on from the inside and pronouncing, 'Hegg,' as I took one out, holding it up for my mother, and she would cook it for me.

# Succumbing to the D

The final straw comes on arrival to Mr Courtier's Religious Education class. Turning up eventually, pale and ghost like on the verge of translucency: limps and spasm of cramps down my left hand side before bowing over a desk and chairs for breath. Eventually enough, even for him to take notice and write me a note to my mother, insisting she take me *urgently* to see a Doctor. Not so urgent, as he would drive me himself, not deserving of dialogue with the School Nurse. No. He is already pissed at me for having so many weeks absent from his Art Department in the run up to the preliminary exams period, through a consistent and personal epidemic of colds, bouts of flu lasting three weeks or longer and virus. Mixing comments on my talent with dismissal of health matters: that he gives his children sweets prescribed by a Witch Doctor to keep their colds at bay. He knows my portfolio will only take me so far, he doesn't believe Mrs Swift has me performing under enough pressure. Urgent I'm like this in his presence, not so urgent to offend his character further: instead he lets me sit the rest of his afternoon, dissolving poverty on a chair and devoid of spirit. Then scrape my ass slowly back home for another half kilometre through the park.

My mother is vexed at this, 'Stupid man's interference,' she takes me off limping, light headed and bursting back through the park gates;

again with these never ending black iron gates, only this time it's to the Doctors directly, which is situated right across from school in the first place. 'Can I have an emergency appointment please? He has been sent home from school with a note.' 'Wit is it *thits* rang way im this time has he goat the cold again?' says the cow behind the desk in monotone unfaltering sequence. "*Tracey*" written on her name-badge, she looks familiar, I've seen her around. My mother creasing her brow, 'Just let me see the Doctor will you?' Hanging off my chair twenty minutes later I observe *Henny* munching through a *Toffee Crisp* and a bottle of *Irn-Bru* awaiting his *Methadone* script; I am finally called *highly nasally accented, 'Paul Cathcart. That's you. GO THROUGH.'* And with a single sniff of my sweet breath, an informed raise of her eyebrow and the prick of my finger, 'Diabetes,' I am denounced forever to a lifetime of exhaustion and discomfort, as she, '*Cackles,*' and commands us off down to the Glasgow Royal Infirmary Hospital and finally we have justification for a taxi. No more walks in the park.

*An old castle-like building, Dr Joseph Lister pioneered the use of Carbolic Acid in the prevention of sepsis, whilst working here back in 1867. A procedure implemented to clean bacteria from the wound, the surgical equipment and surrounding air of the operating theatre: saving the lives of over fifty percent of patients who went under the knife. A procedure, which continues to save countless lives across the world today and the same fundamental solution adapted and prescribed in off-the-shelf mouthwash; helping stop gum disease and freshen breath. – What happened to those kinds of skill sets I don't know?*

Extremely thirsty, I sit and wait the long wait, supping carton after carton of *Capri-Sun* through pokey little straws. Teetering on the end of a paint flecked metal bench and listening to drunks argue with themselves, 'WHAT? IS THIS SEAT TAKEN? WHAT?' the room buzzing, but it's as though I have blocked out the sound, everything has become a numb haze; lights are bright and dull at the same time, all the commotion frantic yet near linear before static, and I'm staring at walls then back on the floor, the stench of the place festering in my nostrils.

A numb shock that feels all too familiar. Though there is relief that I'm going to get better, and I've heard of diabetes before. It was on *'Children's Ward,'* a kid's TV show, on when I was younger. One of the characters; a young boy found out he was not allowed to eat sweets anymore and would have to take a jab each day to stay better. I was ready for that. People often ask, 'What's it like having to jab yourself? Does it no hurt? Does it make you high?' – How ignorant is that? Followed by, 'I couldn'y do that to maself, I don't like needles.' Boo Hoo. For me it was the biggest relief of my life, nothing bitter, no broken promises; by that stage I thought I was going to be like this forever and for the chance to get better, well I would have done anything to get better.

Projectile vomit everywhere, tropical orange and stomach bile splashing white washed walls, my mum, my face and the floor. Very lovely Hospital Cleaners mopping it all up after us with minimal of fuss when a Porter arrives; all smoker's grey skin lost behind navy uniform; with a chair to wheel me down endless corridors following painted green lines adorning subterranean walls and into what seems a giant service freight elevator heading six floors north for the Diabetes Ward. Mum's looking down over me with a face of pure enduring love, anguish and despair. A slight jarring in the elevator; her hand rests lightly on my shoulder, too scared to touch she holds back tears. I was more in control at that point to say I was going to be okay. And as if by chance this friendly enough Porter asks, 'What's it you're in for?' and I reply quite proudly, 'I have diabetes,' to which he condemns, 'Oh kidney problems.' Metallic lift doors open and my heart starts falling through my chest because it's not just giving up sweets anymore, it's really serious.

This guy, why don't they tell these guys to keep their mouths closed? He was the equivalent of getting a medical consultation from a member of the team at *Currys Digital,* and you would have thought the local witch, could have, should have and would have the common sense to instruct so simply not to have any more sugary drinks, saving on the severe vomit scenario. But maybe it's at least almost comforting on some level to know that poor diabetes influence and advice started right from day one and has not been just an occasional lapse in professional judgment throughout the years. Actually no, that's not nearly of any comfort at all.

Now we're in the Diabetes Ward and it's as though a curtain has veiled over my consciousness. We're lucky enough in the first instance though as some nice old fella's given up his private room to us so Mum can stay over. I think it even has a TV. Nurses, Doctors and others come in and go on through the wee small hours; back and forth of swinging doors they prick my fingers over and again to test for sugar levels, whilst filling me with bag after bag of drips and having me pee syrup liquid into grey cartons. Mum strokes back sweat-laced hair from my clammy cold forehead and this comforts me completely, as I ache and cramp and skin burns on the surface, burning against hope and bone. Pillows soaked through in sweat; tucked up and changed. Fluid lines pull back against deep blue veins set beyond translucent skin no longer trying to protect itself before the amber gloom of sleep finally takes over as exhaustion wins over from panic.

Sharp pain as thick needles pierce thin pasty skin on far sides of my fingertips: pushed in hard and deep by a nurse showing all the bedside mannerism of a Rhinoceros. A pain that routinely disturbs me: offering no reassurance. Every fifteen minutes this spike removes me from the solace I have found in unconsciousness. A rhythm only broken by spasms in my hands and retracting calf muscles which interrupt to wince and awaken where I see my mother sat aside; she has clearly not slept a good night's sleep in years, and even now looking down over me as she did when I was a child. Always there for me she grimaces and prays to God that she could only absorb my pain; her empathy connecting to my millions of tiny shattering nerve endings. This is what it means to be a parent.

All so obvious now, my never-ending colds, parched mouth, cramps and weight loss; combined with a growth spurt all largely overlooked by a nervous and highly-strung guardian, agitated and acknowledged instead only as growing pains and natural teenage development. But how; how could she possibly have known how bad this was; how could she possibly have stopped long enough to identify it? She was the one dealing with the everyday countless issues facing us, holding us together and fighting for us to survive.

...

The following day following the longest night; people scuttle, things are tucked in, shutters lift to crisp low winter's sunlight, highlighting an already sterile white room, whiter sheets and plastic furnishings; bedside cabinets, coppers in change and diluting orange the fixtures of the day. My eyes feel awake for the first time in forever, everything is so clear, the detail, the colours so distinct and all so bright and rich. I can almost remember seeing like this, – and just in time to take in a view over the Necropolis. I'm shuffled out onto the main ward with the change of shift, it looks more like a prison yard populated by sick old men coughing, hacking and smelling of buttery mucus. I'll be here for a couple of days at least they let us know, I can't imagine ever getting out. And Mum's not allowed to stay over anymore, not now we're in the open ward in case she excites the old men. I'm shitting myself but when she pops out to go home and change from her tropical vomit tie-dye, I slip into a real deep grateful sleep for what seems like an eternity. Close my consciousness for a little while now, for a long while, let me heal.

Later I'm awoken by two male Nurses; both twice as tired as the other; both far worse off than I, both struggling through day four of four sleep deprived twelve-hour back-to-back sequential shifts. Yet still they manage to make time to chat, still joke, still genuinely care; which combined with being some of the kindest people I have ever met makes me completely calm and all my worries are melting away. They enquire as to how much I know about diabetes and they give me their best shot, to the best of their training; to the best of my understanding, or as much as I can cope at this feathery stage. I ask hypothetically if *me* now eating *Mars Bars* would be the equivalent of someone taking *Speed?* And my knowledge of the drug and others terrifies them. Quickly they take some extra time out of their day; plucked from obscurity to explain with great caution, 'As dangerous as those drugs are for normal people: with your condition they would be ten times more so, so keep very, Very clear of them.' So enamoured am I by their calm and selflessness, the care I feel whilst being under their wings, I draw a picture of them in my sketch pad and even think about becoming a Nurse.

In bed menu selection for the day is doing nothing to win me over, having been carefully edited to remove joy from life, a real *dying faster than I'm living* selection in meeting with the wards special dietary requirements: this being achieved by scoring through with ballpoint pen anything with sweetness, flavour or texture. Not scored out completely; I can clearly see what the others are having; ~~spaghetti bolognese, chicken curry, jelly and ice cream.~~ Nurse Rhino is back doing the rounds; my wounds barely healed, my fingertips perforated like tea bags, my apologies when she makes clear she is in fact Head Sister. Check her out. Has she been using leeches on me? Going on to make it abundantly clear to all; staff included, when overviewing my menu selection: that as a diabetic I would be allowed, 'No treats forever,' for risk of making myself desperately ill. A stark warning of which to concede as I try to console myself with thoughts of, 'It's all for the best, I will regain my health and eventually be gone with these tasty memories.'

Day two and I feel starved, hollow, as I have never been. How I crave for hot dogs and banana ice cream milk shakes. All of the comic books, sketchpads, new PJs, army starched Grandad's handkerchiefs that can stand up by themselves, Sister's tears and hugs from my family can do nothing to distract from the hunger. Though it's great to see my gran and Victor, 'God give me some jelly and a *Mars Bar* please.' Angela does go on to make a good enough effort though, changing my focus momentarily as she tells me the endings to '*Terminator 2*' and '*Home Alone 2*,' both films I had been excited to see all year round. I'm shaking and weak, I need food so badly, anything not consisting of between two and four units of slow release carbohydrate.

# How did this happen?

Night falls with my new comrades; each and every one of these old men has shown me a kindness; a smile of understanding or a few choice supportive words. 'Do you want a *Rolo*?' 'I don't think I'm allowed,' in soft voice. 'I find it's best to have one first, and then ask,' says the Indian man who farts all of the time and the Doctor on rounds is pleased with his farting. – This advice I live on for years to come. Now together we stretch out our necks like baby giraffes to watch a portable TV propped up on a corner table, playing what can only be explained as some kind of personal curse: a Jonathan Ross food special counting down one hundred mouth-watering and delicious recipes, which I will never taste and the one hundred unusual ways I won't *of course* be preparing them. One such meal; a juicy steak with all the trimmings wrapped in foil and cooked against the engine of an American muscle car as it's driven over a rural stretch of Interstate. The resulting feast that lay before them on the bonnet as they delicately unwrap hot foil. I lay there on white cotton feeling oh so sorry for myself. Depressed yet unable to completely resign myself to the echo in my stomach and loss of knowing I would never be allowed, to taste, to touch, to smell, even inhale such gracious meals again: and I'm thinking to myself – quite clearly for once, thinking through the evidence which led me here...

Massive cramps. Cramps in my calf muscles so painful and occurring so frequently, waking me throughout the night. I'd become scared, even to go to sleep. Cramps forcing me to limp upstairs every two minutes when I so desperately had to take a piss and piss some more: thinking on how I pissed so much that mid-way through one piss I would start to need another. 'That's him back in the bathroom,' embarrassed smirk, Angela tells Mum. And guess what they thought I was doing in there, behind a clasped shut bathroom door, age sixteen for twenty minutes at a time? Between pissing, dragging my carcass into the kitchen, drinking vast quantities of anything trying desperately to quench my thirst; brain confused to shit I craved sweetness and invariably went for the sugariest drink available; never quenching my thirst for a moment, only keeping it at bay for the duration of the syrup liquid pouring onto my tongue. Brief cessations through gulp and swallow: I drank tons of the stuff, *Nestle* powdered banana milk shake, mixed listlessly with bottles of *Tizer* as I swayed again back and forth through park gates.

Rab Crowlin whistling up at my living room window for school in the mornings; the week or two before this happened, I ventured down, my eye lids still half shut, 'How you no talking?' He thinks I'm in a huff because he kicked half a puddle over me last I saw him. 'I'm sleeping,' comes my reply, then he laughs, thinking I was being an idiot, and I had similar doubts of myself that day, though now I see why I was trying to capture every bit of rest I could.

Two minutes to nine and frozen through to the bone, desperate to get in doors, already I'd need the toilets and the drinking tap. 'There's the bell,' shout the obvious; my nerves on high alert; was this why I was always so nervous? And first there is French class, or was that in the afternoon; the whole thing an exhausted memory detailed by an out of focus witness.

Weary of lectures on Europe and well versed in the knowledge I was far behind, 'Soooo…?' me nodding my head slightly as if this was the first time and I didn't know what he was on about, just wanting to hide away in a ball somewhere, 'So where are your glasses? Where are they? Why aren't you wearing glasses boy? You get them for free on prescription from the *NHS*. So WHY aren't you wearing them? Why aren't you wearing your glasses BOY?' Fair enough I couldn't see a thing, but that's all I needed, to be picked on for something else. Then being pulled up to the black board, chalking up, and *"Où sont vos lunettes?"* 'Read it out loud boy.' I could never comprehend the writing, no matter how close my table. Maybe it was a white board, marked with green and red pens, either way it all merged with light before reaching me.

Seems that's me now, in amongst a bunch of, 'Unemployable ignoramuses.' Missed the deadline: unable to read and write in fluent French by the end of term. Still put off by the sepia tone nineteen seventies textbooks with their creased cultural portrayal of flowery French families in dirty brown houses drinking from bowls of hot chocolate. 'Quelle heure est-il anyway?' I squinted to watch the class clock, tick tock on by so slowly. – Je m'appelle Paul, Non? Oui?

Periodic table; but as with everything else, nothing connected, no underlying logic no substance. Reasoning is empty and I draped in cramp, surrounded by odds, caught in a hail of *things happening* over which I have little belonging. 'That's pure mental man.' 'Aww no way man, that's pure shockin!' flicking spit balls, 'Whit is it?' 'Ah don't know.' as class teacher, Mr Highbrow Eyebrows enlightens us on how he is a *foremost mind* in the field of Nuclear Physics, of how he knew how to build an A-bomb had he the components; said mere moments before singeing those four-inch long bad boys on the flames of a Bunsen burner. On choosing subjects in the third year I had requested to do Physics or Chemistry to avoid this preordained pish; both of those classes were restricted to students not doing Art. Hey, at least I've learnt how when you mix sand and peas in a jar that they mix together but not on a chemical level, and the dumb arses were kept plenty entertained with time enough to watch salt crystals grow in plastic beakers as I adjusted aching, jumpy, stiff legs onto tall stools.

Pythagoras theorem' and I just didn't know. Math had pretty much stopped making any kind of sense with my high sugar brain restricting problem-solving skills to a complete stand still. Clearly, even now putting green, square blocks into blue triangle spaces and to cap it off; my teacher rattling my nerves, 'I'M A TEACHER NOT A JAILER. You're all *'Muppets'.'* Okay, that's five minutes into class; time for the slap head and Mr Italiano next door to start passing funny notes via ignorant child, clearly comparing students in a game of *'Numpties Top Trumps'.*

Under posters of tortured monkeys and black and white Holocaust trains, *CND* logos and *HR Geiger* fantasy art, Modern Studies fell another tired-thirsty blur. Class maniac JoJo continuing to leave the rest of our group table too scared to learn, except for times when he desperately needed someone to talk to and a shoulder to cry on; when his eyes would well and it blazed apparent that under his bravado of intimidating lunacy, lies a boy, some raw nerves, confused hormones and a violent home from which to stray as much as possible. Playing *Moashey* had put him in grave danger, who would have thought tossing ten pence coins against piss filled doorways to see who could get the closest and a setback of double-or-nothings could surmount to debts of one hundred and forty pounds? He is as sure to be on the end of a knife for that as I was to need to ask the teacher if I could go for a pee for the umpteenth time. JoJo had a plan however: on a run of stealing charity boxes from newsagents along the Shettleston Road to pay his way. I wonder how that's worked out for him.

My mum on requesting I be put up a level, witnessed me being shooed away; in senior explanation, 'Mmmm, – thoughtfulness represented in a hum – although Paul would have space to learn in a higher level class, the difference in learning *difficulty* would be black and white. I understand class C to be a difficult learning environment: you are not the only person to inform me of this. Because Paul has missed too many weeks in absence due to sickness already, he could not possibly catch up.' So I continued; stuck with a Goth for a teacher who applied her white mask on the bus in the morning and bemused us in the afternoons with idioms, 'Pulling out all the stops people. Putting the pedal to the metal. Best foot forward. Against the clock and X marks the spot.' What? – Hello anyone? Really, was it best that I did not learn at all? Modern Studies, what about common sense? Why did none of these people think to look into my health a little more seriously?

Drama class and Mr Thesp taught us how to commit suicide by swallowing handfuls of Paracetamol. Slugging them back in a romance blemished with confusion, 'Whisky is always the way.' Teetering back for a moment on an excuse to stop; it seems they will only sell small quantities of Paracetamol at a time, 'So you will have to walk around the block to a number of local retailers to attain a high enough quantity. Don't worry about quality,' he would say in his deep extra Scottish drawl, 'Then you sit home alone: back straight with stiff nerve you glug it all back. This sends you off into a nice little blasé haze,' – a half puff of smoke gestured from his fingers tips, opening gently toward the sky as he pouts a last breath of unwanted air, absolution in his contented smile. So far removed from his improvised comedy about the deaf in the waiting room of the Doctors Surgery, back when he came to visit us in primary school, 'WHAT? IS THIS SEAT TAKEN? WHAT?' and so on. I got the distinct impression this was all, more a hint to us than a cry for attention by him, but his frequent nervous breakdowns blurred the boundaries and I just didn't know anymore. I don't know much of anything anymore. – I sat quietly, pushing down heartburn and trying to digest school dinner. 'Having to pee, again,' – Anyone?

Art class had become equally tetchy; the only class I ever loved, and a teacher Mrs Swift who loved me in return, from the moment she heard me utter the words, 'I don't like football.' Why I'd begun to snap back at her I didn't know. Why did I speak to her in such a way? Why did it seem so just to do so? – What am I talking about, I didn't even realise I was doing it, or did I? – Till it was too late. Of all the people I should have been working up the nerve to speak back to why did I answer back to her? Why was everyone having a go at me? An entire class held breath in pained anticipation waiting for her to erupt. Mrs Swift, not a teacher for easy dealings. Stooped posture draped in blacks of lace and felt, grey hair brushed and tangled, silver clasped back, jewellery home-made on each and every finger; she shed a wry smile on a small few of us, the rest she kept on tenterhooks but she never reacted to me. She looked over instead. Knew something was deeply-worryingly-wrong, she knows me all too well, let me go because she knew in me that I'm not the type. There was more, something far worse going on and she looked over at me from the other side of the classroom to let me know. Let me away so patiently and I miss her for that. – I needed her to be the one to tell me what it was.

English continued as usual, smiling at Sharon throughout the entire lesson and hinting that I fancied her; the odd bit of footsie under the desk where the combined static of her woollen tights and my nylon trousers could have blown us all up. The cutest little groove trails down on the tip of her nose, even her Cranhill perm, more natural and less Cranhill than all the other girls and sex was never off any of our minds while listening to Rachael bang on about how she was going to lose her virginity, real soon. – Speaking of which, I've not wanked off in ages, maybe next time I do something will come out. As for course work I have no idea, I only attended in hormones and sudden reading difficulty had made all my words jumble on the page. The lights were beginning to dim.

Guidance Counselling is good, they have taken the pains of explaining to us, 'It's *alright* to be *ashamed* and *embarrassed* of your families.' Taken further *personal time* out of their busy day, via an appraisal form, to assess and instruct on our limitations, 'We processed these through a special computer.' It seems I should be ideally suited thus potentially employable as a Fisherman or Miner. With all the mines and oceans in Glasgow, I find it hard to find fault in their persuasion. The fully-fledged Catholic boys got to be Fishermen or Carpenters, and with so many girls already pill popping and sleeping with Taxi Drivers, some are destined to be prostitutes; no one was in any doubt about that.

Ginger haired Counselling person is very pleased to stress, she earns a cool twenty-four thousand pounds per annum, and this is way more than any of our parents could *ever* expect to earn, we would be more than embarrassing ourselves to even hope. Especially all ninety percent of boys just past the age of being scouted for professional football; they and their entire families hopes and ambitions, pinned on a pipe-dream now passed on down through to their younger sibling. 'Look it the baw control and he is only four, he will definitely make it intay the toap eleven in Scotland and then go own-tay play fir *Bayern Munich*, let's no get joabs jist yet.' Let's all stay right in our place and not worry about Europe just yet. There seemed to be something amiss, clearly Mizz Ginger was excluding parents of pupils who drove cars costing more than her home; although obviously drug dealers, maybe they could have got me some medication. Why didn't anybody notice that I was fucking see-through and in agony?

God, not gym class, let's face it I was never bred for sport. I've been brought up primarily by three women: there's been no football in my life or masculine activity of any kind, never has been; we watch '*Mary Poppins*' at Christmas never '*James Bond*,' although Mum has gone through a phase of calling me, 'Mate,' and punching me repeatedly in the arm. That will make a man out of me. – Was she harbouring doubts?

I did once ask the blonde bopped Physical Ed teacher, in her frequent red tracksuit, with statuesque physique of a Russian Short Putter, 'Could I bring a can of *Irn-Bru* into class due to my being so painstakingly thirsty?' she even enquired as to whether I had diabetes. I had no idea what she meant by that, not an inkling, no understanding what-so-ever as to the relevance of her question and she never followed it up. Instead she watched my face contort for weeks on end as I limp-ran along red gravel pitches far behind the rest of class, legs cast of lead, calves on fire, hacking and gasping and rasping for air; all that was missing was the floundering, – it's not far behind. Fat kids with strapped down man boobs and inhaler addicts ran on by. She observed from afar, arms folded with back to the bike sheds along with the rest of the PE department; counting down the hours till they could visit the pub, where they will obviously stand in the same formation discussing what a waste of time we are. And this continued all the way up to class tests where we ran from either side of the gym in time with the beeps, which near killed me as I coughed and near floundered with no fluid in my chest, throat or entire breathing apparatus. 'Not as fast as last time Paul.'

'Here baldy baws,' that will be me, 'His your japs eye gone blind?' Swimming Class, my balls yet to drop and not one single hair, complete humiliation and fear of the showers ensued followed by guess what, more bullying. It seemed angry young men that stab rivals through the lungs with screwdrivers and sexually abuse girls in the playground love nothing more than to stare, compare, comment and in my case laugh in pubic one-upmanship. 'Lick ma baws. Maggot, maggot, get your wee balls kicked. Look it ma big dobber.' Again I was stuck idle; in with the asthmatic, the hairy and the breasted: pre-pubescent me standing shivering flesh draped on bare bone, a rack of meat you wouldn't pick up in the butchers. Wet wooden benches, starch textured towelled: getting dry by removing a layer of skin, watching numpties' throwing inhaler tablets into the pool in desperate hope of altering pH balances' to have class dismissed. – Surely I've got to reach puberty now.

...

All I can remember in sum total are weeks and months if not years of duress. I can't remember being well unless I think way back, way way back. And the thing is; no one at this hospital has really told me what my real symptoms were. I know they point out my dry mouth, point to deep cramps in varying places and weight loss; they are all very forthright concerning me peeing a lot of golden urine, which by all instruction should be clear in a good diabetic (yawn). But they haven't discussed with me my late development; never question my lack of focus or poor behaviour, to them I am just ill. There is no due diligence on concentration waning or on any level the cloud that swallowed me both visually and emotionally through the time leading to diagnosis. Retrospective prognosis to prolonged bouts of colds and flu put down all too simply and too exacting to my pancreas having bouts of stops and starts before eventually switching off for good. Semi functionality causing my immune system to become unstable: vulnerable to attack. Although this I look back on following seventeen years non-characteristic change as being the most inadequate proposal in their pronouncement.

...

Even if I didn't care that they came nowhere near to explaining why; it kills me inside living with today's knowledge that if *they* had put me on the sustenance I live on now, back when under *their* care, *they* could have caught me in the *honeymoon period* and made near escape dependency on insulin injections.

Hypotheticals aside, I was a statistic, a, 'Nobody knows why. It's genetic. Every diabetic is different: like fingerprints,' and in the same breath, 'Here, have the same medication as everyone else.' How to explain to a boy that this was only the beginning, that what I was feeling was only a glimpse of how this condition could ruin me in the future. Nothing personal, no real interest, all experience capped off at the basics, no one under any obligation to look further. My life had been written off entirely as, 'Reasonably bright, absenteeism, poor grades, and best to let him go – Jesus impostor,' leaving me to fall between the cracks. It's terrifying the stuff they left out.

# Honeymoon period

*For anyone happening upon this chapter, whilst navigating throughout to particular points of interest, please do not take much of what has been said here as actual practical advice. In practice, whilst not being so cruel as Health Minister, Manto Tshabalala-Msimang of South Africa prescribing garlic and lemon juice as a cure-all to those suffering from HIV, it is on many levels equally ignorant and the unforeseen source of how many deaths and woes? – I suspect ninety-nine percent of you reading this may also be living off this same advice.

...

I make it through to the following day, having slept soundly without interruption from toilet visits or having unstuck my tongue from the roof of my mouth, and although my legs still feel tired from neuropathy and I'm left hobbling like a cowboy, all fear of cramps has lifted.

Second last day and I see a boy walking around in his pajamas, he is in a bed towards the back of the ward so I pop over to say, 'Hi,' and offer to lend him some of my comic books. His mum by his side, she looks like she is going through a lot, like my mum but not poor; he practically pounces out of bed to say, 'Hi, I'm David,' to someone his own age. 'Are you diabetic now, are you new? It's okay.' He does not talk like a kid; he talks like he is older than me. I'm almost patronised, then I notice up close, he doesn't look all too well. Instinctively, I know that I am recovering more than him. Incredibly sullen skin, he looks like he is a black kid, but his illness is making him grey: very thin, but not in a ragged Glaswegian, third generation Catholic way.

Drawings everywhere; scattered over his bedding, stuck to his bedside cabinet hosting the mandatory bedside orange juice without the orange; stacks of sketch pads filled with all sorts bright and wonderful, the opposite of my silhouettes and obsession with symmetry. 'Do you want to read my comics?' I'm already bringing them over when he pulls out lots also, he has bundles already and is really into drawing from them too, so we smile and we bond and he eats tons of *Beef Hula Hoops* in front of me as I watch in wonder, while his mum is pouring cups of diet lemonade. 'How come you get to eat them?' as I almost bump her out of the way to get to the answer. 'We're allowed diet juice and crisps. You can drink as much diet juice as you like because it's not got any sugar in it, and crisps are just like potatoes, you can measure them like normal food.' 'WHAT?!!!' huge grin on my face, 'Sister Rhino, says no treats. But you're right, crisps are fried potatoes.' My smile is bigger than my head now. They are pleased to have broken the good news, 'Sister Shepherd will tell you, she knows the most. She is really nice.' I can see the love him and his mother have for her.

I'm so chuffed to bits and munching away with David to my heart's content. He is a lot younger than me, but he knows his shit. I have made a friend who also likes comic books, and he is a diabetic: awesome.

...

Another day passes and Sister Shepherd introduces herself to me at the bedside, a Specialist Diabetes Nurse, and absolute angel, she teaches me all about my new condition of *type one diabetes mellitus*, the pancreas, the purpose of insulin, how to inject myself twice a day, and how to test my sugar using a little jabbing gizmo she supplies called the *Soft Touch*. It earns its name well when compared with Sister Rhino. Man's diabetes I call it, proper Clint Eastwood diabetes, none of that American fudge related or Steve Redgrave; row, row, row your boat and have a little tablet diabetes.

'Change your fingertips, don't only use the same one and remember you have two hands. It will get sore and you will end up with calluses, if you don't change around often enough. And don't always inject in the same places,' looking at me in the eye with a big smile to make sure the message gets through, 'It can get comforting to inject in the same area, but the skin builds up resistance and gets lumpy underneath, and then the insulin doesn't get through.' – Now pointing and wagging a thin finger; I smile, confirming the message has got through.

My turn and its questions time, 'Is there a cure? What are the side effects? What happens if I have too much? What happens if someone who isn't diabetic has insulin? Does it go off? What if I inject an air bubble? What if I don't have any? What if my cat drinks it? What is the most you can have? What if I forget and take it twice? Will it kill me?' all in one breath, no gaps in-between for air.

'The experts are working on a cure, they estimate it will take around fifteen years to test and make available to everyone; and the average diabetic life expectancy is reduced by fifteen years. And you will have to sit your driving test every four years in case of eye deterioration.'

'So the average age of a man is seventy-seven, I did that in Modern Studies, and I'll have a cure when I'm thirty-ish? Well before I am sixty; then I won't lose my fifteen years?' Fifteen years is a huge amount of time to say the least, but I can feel it on the horizon and it makes me chirpy knowing that this is not a forever thing.

Coy shrug of the medical shoulders, and not making eye contact on that one; how to tell a child he is absolutely going to die fifteen years earlier than his friends, getting harder now I have pressed on it. Should she be telling me this, without my mum here? I'm thinking to myself. A nervous child already half way to developing a twitch and coming to the end of a serious trauma, this will either be coped with and adjusted to or I was going to scream for weeks. But I could see the purpose of *fact-of-the-matter*; I have to be able to deal with this.

'How will I know what to eat?'

'The *complicated carbohydrate solution*, we just divide everything up by ten to keep it nice and simple. And you can still have one treat every day that's up to six units; a can of juice or a *Mars Bar*, anything up to six units.'

'Or two bars of *Dairy Milks*, they are only three units?'

'Mmmm, well okay.' – Smile.

'Can I really eat crisps and drink diet juice all day?'

'Well, not all day, that wouldn't be healthy for anyone, but you can monitor them like you do with bread or potatoes, so two units per bag of crisps. You know how to do it? Where it says, twenty units of carbohydrates on the back of the packet, you divide that by ten, so you get two units.'

'So I have two units of insulin?'

'Yes, or depending on your body, and we will figure this out in the coming weeks, you may need only two units or maybe three or four, or even only one and a half, depending. Every diabetic is different, diabetes is like fingerprints.'

'So, when my sugar is high do I just have insulin and not eat anything till it comes down?'

'NO, DON'T DO THAT! You must always eat when having insulin. If your sugar gets too low, you can fall into a diabetic coma.'

'Does that kill me?'

'Well, some people never wake out of them, and some wake up different because when they are in a coma, their body cuts off oxygen to the brain.'

'What about the futuristic injections you see on TV, the one that goes, "Schhheee," like opening a backwards can of *Coke*?'

'They have researched them, for people who have phobias of needles, but prolonged use hurts the skin.'

'Don't we just need a machine that measures blood sugar and gives you the correct dosage of insulin throughout the day?'

Further shrug of the medical shoulders, and smile at the little boy, as if I'm talking about spaceships.

'Insulin smells like the inside of hospitals. Can't I just drink it? Yeah you're right, it does taste funny.'

'So you know what you're doing? YES! That's you. You are fine. You will come back again and see us?'

You know what it is like when you're a kid and you are unwell. You don't have it in you to argue back or discuss. You just want to go and lie down, and just figure it out later.

...

I'm out, I'm home clear, I'm days later than I thought I would be and I'm arsed if I know what I'm doing, but I'm so massively relieved still, not to be so ill as I was; I really thought it was going to last forever. Filling my face with so much *Barr's Diet Strike Cola* and bags of *Beef Hula Hoops* to meet the hunger. In fact GT's sister who works in the ice cream van is looking at me funny, because I'm a half-foot taller than I was last week and back at her sliding plastic screen ordering more *Beef Hula Hoops* and *Diet Strike Cola* than any normal human being could want.

On leaving day, Sister Shepherd had invited me to visit her at the *Diabetes Clinic*, housed within a newly developed area of *the Royal* hospital grounds. At first every day, then every second, every week, every month and so on, to get me up on my feet, monitor my progress, support and advise accordingly thus instilling a level of independence. So off I go to visit Sister Shepherd, at first with my mum and then on my own. The cost of bus fare and the additional expense of always having to have, *what if money;* what if I need sugar? What if I get faint and need to come home in a taxi? What if a million reasons flickering through our heads every day? Mum is now having to borrow frequently from Gran, this is taking its toll; it seems that some years prior diabetics received additional welfare to assist with dietary requirements, but the offering had since been withdrawn to new sufferers and we have missed the cut off date. – 'They do however now offer free chiropody!'

...

I'm back the first week with my mum, to discuss some serious concerns we're having about me having a hypo, and quickly reassured that glucose tablets, such as *Dextrose* or *Lucozade* tablets will quickly bring me back up out of it. Chocolate is not so useful because it takes the body so long to process, and a can of *Coke* is great to have at hand because it is easily manageable and reliable not to melt in my pocket or burst in my bag. But glucose tablets are the best to carry around because the powder is absorbed directly by the gums straight into the blood stream. 'Ah!' my mum and I look at each other, 'Like in the movies when the Cops test cocaine by rubbing it on their teeth and gums.' 'I still don't understand why they don't get addicted,' Mum continues, 'Wasn't *'The Godfather'* a diabetic? Was that *'The Godfather'* or *'The Godfather'* part two? I don't think it was part three. Part three was terrible. Your gran and I were left really disappointed. That wee lassie was really stale; she only got the part because of her dad. There you go son, nothing to worry about, *Corleone!'*

Following visit on my own, 'How is your diet getting along? You can also enjoy pizza you know?' big smiles and lots of encouragement, 'The pita bread base is measured in long lasting carbohydrate units, which are good for you, and the cheese doesn't contain any units, then there isn't that much on the topping to worry about. And what Chinese food do you like? Sweet and Sour! – Smiles, I knew you were going to say that,' nodding her head, 'That's the one you're not really meant to have; it's made with too much syrup, do you like noodles? Noodles are okay.' – Just as well because I'm from Glasgow: I live on twenty-five p each or five for a pound noodles.

Back the second week and having a meeting with the Diabetes

Specialist Dietician Nurse to get to the bottom of what is going on with my high sugar(s). She is a bit plump and I'm awkwardly horny, wondering to myself what it might be like having sex with her.

From our meetings she was able to compile a complete diet, prescribed to synchronise exactly with my insulin intake. *Complex* carbohydrates were key; regular and often these would burn slowly along with my insulin to keep me *normalised*, whereas the forbidden fruits of fudge and jam would send my sugar levels sky rocketing then spike down leaving me all higgledy-piggledy. My new diet, photocopied onto numerous pages of A4 with clip art of potatoes and other such starch, taking into account eating habits right down to an allowance for favourite foods: the number of strands of spaghetti, half cupful's of rice and chips allowed on my plate. Not many.

I was delighted though to discover that *McDonald's* was actually good for me, as each burger contains only *trace* carbohydrate in the one hundred percent beef, and has a measured amount of carbohydrate in the bun, which the kind and thoughtful yet health conscious fast food vendors detail in their *McDonald's Healthy Living* leaflets to be found by the side of the tills, 'And plenty are available in the waiting room.' Alcohol is given a mention for future consumption, dealt at a manageable four bottles of *Budweiser* per week, with alternatives such as *Holsten Pils* being advised, as, *"All the sugar turns to alcohol,"* in the brewing process. A small caveat added to this, in that the actual chemical alcohol makes insulin work faster and thus may induce hypos. Although with my background, alcohol is always a fear and not something I would be interested in anyway.

...

In one ear and out the other this all went, as my balls finally dropped and the focus of my life, which until now had been all about becoming an Artist, drawing comic books and designing computer games, is lost; shifting to become only concerned with injections and pissing on sticks to check for levels of ketones. Flushes of pink on the pH like strips meeting with concerns of sweet smelling breath and cramps in my calves.

Ten bags of ten p *Petrified Prawns* crisps to eat at the disgust of the woman sat beside me on the number fifty-one A bus, from Bellrock St to the *Diabetes Clinic* at the far bottom of Alexandra Parade. She would never understand this was essential in meeting with my insulin intake, having run out of *Weetabix* this morning. I wasn't frightened of bumping into Craig Sumbrugh on the journey anymore; his past following me home, petrified, from the swimming baths to take my skateboard, and the time he threatened to make me choke to death on my gob-stopper paled in comparison to what I was handling right now. Besides, I felt maybe a bit more capable to deal with life and stick up for myself now; even understanding he stank of shit because of neglect, as did the kid upstairs who used to kick me on the landing after eating foam from out of the back of his couch because of his iron deficiency making him crazy. I felt mentally stronger to deal with these fucks.

Off the bus, through the tinted glass doors and into the *Lego* looking building; past the shops, the cafes, the magazine and news stand, beyond plastic flowers and over thin green carpeting approaching the lift, always waiting for someone to stop me but no one ever does. Waiting at the lift impatiently on half dead old people who get to go first; trolleyed around, smelling of custard, wrapped in Mary blue knit blankets: eventual further progress with a jarring bump down into "Lower Ground" entering the maze of corridors linking the new to the old building. Following painted coloured lines and taking deep breaths past "*Radioactive Nuclear Medicine*" signs reminding me of being in the car with my dad, and being frightened of *TNT Courier* vans, believing they would explode, taking us with them. Taking a moment to point bewildered visitors in the right direction and finally the last stretch, through the glass and cement corridor connecting to the *Diabetes Clinic*; and to my left, Sister Shepherd's office and my right the waiting room.

*McDonalds Healthy Living* leaflets stacked and fallen on the table in front of me, well thumbed through carb-counting convenience per burger, bun and fries; outnumbering and outshining the two-dozen, two-toned green on blue, diabetes health leaflets by a mile, and I must have read them through cover-to-cover a dozen times. Wish they did *Pizza Hut*.

Can I do a pee? Someone asks. 'Do bears shit in the woods?' I'm sent off for a widdle, down to the men's room; yellow magnolia going with the buttery syrupy piss smell from the previous diabetics in here. Piddling into a tinfoil carton getting warm in my hands, making me think of the Chinese food I shouldn't have; trying so hard not to spray, then I balance it down oh so carefully, wash my hands and dry thoroughly before picking it back up because I don't want anyone to think water from washing my hands is dirty pee. Then I place it as instructed on the ledge beside a hatch, leading to an unoccupied room that smells of *Sugar Puffs* – all very mysterious.

Back into the waiting room, and Sister Shepherd pops her head in. Big smile as always; always delighted to see each other, 'How are you keeping? How is your sugar? Are you keeping a diary yet?' 'Wouldn't I be quicker just coming in through the old building?' 'No, you're not allowed,' she smiles, 'This is all the new modern medicine side of the building.' Clearly I should be more enamoured than I am; my petulance winning over, and she will be back in a moment, going to

77

try and skip me up the queue because I'm young and shouldn't have to wait around in the hospital all day. I don't mind being here though, I'm contented to be here and I like it to be honest, I feel safe here.

Pricking my finger, 'How is your mum? Are you checking for ketones?' Have I been sticking to my diet? Passing me some cotton wool to press upon leftover droplets, I enquire, 'Do you not wear gloves because you are dealing with blood?' difficult question from a little boy. 'I do sometimes, not with you, but I do have some patients who I put on gloves for, if we suspect them of using drugs.' 'Or they're minging and you don't want to touch them?' 'Oh Paul.' The machine reading from my urine has come back, "High," again. 'My blood sugar is usually sixteen when I test it, sometimes twenty-two.' And we are still going over the same questions, as I am looking for reassurance. 'What does the machine with my pee do?' 'It tests for sugar in your body averaging over the course of the week. Your own sugar sticks only test for your immediate sugar. We use them both, and sometimes from taking blood directly from your arm, which tests over the past three months, to build up a better picture. Are you going to start keeping your food diary?' 'No.'

'What are the side effects?' Again, a rather positive response, along the lines of, 'Diabetics are like fingerprints and no two are identical; some people become very obese while others can become very skinny, however this is usually down to poor glucose control rather than anything else and there is no reason for you to fall down this path. Nor with good diet and exercise should you suffer poor eyesight, bad circulation, and heart or kidney disease. Although younger diabetics get away with a lot but this catches up on them in later years. It's around fifteen years before the effects of poor diabetes control are felt. But remember not to panic as there is no need for you to succumb to such ails, with good blood sugar control through moderated insulin, diet and exercise.' 'I must be one of the lucky, skinny diabetics.'

Lastly, 'Will it kill me?' This induces hesitation and slight trepidation, followed by a more negative explanation that diabetic life expectancy is currently fifteen years below normal people, based on a national average, which should however increase in time as the general population are living longer now than they did when the last National Census was taken; not exactly specific to me then but still rounding out to fifteen years less than normal people. I better live fast. I'm also advised that national life expectancy levels should improve with modern medicine, and again, that a lot depends on how well I control my levels. I kept on running the math though, and ultimately they were still saying that I would be cured by the time I was *thirty-two*, and the average man lives until they are seventy-seven, so plenty of time between now and sixty-two to get it all figured out. – BINGO!

'How is David?'

'David is doing okay. He is back home now. We have some of the best *Diabetes Experts* in the world, working in this very hospital, working with him and his family to treat him. I'll tell him you said hello, he is always asking after you.'

...

Am I absolutely sure I don't want to attend a retreat, funded by diabetes charities and no doubt sponsored by the pharmaceutical industries? But photos taken on previous events displayed throughout the hallways and in the waiting room are all of grinning teenagers who often looked a bit goofy and half-witted. I point this out to Sister Shepherd, 'Do they all shop at *BHS*?'

One last try, 'Would you like a free trip, paid for by diabetes charities, sponsored by the nice people who make the medicine?' 'No thanks, I don't want to spend a weekend with sugar junkies and being experimented on!'

...

Another appointment, a fortnight later, and this time Sister Shepherd is stuffed further into the corner of her room by the right of the door on entering; this office has now become a dumping ground for copious cases of *Lucozade*. More like a knock off warehouse in here than a Nurses' Station which seems kind of odd. Maybe she is waiting for an epidemic of hypos or maybe they just got it for free as a promotional tool, and her corner room is being hijacked for unintentional Point-of-Sale advertising.

Sister Shepherd sits me down to explain that David has died. The thing is, David was not a kid younger than me after all, he was twenty-seven years old and as she takes great pains to explain, he did not have regular diabetes like mine, but a rare condition where his body would reject insulin of any kind. This stopped his body from developing fully hence the appearance of a child. 'Experts at the hospital, at the forefront of diabetes research and development, were working closely with him and his family, but could not find a suitable long-term treatment or solution on time. He was suffering a lot towards the end, and he is at peace now.'

'You know he was always into drawing, and everyone thought he was really good?' 'Yes.' 'Well he wasn't.' Sister looks at me with hurt expression, she is hurt for me. I have insulted him because I am angry, I am not angry at him, I am angry because he has died. He is my friend and he has something similar to me and he has died

80

because they couldn't fix him in time.

...

Visiting only every second month now, plans to cycle here have faltered because I do not own a bike. My sugar levels still spiralling way out of control; it is time again for me to see the Dietician, and find out what is going so wrong. 'I am sticking to my food sheets, Mum reads and serves as directed the counted number of chips, or strands of spaghetti and I've not had Chinese Takeaway and only drinking *Diet Strike Cola*. Sticking to my one treat a day, usually a *Mars Bar* because it's got more in it for the units; no jam or fudge, all my carbs on the backs of tins counted.' Why hasn't my blood sugar come down from sixteen?

Working my way back up the tunnels, out of sight of watchful eyes, and washing back my ten pence crisps with a miniature can of *Orange Tango*, I turn the corner and walk straight back into the Dietician Nurse. 'What's this your drinking?' surprise in her chookter's accent, 'DO YOU KNOW HOW MUCH SUGAR IS IN THAT?' 'It only comes to half my daily treat allowance.' She looks suspicious. I didn't know quite what else to say, I just hold it by my side and wait till I'm around the next corridor, on autopilot, and in the lift headed for the exit before enjoying the rest. What else am I not telling them about?

...

Dietician Nurse in full flow, 'Insulin, exercise, fast acting sugars; all factors interfering with blood sugar levels.' And adrenalin, she mentions adrenalin burns away blood sugar and will leave me in a hypo, so to always have some insulin and sugar with me. Adrenalin? Adrenalin burning in *Glasgow* can leave me in a hypo? So every time someone in *Glasgow* gives me a dirty look I am going to need sugar?

That's about every fifteen minutes. I'm going to need to be wrapped up in cotton wool just to make it down Argyle Street. This must be wrong. I can't be the only diabetic in Glasgow; we would be an epidemic of *Irn-Bru* swigging coma patients never out of the news.

The suggestion of keeping a diary of what I'm eating and insulin intake seems a little overboard. I mean, if you're not adjusting dynamically in real time then what's the point of logging years' worth of doing it wrong. It's like wanking, we all enjoy doing it, but at the point where you are keeping a meticulous log, it has become a bit obsessive.

And all the while they could have just put me onto the diet I live on now, and I would never have had to take even a single insulin injection or go through a single diabetic hardship. At least my mum is secretly pleased that I can never be called up for National Service.

...

Now the real honeymoon period; a completely natural phenomena when the pancreas is caught before completely giving up on itself; insulin producing cells, not completely eviscerated are still in action, still functioning on a low key level: still prepared to deal with life as it is meant to be.

To be caught in time however, an accurate social consciousness of the diabetic condition must exist; unified understanding of early warning signs; catching the patient at the end of their tether, of equal importance to picking up on key symptoms of dry mouth, etc.

Our body not in exigency of third hand in-conclusion, lashed in synthetic hormone, but harmony; soul soothing understanding to defend and uphold the soon to be diabetic in their occasion of requisite urgency. A pre-conceived escape plan: equilibrium in *metabolic meditation.*

Hats are off, problem not solved, but handled through a lifetime of natural balance too often mistaken for balancing out; an unmistakable better alternative to injections every day, and emotional trauma that is diabetes.

# A new condition

My arms all covered in bruises, blue where the drip-fed into the topside of my hand. I have the complexion of a bruised banana; fingertips perforated like tea bags; still a touch see through: when I squeeze my finger blood drips from five places making a ladybird. Comforting readings of, "High," on my blood sugar monitor, induced by treating myself to bars of *Cadbury Fudge* are clearly having their wear and strangely now burning the back of my throat. Although still less concerning than the prospect of my blood sugar declining, and machine indicating, "Low," being left on the floor in a diabetic coma; a condition to which I was warned, could result in loss of oxygen to my brain and leave me waking with the mind of a child, or not awakening at all.

'Owwww!' it's gone right through my finger AGAIN. So bloody sharp, it sticks out the other side, under my nail, as if it's supposed to. Keep dropping them too, and they land needle first, making me jump out of the way, but never on time. These insulin pens I have to use twice daily are unwieldy, and too clunky to operate with any level of precision, not helped by the areas in which I have to inject making me frightened. I can handle pressing the needle into the backs of my upper arms, but often imprecision will lead me to inject into muscle by accident. Injecting into the top of my thighs is manageable, but often I clench as realisation of what I'm doing washes over, tension and hesitation heightening the sensation of cold needle deep within my flesh making me cry out. Injections to the stomach are just awful; giving the queasy sensation I am stabbing myself, leaving the only alternative of injecting into my bum cheek. Well this just seems simply impossible, how on earth am I going to stretch around like that with any level of accuracy, injecting with a white plastic pen almost twice as long, four times as wide as and ten times clunkier than any regular pen. How am I honestly supposed to inject myself in the bum cheek with this? Pretty loose metaphor to call this monster a pen if you ask me. Mum and Gran are too squeamish to help, I'm not letting Angela see my bum because she will laugh, and Victor's not getting anywhere near me; did you see *the state he did to my hair* when only supposed to trim my fringe before the school play?

Self-imposed guinea pig-ism is so very hard to deal with, my body racked, and nearly non-existent levels of confidence waver, as I adjust insulin intake to meet with readouts from blood sugar test sticks. *Fray Bentos Pies* and *Heinz Baked Beans*; having to read the backs of the tins over and over because all the words on their labels are jumbling up; they may present one amount of carbohydrate units on the back labels, but my body produces another, and four plus two is often making, "High," whilst six units of insulin will often have seemingly no effect.

Throughout these three weeks or so taken to adjust to my medication and get on top of my new condition, I have also unfortunately missed the prelims to my high school exams and to be honest I never even thought about them. There is no room in my head for anything other than monitoring and adjusting insulin levels to account for and admonish these recurring cramps, which take deeper root into my hands, pulling my pinky finger back like a broken elastic band and leaving me with a claw like sensation. 'Bananas,' I've been advised are a key source of potassium and will help prevent cramps, this trick worked just great but Sister Shepherd's advice on how diabetes would quickly become, 'Instinctive,' still seems a long way off and a long time coming.

...

Three weeks absence from school shortly lapse to four, and we are living in a little world of our own. The most I'm getting done is helping Mum count strands of spaghetti for dinner and wishing I had more space taken up on my plate by chips than tomato sauce. Sitting over the side of the bed one night, my hands start trembling and I know something's wrong; all of a sudden I've become weak and fatigued on the road to fainting while hunger grows in my stomach. Call in my mum to my bedroom and she says I am white as a ghost, so we decide to hurriedly test my blood sugar together: me jabbing at my finger-tips trying to release a drop of blood, dribbling helplessly down the side of my finger so onto jabbing the next as Mum looks on helplessly with a packet of *Dextrose,* a can of *Coke* and a *Marathon* bar ready in her hand. The only sticks I have left are the manual ones, and having ample blood on one, we now have to wait a minute and wipe it back off, and wait another minute for the revealing of the result. One elephant, two elephants... then finally "2.8," – My first hypo! Time to start munching back those *Dextrose,* 'Yuck, give me that *Marathon* instead,' the hunger rising, instinctively, I know I have to eat; in future when I feel this way I will know that I have to eat, 'Glug, glug, glug,' goes the *Cola,* washing back milk chocolate and nuts; what a relief to know that I am able to detect these, and *instinctively* know how to handle them. I have seen both sides of blood sugar now, both high and low, and now I know what to do. A big hug from Mum and a short time to rest, it's time to get life back to normal, and time to get back to the Doctor for another prescription of blood sugar test sticks. – Oh shit, now my blood sugar is reading "16.0," but I can worry about that another time, the priority for now is not being in a coma.

Throughout this period of adjustment the world just passes me by, washed away are all concerns of what the world could do to me, and my attention set instead on what harm I could do to myself. Misdirected injections and repeated injections into the same place now having their impact, although now beyond coming to terms with the initial diabetes; now coming across some of the ramifications. Finger tips become raw and this I grow to deal with, while the stabbing sensation to get that drip of blood; it does feel like getting blood from a stone at times, induces less flinching and the pain a fraction of what it had been. Unable to go near my stomach or bum cheeks; repeated injections in the upper legs taking their toll resulting in the build-up of massive boils with heads the size of fifty pence pieces, sourced from swollen pustules taking over to cover the circumference of my thighs. Crusted and starting to ooze at the tops like cow pats laying heavy on my limbs, impeding my ability to walk straight. But we do walk, all the way through the park to the Doctors, quickly shuffled into see the naive young Nurse, 'OH NO. MY GOD, THAT'S THE BIGGEST BOIL I HAVE EVER SEEN IN MY ENTIRE LIFE,' stepping back, hands crossed over her chest, 'Shriek!' Mum with her hand on my shoulder, nodding her head from left to right, on one hand saying to herself, 'You poor boy,' and on the other saying, 'These fucking people, what the hell is wrong with you fucking people – hopeless.' Anyway Nurse Silly calls in the Doctor who explains it may be the initial reaction and shock to my body of the needles, and this could certainly be compiled with any germs, which may have gotten into my skin along with the repeated use of the same injection site. I would now have to leave these alone no matter how comforting I found it. A combination of antibiotics and poultice prescribed, as they don't know whether my boils will heal up or explode like mustard gas. And sent off limping home with bandages around my two trench warfare legs when an approaching car refuses to slow for the lights, and I hobble as fast as I can manage from one side of Edinburgh Road to the other to avoid being smashed up in a whole other way. 'BASTARDS!' Mum cries out behind them, 'Can they not see you are limping out of the fucking Doctors?' I could see this was starting to hurt her, more than me. Two days later and I awake to the stench of pus, all smothered in fluid down my legs and over a ruined quilt, cat locked out and bedroom windows having to be left open for the next three days to let out the smell.

All that's left to do now is have a sleepless night of high blood sugar, cramps, nausea and general panic resulting in a bus journey back to the *Diabetes Ward* on a Sunday morning, where on asking what to do, my mother and I get barked back out the ward by Sister Rhino bluntly informing us, 'You need to adjust your insulin levels on your own, and ask at the *Diabetes Clinic* for advice on Tuesday, AS MONDAY IS A BANK HOLIDAY!'

...

Tuesday arrives on schedule and I am finally treated to an introduction with the local *Diabetes Expert Consultant*, I have seen him wandering around these corridors, all tall and uber-posh, big red cheeks and dopey looking; suit trousers that are a bit *budgie* around his ankles, and a shirt with dressed down tie. His wife definitely buys his outfits from *BHS*. Hi ho, hi ho, it's off to work he goes. But he couldn't save David, as I look back down on the floor. Everything he said, just going into one ear and out of the other. Something about me being a perfectly healthy, regular diabetic. I want to go home. I peek up, 'Couldn't I use normal needle syringes instead?'

...

Et Voila, what a set of balls on me. Just enough time for a quick handshake with the Devil, and celebrate the first time I came.

...

They say that in any major city you are never more than six feet away from a rat. Fortunately it's the same with *Coca-Cola*, and having a hypo has become far less of a concern.

# Back to school daze

'I don't understand, is it no like asthma? It's pure mental man; he has tae eat pizza fir breakfast and eh gets drunk on *Irn-Bru*! Ad pure love that man, ad be drinkin *Irn-Bru* oh the time. Doon it the ice cream van, "Here mate geeze some *Irn-Bru*, am gonna get steamin." Ah couldn'y inject myself though, it's no like a junkie or nuthin, ah just don't like needles and sometimes ah drink *Coca-Cola* insteed o *Irn-Bru*. Here whit happens when ye drink *Coca-Cola*? Am gonno get mad-wey-it.' — Rab discusses, as we walk on through the park to school.

Back to cheap ass trainers, because I've grown out of the good ones, 'We will be on our feet soon and I'll get you new trainers, again,' loves Mum. All the girls smell of *Peach Dewberry* and the boys of cat piss; their *Nike Air Max* air-bubbles having burst to leak scent from two terms of foot sweat. Teachers are across the board supportive, asking how I am, whist keeping in their desk drawers packets of *just in case Dextrose*, *Bounty Bars* and *Rolos*. Although the School Nurse is clearly well out of her depth and comes nowhere near, nor does my Guidance Counsellor for that matter, and my PE teacher's bemused on enquiry, 'Do you remember that time when you asked me if I was diabetic?' 'Oh you are diabetic now are you?' Keen on herself for guessing it was coming to me, though not taking into consideration she could have saved me a world of pain by looking into things a little further how many months ago?

Classes have become confused; prelim period and exam scheduling mixing class years and pupils in turn; I'm now well aware that the world has continued on without me. I have missed all my prelims over the past few weeks, so seem to be getting slotted into anywhere to keep me on the books but out the way of people who deserve to do well. What have I been doing with my time; haven't I been cramming for exams? The truth; having had so much time on my hands, the only things I did manage to achieve were injecting insulin vials full with air to build up pressure, and launching the plungers of my syringes across the room at my sister when she comes in through the living room door, and defrauding the 'Dandy Comic' by sending in a picture of their characters signed off as, "Paul Cathcart age twelve." The resulting surprise arrived in the form of a t-shirt and poster. The t-shirt slogan, "I'm a Dan fan," wittily translated to, 'I'm a fan-Dan.' by teachers and pupils alike. 'Exams start next week Paul. Do you have your exam timetable? It's time to pull out all the stops; this is no time to be resting on your laurels.'

I'm not feeling very conducive to an academic tenure, standing in this empty classroom; taped up perspex for a window, scabbed layer upon layer of gloss magnolia over radiators surrendered to initials and a Legalise Cannabis Campaign motif. Everything is a bit bright and a bit dark, those CND monkey skulls still scaring the shit out of me; injecting by accident into the muscle of my upper arm. Six units to be precise in the wrong place, not much fat left and easily missed: I am so skinny my face has lines. I already forgot to take it this morning. Blood spec left on my white shirt. – Can't I sit this one out, go home and lose myself in comic books and sketch pads. How can I be

91

expected to perform?

I'll take a wander round to the new sausage van on the grounds of *The Dal* to get some lunch. Kids around me from years below buzzing like flies on *Cola-Cubes*; I won't be allowed them; are smashing each other with strips of plastic pulled from a skip. And I'm barely *here* to move out of the way. I stand in the middle, not losing my place in the queue; more concerned my bag is filled with *just in case* extra vials of insulin, easily breakable, and syringes; *what if* they grab my bag and the lid comes off and one of them gets jabbed? My *Dextrose* already turned to powder; my *Snickers bar* should be okay? But they patiently strike and spit on each other around me. Well a roll in sausage will be two units, the sausage has none. So, 'I'll have two rolls in sausage, one cheeseburger and two bags of pickled onion *Space Raiders* please,' that's about six units as I smear them over in burger relish and brown sauce. Still not had my treat for the day and don't want to eat my *Snickers* just in case, so, 'And I'll have a *Mars Bar* and a can of *Diet Irn-Bru.*' I've never had this much lunch money before.

Now standing in the playground on my own; notice coloured green and orange paper with printed letters taped to the insides of windows, assuming it's something to do with exam organisation. The asthmatic and the breasted are blanking me now; I can't tell if they don't like me anymore or if they are just not bothered because I'm never around. They huddle together at the safe end of the playground in a ball of five or six deep, penguins protecting the intellectual egg; they, over the next few weeks are set to reap reward for sixteen years being called, 'Professor,' and 'Spotty wank.' The hairy, I heard has dropped out early to get a job, his girlfriend is pregnant and they need to save up for a pram. Quite a few girls absent I notice, for falling pregnant, considered a distraction to other pupils more able to get ahead in life, and then I suppose there is the safety aspect. Two junior girls entangled in a hair pulling lock; neither able to release for fear of a smashed head, gouged eyes or torn throat. Some older boy's come over from the gates to pull down both their skirts and pants, revealing two little bushes, to their humiliation and still they can't let go. Some other bunch of girls in fits of tears in the corridor, all woollen black tights irrepressibly distraught; one of their brothers had a machete knife put down the side of his head behind the bike sheds last week; in the same spot where I once felt Sharon's cold bum on a Saturday date. The Police, along with Guidance Counsellors are conducting interviews. And everything is again, a bit bright and a bit dark, but I equally don't care. I have no idea at all what I am doing here anyway, why I'm even out of the house, let alone the hospital. What is the point of this? This is completely ludicrous. I'm standing in the middle of a playground, no one acknowledging me.

Final class of the day is English; half way through when the teacher approaches my desk and enquires, 'Paul, have you ever been knocked down before?' 'No,' I reply in complete indifference, pulled out from my daydream about shagging Kelly LeBrock out of '*Weird Science.*'

The lane that runs between the chip shop and the bookies, teetering over smashed concrete slabs and broken glass; I used to walk home on evenings like this, when it was this cold and turning to get dark so early; I'd go home and watch the '*Ewoks*' cartoon, I think to myself, nearly crying to myself. Spinning over the bonnet, a muffled bundle in unfashionable *LA Raiders* padded jacket, shoulder catches going through the windscreen, curtailing my axis then spinning me up, over, I can see all around me spiralling, 'CRACK,' landing head first onto the curb. I try to get up and walk on in a daze trying to again reach home, all I can think to myself, that this is wrong. Falling back over my left side, sky above within the grass island; on my back and in shock, my arm is not sitting where it is supposed to be, I have it folding over my chest where I can feel it, it should be lifting to help me pick myself back up off the ground because I want to get home, but instead I can see it's flung over to my right; shoulder muscle and bone twisted and torn. This is where my dad used to cry, my consoling thought.

Blood pouring from my scalp, I think I know what's happened, someone passes to me my school bag, someone else tells me to stay still. The Headmaster pops over to see what's all the commotion, I'm bleeding over his deep blue *Armani* suit: he is taking an age to send word for an ambulance. By this time Rab has crossed over the road, scaled the park fence and run through the width of Cranhill Park, is through the gates at the other side, has run over Bellrock St, past my house and up the *Sugarolly Mountains*, over the wall on through the middle flats courtyard, jumped over the wall at the other side, through toward the play park, vaulted that little fence, past the big tunnel, jumped over the final little fence at the other side, entered Longstone high flats, pushed through the security door then leapt and pounced his way up umpteen stories of stairs, pushed through a blue storm door, run through the landing, pushed in through his own storm door, chapped on his front door, waited... and got his father to phone for an ambulance. Clever boy.

Into the ambulance I go as instinct takes over, 'I have diabetes,' I tell the Paramedics, 'Check my sugar?' They do so and give me oxygen, before everything becomes a blur and I'm back to square one, in a hospital bed with my mother and Gran sitting either side of me in tears. My mouth is dry only this time it's because they won't let me eat or drink before surgery. They ask me in the Operating Theatre if I have any concerns before they begin, 'What happens if I have a nightmare when you are operating?' To which they comfort me by explaining, 'This does not happen due to dreams taking place on the

94

verge of being awake; anaesthetic puts you down further into such a deep rest that you no longer feel or dream.' Then ask me to tell them what I smell, on lifting a transparent gas mask over my mouth, counting to ten, 'I can smell new trainers,' the *Nike Air Jordan's* and *Reebok Pumps* I have grown out of so quickly; bought them with the money my gran in Ireland left me when she died, passing them onto Victor, now the trendiest Grandad in Glasgow. 'Three, four, zzzz.'

Awakening to an ice cube being placed in my mouth, and the combined pull of two forces, like the theoretical equation of what happens when an unstoppable force meets with an immoveable object; only this time it's the remainder of high sugar urine forcing its way out against industry strength anaesthetic; the result of which leading Doctors to inform, 'Should you not pee soon, then we will need to insert a catheter tube up through you urethra for fear of internal rupture.' Fifth petrified attempt at compromise and I finally go; what a relief as I fill a litre measured waxed cardboard carton to the brim, handing it scalding hot and froth-bubble topped over through a gap in the curtain, requesting another with open hand and laugh, 'Ahh.'

'What happened?' that's the question and I struggle to recollect, though sure enough when I thought it through long enough; being cold all of the time, I had walked out of school, frozen right through to the bone in a high sugar daze; past students previously absent and disenchanted, vying for supremacy, tossing bricks and shouting along the banks of Edinburgh Road, "You're a fucking dead man," past a smashed car with a *haulfer* sticking through its windshield, then all is blank from here, resulting in a head full of stitches and a disconnected shoulder, screwed back together like something from an old tool shed. Two days later, I'm out and back home, unlike the poor girl in the back seat, who suffering from asthma went into severe shock at the sight of my ugly jacket piling through her mum's *Ford Sierra*, leaving her in the Children's Ward for weeks to come while I miss my exams. 'How is my *'Dandy* t-shirt?' Alas my dear fan-Dan t-shirt never pulled through.

# Fight or flight? Flight

Manifestation of fear to cross roads, conjoined with my fear of leaving plugs in. Getting up during the night to check all the sockets are off, looking behind the TV, down the sides of the electric heater, then opening the fridge door to check there is nothing wrong as I can hear it rattle and hum from my bed. Turn off the light switches, exiting each room, one-by-one, returning to double check the video plug, check that paper wiring diagram has been removed in case it catches on fire. Walking back upstairs and the central heating blows on and off with the pilot light, clicking and igniting, repeating its ritual. Time to sleep because there is nothing else to do; my old *Batman* wallpaper playing tricks on my eyes and Budgie McCulloch is in my kitchen to hurt us, there is a knife and I, 'SCREAM,' back against the kitchen cupboard though no noise comes out of my mouth. I awake cold in sweat, the side of my face covered in blood. Ruby red crusted between my nostrils and patches in my hair. I wipe at my face and the puddle on my pillow of blood mixed with snot as I call for, 'MUM.' Another nose bleed and she removes the pillow case revealing coffee stained blood marks from times before, time for it to go back in the machine and me to go back to school.

I mean what else can you do with a boy who has a few stitches in his head and a shoulder all bandaged up, who has already missed his prelims and now missed his exams? Only this time, every time I cross a road Rab shouts, 'MOTOR!' and I jump through the roof. This does make me laugh though, but laughter never helps dampen wracking pain as my shoulder jolts within its sling; twice the size as it was before, iodine inseparable from bruising and stitches jaggedly poking out over the surface of raw pink flesh unsettled scar tissue, one inch thick and four inches long; though laughter does over time help to ease my nerves. There is not much you can do with a shattered shoulder, except figure out how to take injections with one hand, and get back to regular life while you wait for it to slowly mend the diabetic way, – fifty times slower than *normal* people I'd been informed, 'Not going to heal while your sugar is high.'

...

*Fuck me; can barely get past the gates for half bricks flying by bowed head and Police cars barricading the gates. All stemming from final exam stress, a final, 'You were never welcome; you never have been any good. Even your Social Worker gave up on you by the age of twelve: get the message?' Frustrations rising even higher, the world has given up on you before you had the mind to give up on yourself; sure your rebellion of smoking hash whilst listening to Pink Floyd has been a waste of time, as was scoring your name on every surface and threatening everyone who would take you seriously, as was dousing that boy in lighter fluid then calling out for a light, intent on setting him on fire because nobody cares about you. No point in hanging around the fence crying out for attention any more, no more sniffing Tipp-ex in the bike sheds or going seconds on a cigarette with that girl you fancy; she is off now, getting shagged by a taxi driver.*

*'Punch him, go on punch him, don't let him hit you like that. I telt you punch him....' and as an eight year old boy who already wants to fall apart inside, sniffles and weeps, he tries to make a fist and pushes back, 'Yeah that's it see,*

98

*you've goat to learn to hit them back.' There is a regrettable backward psychology going on in the parent's minds, that if their child learns to hit back now, becomes the aggressor, then this blessed child will swan through life with no problems at all, completely bypassing the life of their parents; killing their own demons in the hands of their children.*

*Freddie Skerryvore has JoJo by the throat against the outside corridor wall. Holding a knife to his face, with JoJo punching out at him, shouting, 'DO IT, DO IT.' and some nasty little bastard has been caught by the opposing faction: escaping blows to run head first into passing traffic. Brendan Devlin storms in high on Diamazepam, pushing teachers into walls and shouting to us all, 'ICF, ICF,' almost clapping his hands in time, staggering farther before his eventual collapse into the tuck shop and calling of an ambulance. Like a violent puppy in its final moments of being put down.*

*Police, long since rejecting any urge to get in harm's way; opting instead to point a camcorder from safe distance, preferably their helicopter; requesting that teachers identify culprits later in the day, to chants of, 'GRASS! GRASS!' Lead offenders instructed via tannoy to reception, and awaiting Officers in the style of a celebrity roll call: laughter roaring throughout the halls, tapered by jeers of admiration in which to bask in notoriety; one last shout back at a system forever banished.*

...

'I don't know if I want you in my Art Class, you have taken too much time off. I can't take you as a serious student.' – Mr Courtier, Head of the Art Department. Thanks for your support. Don't you remember sending me home from school with a note, and me being diagnosed with diabetes? This is the only class I have a hope of getting a decent exam result for. Your Art class is my only link to education through my portfolio and you are taking it away from me. But what to expect from a self-proclaimed religious man, who will deny charity to those who use contraception, in a dry country where famine takes most children and HIV attempts to ruin the rest.

Already missed my prelims and now my exams; physical health completely drained, struggling to come to terms with this new condition, my arm up in plaster and I have nothing to return for. Back to dry mouth and cramps, with the world directly surrounding me seemingly going to self-destruct. I have become helpless with no way of defending myself. I just want to curl up in a ball forever with insulin syringes and sugar tablets.

Going for the short term against the wishes of my mother, "Aim high, and even if you don't reach your dream, you will still be somewhere high up there," and advice of my sister, "Don't drop out of school now, they might be earning one-hundred-and-fifty pounds a week, and that seems like a lot of money when you are just out of school, but they will be on one-hundred-and-fifty pounds forever."

Fucking hell, I can't manage. I can't do this anymore. My world is falling over, I need to sit and rest, to recuperate. Stop pushing me to perform; I'm not normal, I don't feel normal. I feel wounded and want to stop.

Got a two for my Art based on course work, and five for English, sixes for everything else. Still, I'm not going back there to repeat last year and get kicked in. Then there is I, and thoughts on me and I'm not fitting in at all; head full of pus from stitches not dissolved threatening to leave me brain damaged; get me the fuck out of here, please, 'Get these things out of me.' It is without doubt time to bail before I get caught up in this, before I fall as the next undeserving, random victim to a crowd of jackals whose blood is up, grinning in lust, an attempt to prove themselves in the face of others they are deeply afraid of.

So age sixteen I take on a whole new outlook on life; I could die any minute, I've had two near death escapes already, that's more than most people have in a lifetime. Time to grow my hair, dress in black and set the world on fire; an Artist deep inside and I can do it on my own. I quite liked the hairstyle of a boy nick-named *Foxy* in the year above, who is in all the newspapers this summer holiday for being shot-gunned down by rival drug dealers; so on comes the middle shed, growing steadily down my face like curtains.

Dramatic mood change: no more smiles disguising frayed nerves; instead counting stones on the road as I walk and everything is shit. Literally I find no enjoyment in anything, the computer bought with the remainder of my gran's will is shit, I'm back wearing shit trainers, the TV is shit, my family makes me want to scream and even on my own, everything winds me up to a breaking point, where I am banging fists leaving pot holes in paper thin doors. "What happened to my little boy?" – Mother. I don't want to be a scared little kid any more, but more so I cannot understand this torment and rage. So fucking angry, every thought boiling and it hurts inside.

# Life begins at sixteen

# (charming)

Like any teenager I suppose but a whole lot more. I wasn't just dealing with puberty and hormones, and the emotions that go with them; I was struggling to communicate what I was going through, and I used to write these notes in my head for people I desperately wanted to understand. To try and explain what I was going through and they went along the lines of this,

*"Just struggling to let you know what is happening to me and you think I'm being mean all the time. I'm screaming inside and you're telling me I'm just like my dad. She looks at me with the expression she has when she speaks of him, you all do. You have started calling me an arsehole and that is all you ever call him. He has done things, which are in my head, which I don't even know how to think about.*

*You ask me, "What happened to my little boy?" How do you think I feel? You have no idea. I eat food and I scream, I need sugar and I go white, all the blood it's leaving my body. I'm scared and you're not acknowledging me. You tell me that its six o'clock so I'm to have my insulin now and you will put food on in a minute. But it takes more than twenty minutes to make I try to explain, and*

*you won't even get around to starting for twenty minutes and I will be having a*
*hypo by then if I take it now. And yes I am upset, but I'm not like him, I'm not*
*and no one is sticking up for me. My sugar is high and it makes me feel violent,*
*but I'm not going to hit anyone. I'm just pushing you all away to protect myself.*
*Maybe I will be better on my own till I get better then I won't upset you and you*
*won't upset me. BUT I need you and your help because I don't know what I'm*
*doing. I read things wrong, I read the back of the instructions on the tin wrong*
*and you make me feel embarrassed, you dismiss me and you laugh at me and*
*you are ashamed of me because you don't think that I am trying hard enough,*
*and you're upset with me because I'm not this little boy anymore but I am*
*inside.*"

Well that's enough of feeling sorry for myself…

'GET A FUCKING JOB OR GET OUT OF MY HOUSE.' Seven in the
a.m. Irene's clearly not allowing me become a bum, so off to the
*Careers Advice Centre* I go. What was I good at? 'At school? Well I liked
doing Art. What did they train me for at school? Well, they said I
could almost become Jesus.' 'Okay, so we're looking for the perfect
balance between Art and Son of God. How about becoming a *Skill
Seeker?*' Sounds like a good idea to me. Printer by trade, and I get to
spend one day a week at college practicing Art, to build towards my
portfolio and gain a National Certificate, my next step in reaching
my long term goal of getting into Art School. Thirty-six pounds a
week to begin with, forty-six by the end of the two years, minted.

Six spoonful's of *Nescafe* in a mug and fill to half level with boiling
water to dissolve; three heaped tablespoons of sugar to cover my
insulin, stir to taste, and fill to the brim with cold water from the tap:
down the hatch in the one. I call it the '*Caffeine Bomb,*' inspired by the
song on my *Walkman* by the *Wildhearts*. Embark out in the fog
wearing three t-shirts, two long sleeves and three pairs of socks; hair

drawn over my brow so I don't have to make eye-contact with anyone, and a high-sugar-corpse, I coma walk up Bellrock St toward Queenslie Industrial Estate to work. I'm like *'Hansel and Gretel,'* trailing blood sugar test sticks everywhere I go.

Getting there in the dark, coming home in the dark, a glimpse of light in the early afternoon, 'Can I have a *Snickers bar*, a can of *Diet-Coke*, three bags of ten p *Quarter Backs*, a *Biscuit and Raisin Yorkie* and a cheeseburger please?' from the sausage van; whiff of *Body Shop* factory chemicals making every lunch taste like peach soap anyway. Usual head in a daze, mind wandering and freezing cold, 'Has he not ordered a new gas canister yet?' 'His he bollocks.' – John. Blood sugar of seventeen, peeing every twelve minutes; have another injection and repeat till fade. Stirring inks into the wrong *Pantone*; monotonously silk-screen printing t-shirts, putting them through the dryer then checking the ink is set before stacking them into boxes. Three hundred white print on red *Baby Chaos, "Super powered so fuck you,"* T's today all packed and set to go; backs of my fingers all smeared in ink. That's strange.

Insane hypos, cravings for sugar undeniable, can't eat enough to satisfy the hunger. The tuck box in the fridge, start with the good stuff; *Twix, Bounty, Lion Bar*, cans of *Lilt*; 'Here John, do you want anything?' By Wednesday it's, *Whole Nut*, fucking breakfast bars and *Tizer*, 'Am no eating *Turkish Delights*. They are fucking bouthin. Have you eaten aw the *Bounty's* again? Fuck me, you're a gannet,' says John.

Get in from the sausage van, following lunchtime, eyes like a mole; *Baby Chaos* t-shirts being thrown at me, to cries of, 'For fuck sake, how did this happen?' My Boss Adrian, aw he is *fuming*; fortunately John steps in, 'It's that dryer Adrian, I've been tellin ye fir ages, it's fucked.

It dries the *toap* layer and it's still damp underneath, there's nay wiy of tellin without scraping ah the ink aff the t-shirt.' 'Well am fucked with the bill, nobody's going to pay for them.' Adrian storms off, and John waits to hear the door slam, 'Ohhhh Smudge, that was close.' 'Fucking hell, was that me?' 'Was it your hands covered in ink?' He is pissing himself laughing and I'm in belly giggles with a big red face, 'Fuck!' Then he walks over to the side shelf and pulls out a sheet of paper, 'Here, look wit ave been dayin ah day,' big smile on his coupon and reveals a pencil drawing of Princess Diana, with a speech bubble, *"I've been shagged by a cad."* 'What's a cad?' 'Did you no see it own the news? She has been getting pumped by some posh bloke; poor big ears hasn't got a clue. Here, ave also been in Adrian's drawer and seen he has written you up a reference, want tay read it?'

*"RE: Paul Cathcart.*

*To whom it may concern.*

*Paul has been at Print-Trix now for near six months; throughout this time he has shown a keen and proactive approach to all aspects of the printing industry. Punctual, well-mannered and responsible, any company will be fortunate to have him on board.*

*If only I wasn't a twat faced, Flanders look alike with a pig ugly wife, and knew what I was doing, instead of driving around all day while my staff played on the phone. I'd be able to keep my own business and not go bankrupt!*

*Adrian.*

*Director Owner, Print-Trix."*

Then the man comes around late Thursday afternoon to refill the Tuck box, that's twenty pounds out of my pocket at least, just covering insatiable hypos and boredom with over-priced

105

confectionery.

...

Friends from my one-day a week NC course at Cardonald College
have introduced me to other new friends in town on Saturday
afternoons; involving a new kind of friendship, one of equal parts.
Injecting in front of groups of complete strangers who never blink; is
quite cool, it certainly never bothers me; just gives me something to
do before meals and drinking sessions, something to keep an eye on
and yeah I suppose it has become part of my identity. Maybe it brings
some attention, 'It's just a balancing act with my blood sugar. I just
need to keep it level. Food makes it go high, some food makes it
higher than others, like toffee and fudge, some other stuff I shouldn't
have but not much. I don't miss it. I take insulin to burn away the
sugar then sometimes I've not eaten enough for the insulin so I have
to have more sugar like when I was having that can of *Coke* earlier.
It's easy; I don't even bother about it. Guy I was at school with, Frank
Dolan, summed it up best, said me having insulin was like, "Stopping
to have a piss." And it is because sometimes I can't even remember if
I've had it or not. Can you remember how many times you took a piss
today? The best bit is that when my sugar is high, I can't get fat. I'm
a lucky skinny diabetic. It's double beneficial.' 'You're lucky man,
eating chocolate stops you getting fat. I get fat just being near it,'
say's a rather stocky built kid. 'How many times do you need to have
it a day?' A few people gathered around now. 'Twice: once in the
morning with breakfast and at six with dinner. And the other things I
can't do are have a tattoo because I heal slower than normal people,
and I can't have piercings either, but I don't like them anyway so I
couldn'y gee a fuck. It does make me need to piss all the time when
my sugar is high. Can be a total pain in the arse, so I always need to
go into *The Copthorne Hotel* and *Marks & Spencers*.' 'Can you drink

106

*Holsten Pils* because, *"All the sugar turns to alcohol"?* 'Yeah but the bottles are tiny and the chemical alcohol makes insulin work faster, so I need to have sugar with it anyway.' 'That's cool man,' nods of understanding, I nearly get a round of applause.

George Square and Virginia Galleries becomes our scene; a meeting point from Eaglesham to Stirling where rejected rockers unite. The great unwashed, long hair, untidier lengths, miserable denim and all red plaid underneath leather jackets; *GnR* showing heritage, *Nirvana "Smiley Face"* projecting new character, *Concorde, Budweiser, JD* and *Pepsi-Max* mixer: no one ever hurt anyone. One love in Glasgow, 'Fuck the Neds.' Numbers of us, no one would even give a second look, even to group hugs twenty strong and tossing fries at monkey suited charity workers. We had become the punks of my infancy who would guide me back as a toddler towards the arms of my mother when I got too close to the road. I'm refusing to take part in any photographs; trying to make meaning of the loss of past childhood pictorials. When I go there will be no trace of me. And I'm thinking on a letter a girl sent into *'Newsaround'* when I was a kid, asking why people from different lands fight, when we all share the same sky? Today, the world makes perfect sense to me.

Twenty-up *Doc-Martins*, an ankle length black leather coat for winter, black *Levis*, thirty-two inch waist, thirty-two inch leg – I'm a perfect square. Life is so easy I don't even have to try on my clothes anymore. T-shirts and long sleeve black tops speckled in ink taken freely from work; working as a Printer has turned out to be a cool job. Painted blood fountains on our Kurt Cobain t-shirts, and distributing free smudged prints has turned Argyle St momentarily into a red sea of *Baby Chaos*. I find myself speaking of home in the past tense, though I still return there on the late bus, while I have heard a song by a band called *Alice in Chains*, entitled, *'Down in a Hole'* and you know how that feels, as though someone has written a soundtrack to your life.

I hear this guy laughing, telling a story behind me, 'STEVEN, what have you done with the batteries from the smoke alarm?' 'THERE IN MA GUITAR TUNER.' 'That's dangerous Steven, whit if a need thame for the TV remote control?' Steven *'Nolan'* Nolan, has always watering eyes, five feet four at a push and bushy ponytail; holds onto the tip then jumps up to reach, attempting to stretch it out its full length. 'Can he not understand his arms *aren'y* long enough?' smile bemused passers bye. A smile and a warmth about him that couldn't be mistaken or falsified; green bomber jacket and a love of *Fender Guitars*, leads me into the *Guitar Store* as he auditions for piss-taking quantities of time, every Saturday on instruments no one could afford. The close proximity smell of hash, 'You pure reek of that stuff Nolan, and you still give blood? The people who get *you* in their transfusion must be spannered; ahh canny give blood because it might be a bit high on sugar, and you're getting people stoned! How much of that do you actually smoke?'

'Well a hiv,' and his eyes light up as the thought goes in on realisation of how much he actually puffs, 'Ah hiv wan rolled up and waitin for me when ah get oot ah bed in the mornin. Will have wan or two own the toap floor of the bus on my wiy into work, dependin on how long a journey it is. Hiv wan fir ma morning break, wan way ma lunch, wan own ma afternoon tea break,' smiling to himself, 'it helps me to get into the zone with ma work; tune right into the detail own the wallpaper.' Doing the actions with his hands now, even his actions look stoned. 'Get it lined right up *just right*. Spot on mate, Young Painter and Decorator of the Year Award, sponsored by the Glasgow City Council. Hiv wan or two own the bus hame, then another wan when am waiting own ma dinner. Then whoever comes aroon, sit and smoke a few over the evenin and a hiv wan tay maself afore bed,' big smile again, 'An a roll wan ready fir when a get up in the mornin. That is quite a lot isn't it?' 'Everyday? Yes Steven, it fucking is. You smoke more hash in a day than most people smoke in a lifetime.' 'A don't always work the weekends! HA. Here, does that no hurt when you inject yourself?' said with true concern. 'Na mate, you get used to it.'

Bursting I nod into Central Station toilets. Find Ben Longstone begging for change outside, his green face potholed from heroin use, and obviously offering himself up as payment. He looks exactly like the rubber he stole from me, only three or four years ago in primary school. Split from the group down to Buchanan Street, bump straight into Freddie Skerryvore, how did he get to six foot four? How can he run this fast on *jellies*? How am I going to escape him pulling me down a lane round the side of *Cairns Bar* off Miller St? Thank the Goddess Barmaids who come out to save me, informing Freddie they had already phoned the Police after him beating a man to a pulp in this very same spot less than an hour ago. Odd my sugar should fix itself to "8.2" in these times of mass adrenaline. Why am I not flummoxed on the ground, begging strangers to feed me sugar?

# First love and cock rot

'*Words, chatter, more words and smiles,*' we met five minutes ago and she is holding onto my hand; pressed smell of incense, her favourite pretty summer's dress; yellow flowers print on fabric, black para boots and a red star embossed *Smashing Pumpkins* T-shirt over the top. Her friend Monica strides ahead, Cherry and I, we're trying to find somewhere private to go. Nervous excitement and looking at each other all of the time; her hair long, parted in the middle is not dissimilar to mine, her waist tiny and wrists dainty, thick black eye liner and red painted lips. Just the thing to go with my black wardrobe; more smiles and arms around each other, '*Words, chatter, more words and smiles,*' hands still clenching and when I look down she is looking up at me: nothing else matters and that's definitely a black bra.

How come we have never seen each other before? We both hang around the same places; some of her friends seem to know some of mine. She has a friend who has diabetes too, this girl, she injects straight through her jeans. What a cool idea, I'm going to start doing that. Cherry, she has friends just like me. Do I like *The Black Crowes*? I only know one of their songs. *The Smashing Pumpkins*? I like the stuff I have heard but don't know much of it. *Nirvana*? Hell yeah, and best when batteries run out in your *Walkman* because you can't tell the difference. *Alice in Chains?* She knows of them but not so familiar. *Magnapop?* She has never heard. '*The Levellers?* Who the fuck are *The Levellers?*' *Metallica?* Too heavy for the both of us. So we're into the same types of music, well that's easily the most important thing in the world, we promise to loan each other some CD's.

Walked through most of the city centre already; George Square, Argyle St, back up Queen St past the *Art Store,* past the underground and *Forbidden Planet,* onto Suchiehall St. 'Do you know here? They do the best kebabs in the world.' 'Have you been in there?' 'I have been in there once but...' Ex-boyfriends, ex-girlfriends, some laughter and still holding hands, most importantly still holding hands.

'Anniesland? Yeah, there is a skate park there or something?' '*The Temple Church!* That got closed down; some guy got accused aye murder roon there or something.' 'It's Glasgow man, always someone being murdered.'

Plans to start rollerblading into town, 'Ha ha, I wouldn't make it in alive on my skateboard.' 'You don't sound like you're from Cranhill.' 'You don't sound like you work at *Spar.* Where is it anyway? "*So near so far*"?'

'My brother is a Glam, you have probably seen him aboot.' 'My mate *Tears* is a Glam.' 'Tears! He plays bass in my brother's band, *Bleach Meth.*' 'Ah, no way, I've seen your brother play up on the end of Suchiehall St, that pub with all the bad drawings of Jim Morrison on the walls.' '*Speaker's Corner,* ha, it's pure shite in there.'

...

'Can I leave my insulin in your fridge?' 'Sure. Keep it in the flappy shelf bit for the eggs.' 'Is your mum addicted to vacuuming? Your house is spotless.' Smell of incense tickling my nostrils at the foot of

111

hollow stairs; Jesus, those are some ugly baby photos on the walls. – I'll keep that one to myself; then reaching a bedroom door identical to all other doors on the landing, instinctively scanning around memorising my way to the toilet and back from these now thick fumes of sandalwood, 'See idiots trying to smoke incense sticks in phone boxes all the time.' Cherry smirks. 'You have tried it haven't you? Idiot! Ha ha.'

Box room, empty window ledge, all other surfaces covered in posters of *Pearl Jam 'Ten'* and cut outs from *'Kerrang Magazine'* pieced together with *Sellotape*. Six foot tall of *"Kurt Cobain RIP 1967 – 1994"* in monochrome, looking down over the smallest single bed I have laid eyes upon. Kurt's puppy dog eyes and gloom, taking reflection of summer's dusk from a slither of mirror leaning up against the side wall, still more than wide enough to take in her slender form, and I'm still recovering from the world's most ugly baby photos on the way up the hall stairs. Hi-fi unit propped up on a corner shelf; scattered tapes, *Pearl Jam's 'We're Gonna Hungry'* limited edition and numbered bootleg CD, *Smashing Pumpkins* vinyl *'Disarm'* on near repeat. *The Levellers* on cassette; hide that. And her clothes come off. I lie on top of her; never felt anything like this, 'Aoww,' she is caught in my hair, I'm all elbows on hers, 'Ahhhhh.' 'YYAAhhhoww!' 'Sorry.' 'You okay?' 'Kiss, smile,' still never felt anything like this. She tells me I am beautiful; I have never felt such confidence before. 'My friend Jane is an Artist, she is much better than you, she won a trip to America and the only reason she never made it into Art School this year is because she is still seventeen and they want her to take a year out to get more life experience.' I have never felt such lack of confidence. Her brother draws comic books in his spare time, he is also better than me; there is nothing of me left. Do I want a *Marlie Medium*? I'm strongly considering it. Fuck I'm fragile, 'Right, I'm off up the road.' 'What's wrong? You look totally pissed off. Please stay?' She looks upset, 'Okay.'

Sleeping over at Cherry's almost every night, I wake myself up from laughing intrinsic in my sleep. Her eyelashes fall out when she is sad and I hold her breasts to comfort her. Her dad comes home to his classic cul-de-sac red brick, in from work on a curry Wednesday at the ship yards to find I have eaten all his food; going to bed at night knowing I am next door shagging his little girl, through a paper thin wall; my body clock waking me at near dawn every morning for a poo, then he goes into shave for work a moment later. Sunday mornings, and her mum always shouting about there being no *Penguin* biscuits left, banging her hoover against the bedroom door as we untie stockings from the headboard. Every cheese toastie we share, every overly milky cup of tea, taking LSD together over in the sports fields, watching the clouds form into numerals, and trying to get drunk but falling asleep instead, I completely love her.

...

I'm crawling my way out of the world's most cramped bed in the morning to get back to work. 'Where did you go to last night?' 'I was at the garage getting sugar, because your friends had none.' 'What was that bottle of orange, would that not do?' 'No, that was tramp piss 20/20. I want to vomit again just thinking about it. Think Liza and Lance drank it in the end.' 'Was the garage not dangerous?' 'No, the little boy with the stick was actually quite nice. I bought him some orange juice. How much fucking *East 17* did we listen to last night? Are you not going to work?' 'No, I've decided last night that I'm going to go back to college, do you want to come?' 'Yeah all right then; see you later.' 'I love you.' 'I love you too.'

Just enough juice left in the *Walkman* for my bus ride back to work, *Alice in Chains*, '*Rain when I die*' all the way. Sunny day, and I'm how

113

late? John changes radio stations over to something more suitable and Adrian can go fuck himself, because I'm going to college full-time. I don't know what college or what I'm going to study, but we've decided I'm going.

'Ohhhh! Smudge has got a girlfriend. Still that wee hippy bird?'

'Yeah.'

'Dirty, lucky bastard; ave no hid ma hole fir six weeks.'

'We're about ten times a day,' as I pilfer the tuck box of *Bounty Bars*.

'Nay wonder you need so much chocolate.'

'Met some of her other friends last night.'

'Whit were they like? A bunch of *East 17* fans?'

'How the fuck did you guess that?'

'They always are mate. They always are. They think that's rap music.'

'Are you fucking joking? Where you there? I wish you were; they were doing the dance and everything. It was fucking horrible.'

'Whit were you drinkin, you're stinkin aye booze?'

'Mostly everything! Offered out some of my *Labatt's Ice last night*, but they were all, "We only drink *Miller*," then one of the fat fucks had two bottles and fell through a couch.'

'Fat virgin, till he is at least twenty-five. There's wan at every party.'

'Definitely. He probably ate all the sugar. They didn't even have any sugar in their entire house. Not even sugar in a bowl for tea. Some idiot offered me a bottle of *Mad Dog 20/20* thinking it was orange juice. I had to go the petrol station by myself at two in the morning for *Pot Noodles* and *Coke*. They were all too shittin it to come with me because of the local gang, get this, *The Young Temple Scurvy*.'

'The YTS, the Youth Train Scheme like you! Wankers. I'd gee anything to see wan a they wee posh gangs walk doon into Bridgeton.'

'Nice people though, easy going but falling apart at the seams. Two of them got a *Volvo* for a seventeenth!'

'A *Volvo*; the safest car you can get, so he or she doesn't sprain an ankle on their way to the shoaps. I'm tellin ye *Smudge*, the middle class canny handle it.'

'I know; one of their friends jumped off a bridge. Fuck, and some other girl in their class tried to overdose, and another girl who didn't make her exam results has gone mad. Nothing happens to them all their entire lives and when it does they explode, – the girl over the street from her has randomly got into skag.'

'Deliverin chinkys in her boyfriend's motor to piy fir it?'

'How the fuck could you know that?'

'It's the same as everywhere; they're no made to handle the real world. Just remember never tay say "*sorry*" tay any of her boyfriends mates, they take that as a sign of weakness. Yeh listenin Smudge? Never let them hear you say you're sorry. That's when they attack you.'

'I know, but I wish I never said anything about it out loud. Last thing I remember is walking back to Cherry's after drinking two bottles of *Thunderbird*, saying, "Save me, save me," then being sick into a cup of sugary tea and all the tea spilling out onto the table and the cup filling up with sick, it was bogin. And flashes of some girl called Liza, kept sitting in front of me with her legs crossed, I could see her bush sticking out the sides of her pants.'

'Fuck sake, should have invited me. Whit aboot that we Goth bird, you were sick on her shoes.'

'No, that was last week.'

'Wish a wiz there. Ah was dreamin again aboot being here. I keep coming to work then going home tay sleep, then dreamin aboot workin and printin these fuckin t-shirts, then wakin up and coming back into here to print mare t-shirts.'

'Jesus, you must be cracking up.'

'We'll be oot of here soon, I'll tell ye after ave been for a pish.' John returns, pointing at me and laughing, 'Wit's going own with theme t-shirts?'

'Cherry's cut all the sleeves off of all my tops. I know, bad enough having long hair around here. I'll end up getting stabbed dressed like this.'

'Here! Debt collectors were in earlier looking for Adrian; leather jackets the lot.'

'No way.'

That's why he is never in here anymare, dowin aw they wee cash in hawn joabs, auf the books.'

'I, on my college day, they said he hadn't paid for me in months, but it was too late to take me out and place me somewhere else.'

No Adrian around today then, I'm phoning her for an all-afternoon chat. Then when four o'clock comes, I'm out of here, getting the fifty-one A back to hers; goes right from Easterhouse to Anniesland; it's meant to be.

...

My Boss has dropped all communication with college, so I have dropped all communication with work over this summer's holiday; to enjoy what I feel is a well-deserved six-week summer break with Cherry; who is now on the pill, her breasts have blossomed to a "b" cup and I'm in heaven. We stand outside of *Asda's* cash point every Thursday night from a quarter to twelve; pensive expectation, checking my account balance to see if the forty-six pounds has gone in. 'I can't believe they are still paying me,' and down to the *BP Garage* for some excitable late night munchies, of *Cheese and Chive Pringles*, *Bacon Frazzles*, massive bags of *Prawn Cocktail Shells*, *Diet Cherry-Aid* and twenty *Marlboro Mediums*; aware that the week ahead is going to be a cinch.

Injecting through my jeans all of the time; I have completely given up on testing blood sugar levels, as far as I am concerned it has all become a thing of instinct. I know when I'm having a hypo because I become all weak and shaky, I know when my sugar is high because my mouth becomes dry and I'm really thirsty. I know I am doing well overall because I'm not missing any of my injections and carefully living on the foods I am allowed; *Smash Potato* mixed in a bowl with gravy and *Beef Hula-Hoops*, *Pasta Parcels* and *Pot Noodles* for breakfast, lunch and dinner; only benefitting from hypos to allow extra treats beyond my one-per-day and even then only sugary cups of tea and half a packet of *Penguin* biscuits. Cherry even got me a *Soda-Stream* for Christmas, so I can finally get my hands on some Diet American

Cream Soda, and turn my *"no added sugar"* cordial, *Robinsons Summer Fruits* fizzy to make it more fun.

So skinny that my bony hips dig in and bruise her inner thighs when we shag. Started sweating profusely down my back, chest and forehead in clammy weather; sheets of salt running over, stinging in my eyes, clothes clinging to skin on my back, getting progressively worse; spots, small boils and deep black heads all ready to burst, and I don't know why I am getting all wound up all of the time. 'Stop being so contrary,' she says, and I'm to the point of storming off home or going quiet for ages. People around me, are just plain pissing me off. Started having baths with capful's of *Dettol* in to kill spots now all up my neck. Night-time, acid indigestion bypassing my chest, coming straight out of my gob; standing over the sink with mouth open, drooling out from under my tongue for twenty-minutes at a time: the only way I can get it to relent is to stop letting it out and swallow it back down. Concentration has completely gone again, and I'm thinking of skipping college after summer because I can't manage to fill out the application forms, but Cherry helps.

The skin around the end of my cock has started to peel, gotten really tight and gone pink then white. Rubbing it, the skin breaks away, rolling into putrid little pellets. Tightness breaking through to the point of cutting under and around the tip of my foreskin, like paper cuts it kills when I pull back to pee. The end of my foreskin now having become so tight, it does not fit anymore, so I can't adjust it back and have to sit down to stop pee from going everywhere. 'I need to see a Doctor.' 'Yeah. What do you think it is?' 'I think I may have burnt the skin with too much *Dettol* in my baths. I think I've burnt my dick off.' 'We need to start using condoms, and I have been forgetting to take my pill,' she says.

118

...

I have a class of Junior Doctors queuing up to feel lumpy glands on the back of my cranium. I'm the unusual proof positive, with distinctive side effects; measles can return a second time. Now back to Sister Shepherd's corner room, her desk pushed almost entirely into the corridor from all the cases of *Lucozade* continually stock piled behind her. Acting like that's of no concern, touching my feet with long straws to check I can still feel them, 'Yes it tickles.' Looking up at me with a warm smile, 'Are you absolutely sure? Can I not tempt you with a free diabetes trip?' pointing to the notice board above decorated with still more photos of this season's smiling idiots in primary colours. 'No thanks,' bigger smile and I think she is beginning to appreciate my cynicism as a coping mechanism. As for my sugar being out of control, it seems too much insulin is causing my body to create more sugar, pulled from fat stores, and the solution is to increase from two injections per day, to four? I'm baffled, 'She is quite pretty though,' pointing up at a girl on the notice board, 'I never see her in the waiting room, when is her next appointment?' even bigger smile. 'Oh, and I was going to ask. Can I see a *male* Doctor please?'

Now shuffled into a Consultation Room; back in with Chief Consultant Dopey with his big pink cheeks; a lovely man, he is explaining to me how natural bacteria on my skin are feasting on high sugar, which my body is pushing out as sweat, and this is what's causing the outbreaks of spots on my back and the tight broken white skin around my penis, 'There's no sign of a yeast infection. It's perfectly common in male diabetics, women tend to get thrush.' 'I was worried my girlfriend had given me something.' 'No, no,' smile, 'It's very common for diabetics to be circumcised for this reason; try this cream and if it doesn't work in a couple of weeks come back and we

119

will have to circumcise you.' '*Throat noise of terror.*'

...

'So I think it's because my sugar is too high all the time that I'm sweating to push out the sugar, and the sugar in my sweat is feeding the natural bacteria that everyone has, but mine is going nuts with all the extra sugar and causing spots. That's why my skin's got all dried up and all sore. It is the same with the skin here on the side of my mouth starting to split. So they have given me different insulin, and now I'm having four injections a day instead of two. – *This is awful.* And you know how, my skin is all sore and broken there? That's the same as with the spots on my back, and he says I've to use this cream and if it's not better within two weeks then I'll need to be circumcised because the tight skin can cut off blood flow. So I've got to use this now and give it a rest from friction, – basically shagging too much.' And she replies, 'Well I'm not going without it for two weeks.'

...

Cherry sleeps upstairs, too much *Jack Daniel's*; got his number from his brother, easily found by a Telephone Operator and quickly passed through to the Reception of his old insurance company. Ever so helpful on mentioning my surname and blue ink on yellow *Post-its* I have in my hand and dialling now the number of my father, whom I'm assured, 'Is sober; a bit down on his luck and struggling to find work but sober.'

Tears of joy on hearing my voice; the boy long returning to his dad, forever in their thoughts, or tears of relief wanting to get him off their clean hands? Typically Christian or otherwise, I wanted to find someone, understand something. Maybe he will be pleased to hear

120

from me, be like how it was when taking me for hot dogs with mustard and ketchup, washed down with banana milk shakes. A down and out's voice answers my call, 'Hello, who is that? Is that you?' It's a woman's voice, sounds as though she wants it to be somebody, sounds bruised, and for him to even be with someone in this state, he definitely isn't sober; heads in the sand, he must be worse than he was before; bad enough Greta exposing herself to me, his last drunken casualty.

'Is Stuart there?' 'Stuart? Stuart?' goes on the drunken denial, aggrieved building to abuse, more probably abused, this phone call not for her, not who she needs it to be. 'Is my dad there? Stuart Cathcart?' 'Stuart, Stuart, its you,' says the vanquished tone moved distant from the line, perhaps a hall or only a room away. I see the white banister of a communal hallway in Irvine, smell nicotine stains and closed windows, feel the tears on my face of a girl he is molesting, noises breaking my sleep, didn't know what they were; waking on a wet patch of urine that did not belong to me. I was playing on my bike with her yesterday, in the car park out front of this, her parent's bed and breakfast. I don't know why they let her stay over to play with me in the room with this man who had only been renting here for no period of time, when her bedroom was only downstairs. Smell vodka in Kilmarnock as I hold closed my eyes, turned away and pretending I am asleep as he is fucking a woman by the side of the bed. 'Who's that?' 'It's Paul.' 'Paul, Paul, is that you son?' come the voice of, I'm still here son, I'm still your dad son. 'Are you hitting her? Are you hitting her as you did my mum?' 'I, I,' stammer, 'I never raised my hand to your mother.' 'You made my sister hold onto your cigarettes so you could punch into her.' The line goes dead but not hung up. Silence and I know the receiver has been left down. Him on the other end, I expect in shock, 'I FUCKING

HATE YOU.'

I call my uncle, I want to speak with my uncle; perhaps he can explain something. A woman answers; frail, tired, he is not there, convenient. I am drunk, I should go to sleep, she doesn't know anything and I have awoken her at near two thirty in the a.m. I am embarrassed; I come off the phone with an apology. Now she is going to think I am a no good drunk like my father. I only want them to want to know me. I could just stop having sugar... but I hear the birds chirping outside, it's already getting light and it's beautiful out there. I go wandering off into a balmy Anniesland. Will this summer ever end?

...

Cherry passes me a cut out article from 'Kerrang,' on Chris Cornell from Soundgarden discovering his voice, and I wish I could draw. I wish something like that would happen to me. Wish I could suddenly discover my voice to become an incredible Artist, but I take solace in the understanding that I can only get better, and by the time I am sixty I will be amazing with still two years left at least. I give Cherry a page from the idea I have been sketching out for my comic book. The penultimate scene; of a boy with not too dissimilar hair to mine, struggling to place an antique gun against his right temple; sunlight reflected into his eyes and the text block says, "All I ever wanted was to be an angel." Frame by frame horror in his expression highlighted in the reflection of sunlight from the pistol. A Mother God figurine falls from a thin tan leather strap, which had been around his neck into the ocean below. Rain pours; the boy is taken by sand to screams of the Roma people he has saved. She says she will keep it.

...

Christmas Eve and meeting with Daniel and his friend who never takes his *Pearl Jam* t-shirt off, down at the *13th Note* for drinks and celebration but mostly to get out of the house because I can't stand my own company and have never felt this lonely. I have literally nothing to say, but I don't have to, because it's Christmas Eve and everyone is so fucking chirpy. *PJ* boy can't sit still, popping his head up like a Meerkat from his chair every two moments; *tonight's the night* he is going to ask his girlfriend of two weeks to marry him; arranged eyebrow piercings as engagement rings and everything: asshole. Everyone in here is coupling tonight; everyone except Daniel who never brings his girlfriend out ever, everyone except Daniel is outside in the cold sharing scarfs, everyone falling out about money. I'd give anything to be falling out right about now; to storm away like I always do and for someone to want me to come back. Jesus, my heart is sinking through my chest and I feel someone has actually grabbed and ripped out my guts. How can a human being possibly be this upset? How am I going to get over this? I know it sounds so stupid, I really don't know how I can live without her. Daniel offers up some great advice, 'I know how you're feeling man. It took me three years to get over Carla.' Three years, that's comforting. Only three more years, I reckon I can do it in three months; tops.

She pulled her woollen hat down over her eyebrows, peered up at me, 'Do I look cute?' 'Cutest thing in the world, I absolutely love you.' 'Forever?' 'And ever.' Laughed practically in the face of that other boy whose heart she had broken; that could never happen to me. Jeered about how I had such a beautiful cock and he couldn't manage to pull his foreskin back over his purple knob properly. He is at Glasgow University now, some kind of genius and world class musician and I'm here listening to *PJ* boy banging on, rubbing his hands together in glee: I'm giving it two months tops. He doesn't deserve love and she must be some kind of mutt.

I'd give anything for Cherry to want me; she is out there being happier with someone else, what happened to it being forever? Loving me forever and ever? This time last year we were trying to get over not seeing each other for only one day; a single day; agreeing with smiles to masturbate at the same time in the afternoon and the evening, detailing what we would be thinking about doing to each other. Really wished we had a phone at our house then. As I understand it, she is now doing all those things with someone else. Fucking hell, why doesn't she want me? How can somebody I love this much not want me? I awoke this morning to an empty mind of bliss, lasted the duration of a shooting star then crumbled onto her leaving me. I was happy then I remembered she could, 'Do without it.'

'Are we going to the *Rat Trap* then?' – Daniel. 'Well I have exactly fuck all else to do.' In the forefront of my mind, she doesn't want me anymore is all I can think on repeat as we walk. Argyle St; Christmas lights stirring at emotion, hold it together man, couple of months and I'll be over the worst of it. 'Uhh,' that gutting feelings growing again in my heart and my organs at the thought she may walk in there with someone else. 'I can't do without anything.'

Get to the *Rat Trap* door; have passed under the bridge at Central Station, walked through the heavy stench of greasy chips, past the prostitutes freezing in belt length skirts and shammy mittens, and now stand behind a queue of couples; fifteen pounds to get in and a free *Budweiser* on entry. Piss water, I'm not drinking that. Drunk and I don't know anyone. *'Congratulations,'* she has said yes and they are all smiles; she is fucking beautiful; last time I was here I took a girl home, she took her clothes off in my bed and just when revealing her huge tits she started to sneeze; eyes red and allergic to my cat, expensive taxi home. Time before was my eighteenth birthday, a woman in her thirties asked me if it really was my birthday and like magic the fire alarm sounds at deafening proportions, she took me off into a car park and gave me a quickie. I've had enough, all thought jumbling into one, I've drunk enough; nothing magical is going to happen tonight. I'm drunk and babbling. I'm going home.

My heart hurts, physically bemoans her; or is that from smoking at minus four degrees; breeze rushing off a black glassy Clyde into my ribs? The surface of Glasgow is all misty; sparkling everywhere, surface over car bonnets and concrete bringing everything together. It's quite beautiful: sky is clear dark blue near pitch black going on forever, continuing the shimmer infinite. How can it be infinite? How can it go on forever? Of course it does. Why shouldn't it?

Christmas Eve and only a handful of cars, a handful of revellers and a single scratched girl; she must be trying to draw back memories of better Christmases past. 'You goat a light?' 'Yeah, sure; have some of these,' I deal her out a few from my packet into thin porcelain hands, shiny in the middle, dirty around the edges; as with her pretty face and bare shoulders. Clear she is trying to keep clean. Can't take her home, can't keep her warm; can't help her, can't make her change, we stand under a thousand clasped shut windows, 'Hiv yey no goat a girlfriend?' 'Not anymore.' 'You should be home; it's the death ou cold oot here. Am used to it.' 'Yeah.' 'Are you looking for business?' 'No. No thanks. But here,' and I reach into my coat pocket giving her the twelve pound odds I can spare so she can get high and find something resembling peace, and I still get my taxi home, 'Take care of yourself, please.'

Surely she is the one looking for business, I think to myself, a few blocks further down past some fencing surrounding waste ground that has always been fencing surrounding waste ground as far back as I can remember. Aww fuck, I can feel the low sugar lunge kicking in, and up ahead the glow from the tunnel of greasy chips I so depend upon has gone out. To my right, past *Missing Records*, some club I've never set foot in for as many reasons. 'Not tonight Pal, you're hammered.' 'No, am going up the road, I'm diabetic, I've run out of sugar.' 'Aw here, haud own, stiy there,' says the fat possibly diabetic bouncer as he shoots inside a forever swinging door and reaches out to me before the rest of him has made it back out. 'Will these day ye?' handing me two of the biggest handful of *Quality Street*, 'Thanks man. You're a star.'

'Pure quality man, *Quality Street*,' as I thumb through the foils looking for the yellow toffee ones and raspberry fondant. Hope they are in here and that's not *Roses*. Purple ones are Angela and Mum's favourites, I think they are stinking; here's a wee caramel barrel. Looking down through the Central Station tunnel, have never seen her so empty or heard her silent before. No trains thumping overhead, fog of car fumes a lingering memory, holly green painted metal as though decorated just for tonight. Christmas Eve and I'm heart broken, round doors begging for food, and walking alone in the twilight in search of a no-chance taxi, it's not so bad, 'HAPPY BIRTHDAY JESUS!' goes echoing on up ahead: I need a fucking hug.

Thank God we don't have a telephone; surely the best thing about ex-girlfriends is not having to talk to them, I'm thinking, banking left at the end of the tunnel; follow the perimeter blonde sandstone. Buildings so beautiful, if only we would look up; turn right from Gordon St, into Buchanan St and George Square, remembering a '*Long Gone Day*' with Titch and Nolan; playing football down here at one in the morning and Nolan running up and banging on the sleeping Night Bus Driver's window, scaring him shitless as we fell about laughing. Looking up to the windows of a top floor corner building above *Greggs Baker*, where Mum used to work in the basement *Toastie*. Dream I could one day own a place there. Finally the night bus arrives, 'Ahhhh Angie, there's your wee brother.' 'Here Paul, wit you dain oot here?' smile, it's my sister, her boyfriend and his brother. 'Here, smell Frazer, that's what I goat you for Christmas.' 'Wit, cheap cider?' – Frazer. 'No, that aftershave.' I sit down on the row in front for the journey home; she looks at me with concern, 'Are you alright?' ' Yeah,' handing her from my pocket a purple *Quality Street*. 'Houww you two, nay poacket munchin. Pass the *Quality Street*, pure quality. Where did you get thame?' I'm saying shit, and just being around her is the biggest hug in the world.

'*Alice in Chains Unplugged*' in the hi-fi, skip to track five, '*Down in a Hole*' check my blood sugar, "17.0" some insulin and cry myself to sleep.

...

Listening to music together at four in the a.m. those had become our hours. She loved you with those words and you loved her, you believed her; she needed you with her crocodile tears and you held onto that. She left you with that look and it took you years to recover from. She never taught you anything, never encouraged you, never made you happy when you were down and never blinked an eye when she said she could, 'Do without it.' She never wanted you back and you never wanted for anything more; she forgot and you remembered, she left, she changed and you had to wait for the world to change while you stayed the same. It's like being killed over and over again. Why did I get back with her ten months later, just as I was starting to feel good again? I had to wait for the earth to orbit the sun three more times and she just walked away. At least I got to keep my dick.

# The 13th Note (belong)

*'Here's to the people we love the most, who hurt us the most.' nineteen to twenty-two, 'and even the people we hate, we love. Cheers!'*

You don't have to be alone in the pub, that's the simple law of man. Escape from any social vacuum, into a world of arts, music and alcohol; more friendships that would last forever? Who cares, I've got enough money left over for either a veggie burger with fries or another two pints of *Guinness*; they both contain to my estimation roughly the same amount of sugar. Being served at the bar, I enquire, 'Is there any chance I can keep my insulin bottle in one of your fridges? It's completely sealed and it's getting too warm to use in my pocket.' 'Diabeeedic my ass,' overly pronounces the Canadian Barman in reply; fuck you then, pronounces the look on my face. 'Fuck's that all about?' says the face of his colleague, her demeanour in my favour. Think I'll go for the *Guinness* this time, 'A pint of *Guinness* please, and have you got any matches?' as she picks them up from beside the till, right in front of me.

Cold enough for condensation to cling to glass, and a head like an ice cream cone, with the always-open invitation to, 'Bring it back up when it has settled and I'll top it up,' said with plain smile. Feels a bit off requesting she need make amends four times in an evening, even if she can't pour a pint to save herself.

Still, looks great on the table with my *Red Marlies* under near orange sunlight; the closing of autumn projecting over neighbouring rooftops, highlighting within reason and cigarette smoke our vagabond group in dress of anti-establishment garb; enthusiasm motions naivety, gestures of fear, expressions of belonging, we gather together knowing this is *our time*. Last reaches of sun coming up from Argyle St, making Glasford St, stroking our faces when we watch through *Blue-Tack* and *Sellotape* marks those workers who bemoan the commute home. Final shards of heavy amber over a gantry reminiscing, bringing to life wooden floorboards as in oil paintings of bread and bottles of wine; continuing throughout to illuminate and identify every speck of dust caught up in the air. Elevating our belief that we do belong, that this world is ours for the taking when we are ready, when the time comes, but not now, no yet willing to move beyond playing saxophone in curry houses or busking to repay parental debts, not quite ready to dress in formal manner befitting of full time employment.

I feel lucky to be here among them, Alana is smiling, 'That's awful,' and Mo, sitting pretty in his ginger ponytail, is laughing in disgust; at a dash of blood from my finger tip, dripped via a blood sugar test into that overly frothy head to deter pint thieves; turning the stomachs of those less gothic around us. And I'm smoking my first cigar when silent heckles released from behind the bar; switch from Beck's '*Odelay*' to the '*Hamlet*' theme song. Embarrassed, four of us put them out. Now he is over clearing ashtrays and lighting candles, 'You're so neegadtive Paul.' 'What's his problem?' we all think, 'Used to be alright as well.' People come and go, conversations drift to those floating around us; eventual sun has fallen to candles glow.

'There's no wiy. No wiy did that just happen. Ah wiz like that man, no wiy!'

'Mind Cass? Hear he goat his baws booted? Own the phone way Shaun fay the phone boax in Cranhill, and just as Shaun's siying goodbye, aw he hears is, "Ahhhh, ahhhhh, ma baws, ma baws, ahhh," and Shaun's shouting, "Alex are you ahright? Whit's rang? Wit's happenin Alex? I love you." And awh he can here is people shouting, "Yah fuckin hippy, smack, smack!"'

'*Quality Street.* That's pure quality man.'

'Ah know the guy.'

'Hiv you seen his da's arm? Goat it caught in a machine at work. Looks like a chicken wing.'

'And ah wis like that, and he wis like that, an ah wis like that, an he wis like that, then a wis like that, and he wis like, WIT!' – Always some wanker pretends to have been in a fight: our whole table nodding our heads in condemnation.

'Left ooer band to join their band, noo he's a dancer.'

'How can you be into Gangster Rapp, when you come fay Glasgow? It disney make any sense. Heavy Metal, I, angry and pure fucked off, ah understand that. Grunge music, I, it's heroin music, I've been around it forever, I get it. Techno, pure pish man, but fair enough and Industrial music is good. But Gangster Rapp?' we interrogate the unfortunate *Straight Edger* at the table, fresh from his attempted overdose on anti-depressants, 'Have ye ever seen a drive-by shootin in Glasgow?' 'No, but I seen a guy throw a brick at a bus once.'

'Crunch, that fly was in my *Federation Space.*'

131

Daniel stops half way through a conversation about a party he has been excluded from and enquires, 'Does nothing ever wind you up? You just let everything brush you by, nothing ever gets you down.' I guess I had been through enough shit already, the grievances of my late teenage and early twenties were paling in comparison. But God it's amazing how people see one thing on the outside when you are crumbling on the inside.

'See you later Paul, I'm popping out for fags,' – Ratty.

...

*Hash, alcohol, acid-tabs, speed and vallies; jellies are for Neds, ecstasy is for dance music; handful of undefined pills, none reaching far enough to meet with an infinite void. Amber glow long gone, smiles undelivered. Attracted through necessity to a bowel cancer scary character, kidneys shot, skin gone rotten under the eyes, would never normally acknowledge this old man other than wonder what he is doing in here. Started with a friendly nod. Drinking himself to death, seems so much farther into the journey complete than I. People are looking over, what's he doing with him? People who belong to each other, they all have something to do tomorrow. 'Do you want a cigarette? How are you getting on? What meds do you take? How does that work? Can you slide me one under the table and I'll get your drinks in? Yeah fifteen quid's fine. How do I? I just break the vial and drink it or inject.'*

*Pushing into a toilet stall, white door, terracotta tiles impossibly tidy, too small, packed together, rushing him; an excitement, introversion, a drunken gloom – head already falling; escape, what is on the other side? Music would understand this as a time for silence. A single comforting glow, it has got to be in here, broken vial, fractions of glass fallen into itself. An insulin syringe revealed. Careful pointing of needle into clear simple liquid reflects ceiling lights, pulling back the stopper filling to the first forty units' line. A close eye view of its silken contents, no fabled air bubbles, now where to inject? Trousers to ankles, cold porcelain, it wouldn't be so cold anymore. Light blue lines tap vague between thin bones, contents are met; a drip of blood and it's deep enough in? Plunged in uncertainty; sick from the stomach, removing the needle as carefully as a staggering boy can. Yellow not what he is expecting it to be he vomits love, warm and conducive to infinity a connection to those who do not want him: the connection between his consciousness and soul, he would believe in anything with this God. Padding down rolls of toilet paper, making steps in warmth; wishes someone else were here. Best to be alone; looking into the blue unknown, held in green, waiting on purple fear; it doesn't take, neither orange anger nor the poppy red of passion. Wishing someone else was here. Back on the toilet seat, more holes to find, more engulfing liquid in broken glass to extract and spread throughout legs or arms now sparkled in unfulfilled marks. Wishing someone was here.*

...

'Geeze a wee haun a minute,' Haggis nudges discreetly. 'Yeah no worries,' following the man with dreadlocks, shorn hair round the sides and enormously stretched out ear lobes cast in metal hoops, through into the gents, wondering, should I be surprised or frightened? 'Goon has locked himself in a stall,' I'm thinking what the fuck, is he dead? We push until his knees finally give in from the door, enough so Haggis can clamber over into this nest Goon has laid for himself; reams of toilet paper in a circular formation. An astounding feat of environmental art, a nodding bearded haze, full grown man in a man-sized nest, rested on his left side with praying hands; looking up, blinkering, cowering as though light were being shone down on him. 'Get up, fuck, yeh canny day that in here,' says Haggis, sending me off back to my table, assisting Goon peacefully to the door, sending him off to stoop down by his usual favourite haunt by the banks of the Clyde Side, where on sunny afternoons he famously wears a found boating hat and rowing club t-shirt. Cheap bottle of wine and roll ups in hand, waving on to athletes as they perform back and forth, waving back mistaking him as one of their own.

Recreational drug use amongst experimental friends, not because they felt a need to escape, not because they were sleeping in car parks; simply venturing into experience they sought control over; naïve enough to believe they were about to touch a higher ground. Inspiration from musicians aspired to and the sexy danger of it all. Well, other than sticking myself with needles all day anyway; although some thought this would make it an easier step; I had already been surrounded by stupid cunts like this lot my whole life and I'm fucked if I'm going down that road. Truth is, the only reason I am here all the time at twenty-one is because I still can't stand to be alone.

'Ahrigth man, can you get us a Guinness?' Ratty's back, having been around Central Station asking everyone for a cigarette, twenty minutes and he has returned with a full deck: the Barman guessing what he is up to and deciding to smile.

...

Past closing and I'm standing at a bus stop facing toward Duke St, as all too often waiting in the frozen rain, thinking on with solace my odd predicament; if I can't account for having company at least four days in advance, I will fall into panic then a slump. My mind won't switch off and I'll over analyse every thought, every expression, transcript, turn of phrase, pointed finger reduced down to, do they like me? They call me by my first name; smile when they see me; why is it I look for negative space in everything? Why aren't I calm? And when I find calm, and test my sugar, my sugar is always level at that point. It can't only be coincidence. Even on a good day, I awaken with a grin, shake my head, and then remembering as I am; depressed a massive cloud to bear down over me. I miss her that is for sure; gutted, my heart physically aches and everything so empty. God if only she wanted me in return. I believe everything will be better if she wants to be with me in return. I start to go a bit manic, and then the euphoria that comes with it; infinite confidence over a moment's thought, finding humour and joy in the simplest concrete blocks. Looking up to find I am counting the number of buildings ahead of me, begin to estimate how many of you on the road complete, how many floors, how many flats within each floor, how many rooms tucked in each flat and surmise, 'Fuck me, that's a hell of a lot of shagging, gone on in this road.'

...

Here to get my insulin prescription, keep thinking to ask but I never do until this week when listening to '*Radio 1's*' '*Mental Health Awareness Campaign*' and fitting all criteria.

In the surgery, and he still has the cauliflower ear he always had when I was a child; in and out of here every two weeks with a sore belly, a flu that wouldn't shift or a cold sore. Sometimes it would fade, returning in part to a normal ear, but mostly he had been smacked hard playing rugby and he wasn't going to allow that to bother him. He probably remembers me staring at it, while telling my mum it was just another tummy bug going around. Reminding me that peculiar under the weather feeling of childhood is exactly how I feel now with high sugar.

What could he do for me? 'I *think* that I am depressed?' He looks at me seriously and gently, and I'm glad to be treated seriously because I don't know what is going on or if it's just me. 'Take me through what is going on with how you feel?' 'I don't feel depressed just now; I think that's because I have something to do and someone to talk with. But I'll go home and I'll crumble, and I can't be on my own. And when I sleep I am fine, then I wake up and feel good at first, then my head falls down again and I'm ungodly unhappy,' now my hand is over my mouth, 'It happens more when I don't have anything to do, like just now during college holidays. I'm at college doing art, I've been accepted to do my Higher National Diploma, my mum has managed to buy a flat in Dennistoun getting us out of Cranhill; I don't know why I feel like this when I should be happy.' 'How is your sleeping pattern?' 'Well, yeah, I can sleep all the time. That's the thing because I know you're not supposed to be able to sleep when you're depressed; I don't know if this is depression. And then later, about once or two times a day I'll be ecstatically happy and I don't think I'll ever feel sad again, but I do.' 'Okay,' and he picks up a pen with a notepad, starts scribbling down "*sad*" on the left "*happy*" to the right; draws a line even down the middle and a curve motion between both words. 'Most people are here,' scribbling a mark in the centre line, 'From here they reach happy, and then go back to the middle and from there to sad, balancing between like a pendulum in an old clock. What's happening to you,' and God, just because he knows, my heart is lifting, 'You are jumping directly from one to the other.' Jesus, yes that is exactly what is happening to me. I nod full understanding. 'That's fairly natural and extremely common in boys your age. Chemicals in the body and the brain, levels can go up and down; one chemical in particular shown to be commonly running at a lower level in the brain is called Serotonin, this is what is making you feel how you are. Now you could wait and let the body balance out naturally, or you could,' whatever this is, I'm taking it, 'Go on a course of medication that will help to top up your Serotonin levels and give you a short cut?' I'm in like *Flynn*. 'Are they dangerous or addictive?' 'No, not at the very small levels you would be taking them.

136

It's one tablet per day; it will be two to three weeks before you feel any benefits; hopefully you will start to feel much better.' Scribbling into the centre of the pendulum, nodding with his head to hold my full attention, 'From there you would have to continue taking the pills for a minimum of three months to keep your levels topped up, if you stop right away when you feel better, then your levels will drop back down again, your brain will not have had a chance to maintain levels where they need to be.' I know what this is; this is going to be *Prozac.* That's a bit scary. 'I will want you back here seeing me in two weeks' time to see how you get on, then on a month by month basis; coming off of them we reduce the dosage to one tablet every second day to wean your body off.' Overjoyed, this all makes perfect sense. Do I have any questions? Can I have that picture of the pendulum? No I won't ask for that but I really want it. Then he will see me again in two weeks, tap of the keyboard and prints off a green prescription handed to me with a smile suitable for acknowledging and respecting a young man.

Should I feel embarrassed to be put on them? Oh fuck I don't know, but I'm not stupid enough to think they would give someone on anti-depressants pills they could overdose on. Though I have forgotten my prescription for blood sugar test strips, and now I'm standing at the bus stop outside of a purple-signed *Haddows Off Sales* on Edinburgh Road, across the traffic lights from where Dad used to embarrass us, looking up to the spot where I got knocked over; wonder whether that girl in the backseat who had the massive asthma attack is okay? Please hurry up with the bus before I bump into any number of cunts I grew up with or get stones thrown at me for having long hair. Fucking sleeveless t-shirt will be the death of me around here.

Headphones on, I'll stay on the bus straight through to the chemists on Argyle St, collect my *anti-depressants* and go for a pint in the *13th*

*Note.* God, just thinking the term anti-depressants spells madness to me, though already I'm one hundred times better, knowing the Doctor understood, just knowing it's natural at my age, comforting knowledge that it's going to be okay.

Chemist lady behind the counter, bagging my prescription and the usual address check followed by an eye contact that says, it's okay to talk about this, and questions, 'Have you taken these before?' 'No,' and I clearly don't know what I'm doing, although she can only repeat what the Doctor had said and reminds me that the instructions are printed on the packaging. I'll have enough on my plate hiding these from my mum, though I've made the decision to tell Alana and Mo, I've got to tell someone, they deserve to know why I keep bursting into tears.

'Ayyyye. How ye didlin?' Comes Haggis's special smile, beaming from a wooden booth, nursing a pint before his shift on the door tonight begins. I join him for another and I need to get it out of my system so I tell him, 'The Doctor has put me on these *Prozac* tablets.' And he looks at me with such a complete understanding, warmth as though he is looking at his own child, taking me through how he was in exactly the same situation at my age. Twice in one day and it makes all of the difference in the world, twice, when you know you're not in it alone. 'It's when yeh canny see the light at the end of the tunnel, that's what it is.' 'Jesus, you're exactly right, that's exactly what it is. I'll get the beers in.' 'You might want to not be drinking too much way thame.'

*Guinness* and *Red Marlies*, it's getting dark, there is a brisk chill at the other side of the glass and the conversation moves on. 'I seen you sittin with a braw smile own the other night, some wee girl braidin your hair.' 'Yeah, over there, she was stroking my hair for hours.

Couldn't believe it was down to my waist and couldn't leave it alone.'
'When a hid ma long dreadlocks, I'd have awh these wee lasses comin
up to me way their maws at *Tesco*, sayin, "How do you get your hair
that wiy?" an ad say, "Ah just hivney washed it in three year and it
goes like that by itself." They'd look at their mas terrified and they'd
both run away. I think they thought I'd been to a salon.' We're sitting
laughing when Dan and his brother Nelson join us, Dan still pale
from his lung collapsing and the combined weight of being a pacifist
when watching his friend getting stabbed on Suchiehall St whilst
busking together some months past. 'Haggis, is the red heeded
barmaid own tonight; you still hankering?' – Nelson. 'I'd like to come
hame tay her in ma kilt, fresh fay poachin, carryin a grouse and is
many trout, and she'd be standing there way her beautiful long reed
hair in braids, waitin own me to come hame, holding oot a basket of
tatties,' we're all on the floor howling, 'And wan aye you bastards told
her that was my dream and now a canny look at her withoot ma face
goin bright red.'

'I mean, how else are we going to understand a painting by *Van Gogh*,
a beautifully tortured piece of music, a love story, or what's going on
in the hearts of people we love. We all have to be heartbroken at
some time.' Heartbreak is all there is, I am now officially alive.

'He just buys three pair aw socks fir a pound and throws them away
every three days. Never has to do any washin!'

...

Knew I was feeling better when you could have locked me in a dark
cupboard on those tablets and I would have sat there with a smile on
my face. Knew I was better when I kept on forgetting to take them,
struggled to remember the every second day and happy to be off
completely. Slight lull during an Easter break, but I knew what was

bothering me, and huge celebration on my twenty-second birthday; near a year of not being on them and knowing I would never have to go back to that black place with no light at the end of its tunnel.

I have got no idea what I'm doing in life at the moment, and for me, for once, that is a good place to be. I'll have some more insulin now, to sober up.

# College

I'm fitting right in here; the world has become one massive opportunity, with diabetes yet to show any kind of scar. A free spirit with cold feet; how fortunate my life needn't be shit. Economic prosperity at the dawn of the Internet: yet simple theories often seem confusing and I'm reading them over-and-over, perhaps my sugar is high? Higher National Diploma in Design With New Technologies, at Glasgow's, Central College of Commerce – very swanky; three of us cowering over a single screen, avoiding *any* eye contact with Librarians; browsing the web for the first time, trying to outguess a firewall, 'I've never seen a *lady* do that before.' 'Hold on, you've typed in *laddies*.' 'SHIT, turn it off. No Andy, don't press print!' Again, I'm going all dyslexic with high sugar.

*Courried-in* beside stairwells on Virginia Street, back to stone, my knees rest as an easel, catching winter's afternoon cold light. Yellow pale sun is filling in under my eyelids, hands held half way up my cuffs, sketching line decals in fine nib pen with a smile on my face in admiration of stone from a tobacconist's age heralding decorative rooftops. A woman walks by and smiles down; I don't want to sleep with her; I recognise in me that I must be growing up; raindrops falling on plain page running with ink to make far prettier marks than I am. So cold inside, around my kidneys are seizing up under the many tucked in layers; giving pause to remember Cairnsey and how we inverted our jackets with hands and waist tucked firmly in. Jumping against gale-force winds to catch and be caught, to fly one tenth of an inch: all we wanted was to live, and here I am now.

Cracked dry lips and cold feet, wondering what happened to summer; standing outside our college block on Cathedral St; having cigarettes, listening to pretentious piss. Everything has to be, 'In-situ, eclectic, zeitgeist,' it had to be 'Juxtaposed,' or it wasn't getting in. Aww the, 'Epoch,' couldn't get out of bed without the epoch, and the, 'Visceral,' bless the visceral. 'If a tree falls down in the woods and no one is aware to hear it fall, will it still make a sound?' proclaims a soon to be pseudo-intellectual, currently a big guy in a black trench coat. 'Of course it would. Do you think when you blink the sun goes off? Or maybe you stop talking shit when in the company of the deaf. Don't start on about the dead cats in boxes.' I'm getting a touch *tetchy* at the words *Bauhaus* and *Le Corbusier* being thrown in at every half conversation; I'm freezing my balls off and it feels as though someone has turned off my internal pilot light, on top of that I took my night-time insulin twice by accident last night. I've never had to drink so much juice throughout the day.

I have preference to study Pop Art, magnification and duplicate images of burgers and *Cokes* to highlight darkness ingrained within society; *Benday-Dots* fathomed together, building brighter colours, compressed giving response to the illusion someone is behind you. Between evenings ushering at the *Glasgow Film Theatre* to pay for drinks, topping up student loans; cutting class to attend the Student Union and lunch down at the *13th Note*; returning late afternoon to prey on Beauticians, dressed in all-whites, who flock in like seagulls to the canteen area: the prettier ones queuing up at the toilets as laxative chocolates have taken their desired effect. Confidence meandering between cheap drinks and the boil spots on my neck which Wee Alan points out, 'They're mare like eye-balls sticking oot than spots,' going home early, now-and-again, with cramps in my chest. 'Paul, you should have let someone know you have diabetes,' – my tutor David. I don't know why I have fallen shy of the idea; and somewhere in between, two years of completing thirteen-week blocks concentrating on everything from multimedia, architecture, life drawing and mise-en-scène. Yet still no amount of partying seemed to be touching the sides of my diabetes.

...

Lights to the world come on; crystal clear, sunny day, blue sky, illuminating both a city and her inhabitants; breadth of her streets allowing sunlight to pass truth of her mouth-watering fruit from across Las Ramblas; visible through static forms of street Artists. Greeted by none other than Antoni Gaudi, welcoming and telling us who we are and what we aspire to. Locals cast alive, beings openly inspired by art; this is real culture as to be the opposite of being alone. I have never witnessed anything like this through near two decades conformed in pessimism, and it is worth the weight of my soul.

*"Sin azúcar,"* on the back of every *light* can; so simple to slip into life here with barely a second thought. Not a second look when testing my sugar, a general populous well versed in common knowledge, diabetes a warmly received, internationally recognised condition; only hesitating to waste *Jack Daniel's* on a mixer with anything-*light*. Entering a nightclub at nine p.m. with no understanding of local customs, a sign behind the bar translating to roughly, *"No cigarettes to be sold to anyone under the age of twelve."* These children spark a conversation with us over the background of *Snoop Dog, an* album being played out in its entirety, 'Spanish?' 'No.' 'Italian?' 'No.'

'German?' 'Eh, no.' 'French?' as she shrugs her shoulders and grunts. What a bunch of ignorant fucks we are.

Oranges are actually orange, the fish, fresh and I'm digesting without thinking; beer is *thirty pence a litre* and the cigarettes are so cheap, it'd be a sin not to smoke. Public squares host fountains, where water plays as sculpture and palm trees catch raindrops before they evaporate above dust, where we stick out like favourable sore thumbs in our t-shirts and linen jeans, contrasting acclimatised March attire of dramatic local black coats and scarves. Though Andy for some reason has come dressed head to toe in apple green denim; pointing up and shouting, 'SHEEPDOG!' every time he gets excited, – which is about every four seconds.

'Watch this. See if they understand ma accent,' the world greets Andy, 'Aaah *Big Mac*, eh Large Fries, show-us-yer-tits, a Banana milk shake, naow Strawberry, make that Strawberry hen? I Strawberry, reed things that taste like Strawberries. I, nice arse and that's aww thanks.' Big smile and I'm nearly on the floor. Girl behind the counter senses something is up, turns to collect the boxed burgers, her pants sticking up out her uniform trousers and here we go, 'Look it the size ay they pants! They've goat Strawberries own them. How can she no know whit a Strawberry milk shake is when she's wearin theame!' 'Andy. Stop. Shut up. Please stop?' my sides splitting. 'Whit's she so miserable fir anywiys? Miserable moo. MOOOO, MOOooo.' *She* pauses, pushes a tray forward, face furious, Andy holds it straight. I don't know where to look, trying to explain to him, 'Andy, cows make the same noises over here that they do in Scotland. Your accent isn't hiding it very well.' 'AWWW FUCK, MOOOOOOOOOO.'

All of that hosing down the streets at dusk has got me bursting for a pee. 'Pop in there, Paul man,' says Big George convincingly, pointing to what I thought was a bank machine in the middle of the road. 'Aww cool man, just stick my coin in here and go for a wazz,' too much walking around drinking *Sin azúcar,* falling in love every fifteen minutes because the girls here are so beautiful and I'm totally bursting, 'Ahhh that's better, much better,' hold on something's not right, shit, the door is still closing in slow motion behind me and the whole of Las Ramblas can witness me tinkle.

'You whon hashish?' the stranger on a bike pulls over and asks in a thick Catalan accent. 'Excellent, I've won hashish? I better not take it though, the Police around here carry guns and we just witnessed them whip the fuck out of someone.

*'First we have Woman-Woman, then we have Man-Woman, and then we have PARTICIPATION!'* This is heaven, but I'm too scared to go in. 'Oh, so sad, so sad!' – Andy.

Simple diet of *people's food*, resting in a class shared room; jar of *Nutella and* freshly baked bread to scoop over, fresh fruit and banana milk shake to stave off midnight hypos, *'Gag, spit, cough, spit, boak,* water fast hurry. *Sick, uuggggg.'* 'That's right Paul man; they use goat's milk in their milk shakes over here. HA HA HA.' 'Thanks George.' 'ARE YOU HAPPY NOW? ARE YOU HAPPY NOW, YOU'VE GOT YOUR CHEESY BALLS?' – Andy.

Abstract reflections of sky rendering over water, reminding me of the wall of glass in my Catholic Primary School; I'm not stuck in that world anymore; I can do anything with my life. I can go anywhere, be anything I want to be, just so long as I remember to carry my insulin in my pockets, I will be fine.

Fear of flying? More scared I have to go through customs with my

145

syringes; twenty pounds for a bloody Doctors letter stating I have diabetes, to allow me onto the flight in the first place. What a rip off. Being too nervous to present it at Customs and having to ask my Tutor, Bobby Digital to take me over for support.

...

Four nights a week working at the *GFT*, three nights working behind a seventies theme bar wearing flares and a wig: College, through to Caledonian University and I can't believe I have even got in. Learning to think of the world as architecture, whilst passing blood in my stool and picking conjunctivitis from my eyelids. Thursdays, always a no show, and Tuesday mornings a wash out as I can understand barely a word of the tutor's accent; his *Digital Audio* class by default removed from the list of questions I will be answering come exam season. I just need to be awake enough tomorrow to get into class. When I do finally get there, a lot of what should be common sense seems an odd sense of, not so much over-whelming, not really overly complicated but not going into my head anyway. No amount of partying seemed to even be touching the sides of my diabetes. I don't know if that is true anymore.

# GFT

It seems the natural progression to come here and ask for a job; my mum would bring me here when I was in my early teens to keep her company and sit through some French films. In return I got a *McDonalds* on the way home, had a nap during the boring bits and woke to see lots of boobs and bums, 'You get to see a lot more in French twelve certificates than you do in American ones.' Constant peachy arses and deep cello to cutaways of bleak countryside, depression, suicide and more intimate depiction of Gérard Depardieu's bits than I could shake a stick at. 'And I'm learning.'

On seeing me rap my knuckles unsuccessfully trying to make a noise, frailty in a purple knit cardigan with tea-cup in hand unlocks heavy glass doors under traditional cinema deco setting, 'Hi, do you know if they are looking for anyone?' So easy to ask a lady resembling so closely in nature and station my own gran. She replies fresh from a cigarette, 'I don't know son. I'll go find oot. You wait there,' inviting me in, left to pause within magical surroundings, under tiny, ever-changing coloured optics, by a vending machine and slither of couch sculpted into smooth corner wall that's comfortable enough for about an hour, under, *"Tonight's performances."*

Call my mum, reverse charges from a booth on Suchiehall Street, 'You know you told me this morning I would have to get a job because

147

we're fucked? Well I got one just now at the *Glasgow Film Theatre.*' 'The *GFT?*' 'Yes.' 'My *GFT?*' 'Mine now.' 'You lucky wee shite, I'd love to work there. Am I getting free tickets?' Great to hear her smile, she was drinking from a cup of anxiety this morning. – Me with a job, we will be on our feet soon.

...

From my assigned perspective at front of house in the most romantic place in Glasgow; populated by the *culture vulture* and the romantic; I sit back and observe this tiny ecosystem of love and friendship, greetings, held hands and long dreamy stares taking place. Stacking leaflets and saying, 'Hello,' and 'Cinema Two is downstairs,' I'm good at this.

Between evening showings, I sit by the door, keeping an eye out for drug abusers coming in off the damp street while flicking through the works of *Nietzsche* and *Ennis*, as left behind by a budding PHD studying colleague whom fixates on cold *cans* of *Coca-Cola*. A famous work in one hand and the equally famous *Oxford English Dictionary* in the other, I read the same paragraphs over-and-over trying to make it fit in my head.

Nietzsche seemed to say; that we only live one life, and there is no truth in perceptions of *good or bad.* Leading a single life, we should not indulge in nor be held back by guilt or responsibility; we must be completely independent of concern and morality to achieve true free will. Garth Ennis seemed to be saying; we're all a bunch of hopeless fucks and should be making the most it, while we can. And the '*Big Issue*' seller, sweeping in and out, suspiciously requesting to use the toilet, is communicating in the form of printed poetry, "*Happy, happy, clouds, smiles, balloon animals. Then Daddy came home. Hiding under the stairs, weeping.*" Protesting innocence, he asks we remember he is still

148

here; he needs us to know that it's not all his fault. Wanting love but settling for coffee in *Styrofoam* cups to keep hands warm until the next hit.

Half past ten and closing up time; having updated letter by missing letter, *"Tonight's performance,"* for tomorrow, and stuck back on with *Blu-Tack* the *THX* Certification. I duck back into the broom closet behind life giving vending machine to assess my blood sugar one last time, have my night-time insulin, then question the projectionist boys, 'Who have we managed to chat up today?' Free tickets to give away to the pretty ones; meeting for last orders in the *Brunswick Cellars* with the loose ones, the French girls, the German girls and the Portuguese girl; *ah Sophia, who put milk in your herbal tea, why did you not want me?*

...

Dashing in from late lectures, into the broom closet, off with the jumper and on with the white shirt, I duck on quickly from stage right, 'Applause erupts.' the crowd go wild, but I'm not famous, I'm only here to place his water on the lectern. I laugh to myself as I exit stage right and think how far I've come, how safe I feel.

Working every shift I can find this summer, front of house and ushering; got it in my mind to visit Paris; seen it in the paper too, *"Pay for two, get the third night's stay for free, hotel, breakfast, flights the lot."* I'm going to venture out on my own, see *The Dying Slave* for real, spend my days in the *Louvre* and spend my pittance remaining on, 'Black coffee s'il vous plait,' and the sweet baked bread my French teacher was always banging on about. I can feel my horizons broaden to think about it: out there in the world on my own.

We sneak up to the rooftop mid showing of some Woody Allen flic, this gorgeous summer's early afternoon; cigarettes, laughter and nerve endings waiting on our Manager to catch us up, these sneaking staircases are made for exactly that. Some Usher girl asks, 'Why is it Paul that you always have to be having a better time than everyone else?' Why did she have to ask that I wondered? But most importantly, for the first time in my life I'm not scared anymore and have not a care in the world. Better get back downstairs, so Steven can change the last roll of film and we are all in formation to open doors for old biddies grossly offended by the use of crude language, always in the final fifteen minutes. Full refunds as way of an apology, 'See you the same time next week.'

...

Life is Peachy. Seasons come and go; Art Students form into pupa before full metamorphoses in term three, where they hang upside down from their Charles Rennie MacKintosh chrysalis, pumping cider and black current juice into their wings to emerge fully formed into, – 'Art-Wank, Woo-hoo,' we whistle in passing over cream mosaic tiles, dossing around within this art house cinema.

International opinion on our doorstep; Prime Minister Tony Blair gives audience to girls selected from schools all across Scotland. Not quite clear on why these girls have been chosen based upon appearance rather than intellect, as 'St Trinian's' punctuated by *Montessori* Bomb Dogs and undercover *femme-fatale* Security Operatives; easily identifiable by calf muscles like rugby players; revive our once still place of work. Three action men in balaclava's, struggling to open a poster cabinet, 'Can I help you with that? It's got a bit of a knack.' The Door Men and I, we stare at the ground, chuckling, 'How does Tony get away with this when Cherie is upstairs using the Cleaners' toilets?' What the head of our

Government looked to achieve in Cinema One I have no idea. No wonder we are all fucked.

This morning I woke up so drunk, I was trying to chat up the television presenter, and now to face the world. 'What does one do, when one requires a sandwich?' as they stand oblivious facing a vending machine filled with sandwiches, jangling a pocket filled with change. And these are the men influencing Governments throughout the world on the quandaries of society. – I'm surrounded by esteemed thinkers throughout the Quads of Glasgow University, helping out fellow *GFT* Door Man and soon to be Dr Pugs with his International Conference on Sociology. Basically, I copy and hand over floppy discs with essays on to academic men in beards, with fifteen PHD's, who skulk around to pontificate at set intervals, 'Sociology is a self-fulfilling prophecy, where the student becomes the teacher and so on.' Well on that inference so is racism. Before I'm asked on the final day, 'Do you want to arrange your own tax?' for a cash envelope holding three days wages. 'Yeah go on then.' No wonder we are all fucked.

Now I'm seeing my first middle-class girlfriend who buys two-for-one bags of oranges from *Sainsbury's* and only takes the one home because she'll never finish them. Claims to be poor but her mum has a cleaner in two days a week to help around the house; never mind how her taste for *chart* music offends me; as does her looking at me funny for licking the lid of my yoghurt pot. I don't get it.

Total culture shock, this world I now inhabit; they seem to be working together though uncoordinated to tear the soul out from *our fair city*; removing books from our most proud standing library, to replace with papier-mâché statues of Diana. Their understanding, in no way connecting the soul with the consciousness, stands proof of nothing; in no way inspiring the people it betrays. No wonder we are all fucked.

Surrounded in environmental art, completely unaware of its surrounding; single parent mothers cannot take their children into the Gallery of Modern Art to stay warm, while awaiting emergency accommodation; our streets littered with illiteracy, can they not recognise this?

Standing at the bar wearing Netty's purple knit cardigan, *'I'll tell you of the times we live in. I was sitting on the sofa this morning watching Beethoven and eating an Octopus, as Tony Blair ignored the calls of one million of his own people, in protest not to drop bombs on a foreign land of whose culture we have little understanding, for an inheritance of fear. – We look down or we look away, aspiring to advertising. These are precisely the times we live in. Café culture and cretin art leaves covered in soot the yearning of an unaware public. It does not reach for the better man.'* – Back to some subtitled films so we can all pretend to be clever.

...

Recognising a face in the crowded foyer, too shy to be forthcoming, I wave over, 'Hey, you alright? Enjoy the film?' 'Yeah it was alright.' 'Well I suppose that's our kiss at the school disco never going to be rekindled then?' I nod hello to her girlfriend. 'This is Paul; I was at school with him,' like I've got the plague or she is unsure to let me guess she likes girls. 'Everyone comes here,' I assure her. 'I, ah see them aww doon at *Bennetts*.' Nothing more stunning than a Glaswegian lesbian I tell myself – HA. 'It's crazy how many people in our year turned out to be gay.' then she starts reeling off names, the only one suspiciously absent for me being the kid with asthma who used to get up and open then close repeatedly the class closet doors during attacks. Turns out he choked to death on his own tongue. Well that's a cheery way to end the conversation, 'Have a good night.'

152

Jesus, it's so cool to be gay, but it's seen as a sin to acknowledge me.

...

Payday tomorrow, but I'm too late for Paris; time has moved on into peak tourist season, my wages wouldn't cover the return flights. Dreams of the girl I might meet out there, my real life crossing of Pont-Neuf bridge put on hold indefinitely. I may as well piss it up against the wall in Glasgow.

Someone has noticed my sad face; advice from my Bosses' Boss to stick in at uni no matter how tired it gets, or how pointless it can feel at times; her son has made it and Marian thinks I can too. Then she indicates down with a nod to show me she is wearing two different coloured shoes, laughs and heads back upstairs to her office. – Something is going on. 'Hey Paul man,' comes a familiar, overly pronounced accent, simultaneously tapping on my left shoulder, 'I was playing a gig in America last week man,' so smug I feel sick, 'Filling in for a friends band. We played to four-thousand people man it was awesome!' Can't believe this guy is going out with one of the girls behind the bar, and I need to put up with his face. 'You're so neeegadive.' – And there it is.

# Part time jobs and full time

# social life

Popping up to a flat, over from the *ABC Cinema*, having a bit of a fling with an ex Beauty Therapist who quite peculiarly likes me to ejaculate over her face. Incredibly good fun though, and back off downstairs to catch the last bus home, but I've missed it. Walking home instead, balmy night with some of her left over cigarettes, thinking on missed lectures and I need to be awake tomorrow, just enough to make it into class; the tutor is taking my constant absence personally.

Chuckling to myself; most people when they think of university, they think of incredibly bright young minds, whereas I'm at *Caledonian Uni*, with one guy who ejaculated in his own eye, another who is type one diabetic, as signified by the massive boils always sticking out from his chest and a red face of high blood pressure hell. Got the shit punched out of him when he flipped out last week. A guy whose flat is so cold he just leaves all of the windows open because he, "Might as well have the fresh air," and his mate who has the most severe outbreaks of genital herpes all over his lips. Conversations only going along the lines of, "Fuck you." "No, fuck you." "No, fuck you." "No, fuck you." "Fuck you," in the harshest Glasgow accents achievable, followed by interruptions to anything serious, "A horse walks into a bar," "Fuck you." "This horse right; walks into a bar." – Headphones on and smiling, always smiling, life is so good. I look up now to see the Diabetes Ward; that seems like yesterday and such a long time ago at the same time.

Other people in my year having flats rented for them by their parents, all fresh and bushy tailed every morning but no work ethic; it's nice when the competition wipes itself out. I'm pulling forty hours plus and living from a box room, on a futon beside a desktop PC that I'll be paying off forever, just to get me through this term. No space for my old Gothic burgundy drape curtains I was warned when Mum bought the place; warming me toward a larger cupboard off the kitchen with no windows. On the door we now communicate via scribbled notes ending, "*I love you*," time division multiplexing our residence.

What a geek; I'm sniggering to myself when I hear from behind, 'Here mate, whit ye up tay? Where ye oftay?' said slowly, in control and analytical. Two junkies starting conversation past safer ground of the late night serving sausage van; fuck me; I'd better pay more attention. 'Here mate, whit ye up tay? Where ye oftay?' They only need one sentence, sussing me out, a coward or not. I've been assessed as a safe victim. Their opening salvo to see if I will buckle and say, 'Sorry,' it starts where they intend it to, well practiced, at the point of no return in the grounds of *the Royal*, verging on and into the tunnel under the dual carriageway. 'Where were you tonight?' I offer up as conversation, giving nothing; like a cat in a box and he gets to decide. 'Just oot the toon, where wir you?' drawing me in, a dagger on his face. 'At work; what pubs were you in?' 'Nay pubs, just walkin aroon.' I am fucked. I'm going to get done in. Even worse, the other is silent, so he is waiting on this one, the nasty one, to pounce. 'What about you, you hiv a good night?' I enquire to the quiet one, hoping he will be the reasonable one. Nothing back, I start walking a bit faster, a bit further, they let me stride on a moment, they have something to discuss. I'm dead.

Near jogging trying to reach the light of the car park, reaching for safe distance, get clear of the underpass, 'Where you goin?' 'Up the road,' don't know why I'm answering facing the other direction. 'Come 'ere. A said come 'ere,' angry, he is used to people being too petrified to move, and I turn to face them, see how far they are and see my chances of escape, 'Fuckin come here,' and he is reaching into the back of his trackie bottoms, – no doubt it's a knife and I'm running like fuck. My *Walkman* flying out my pocket, I hear its plastic shell crash to the floor; I don't hesitate to consider stopping to pick it up, running like a Whippet through the car park toward the main road. I can hear him shouting something like, 'Come 'ere and get it,' tucking his knife back into the back of his rolled up wrong sized trackie bottoms when I turn around. 'Fuck you ya junkie prick. Ya dirty junkie bastard!' amazingly brave from safe distance, and he makes a pointless lunge; I'm long gone toward the *Shell Garage* on Alexandra Parade and thank God he stopped to pick up that *Walkman* or I wouldn't have a face left; never mind the hepatitis. – Odd that my sugar should fix again at "8.2" in these times of mass adrenaline. Why am I not flummoxed in a puddle, begging a stranger to feed me sugar? I suspect in these times of harsher reality nature more advocates to look after itself than is given credit.

...

Relentless, Christmas drinking season on the horizon, and it's all becoming a repetitive haze; *Brunswick Cellars, 13th Note Club*, late night Chinese restaurant on payday, eight of us waking up scattered over my bedroom floor twice a week. A few of us plan for a New Year celebration together, but to be honest, I think we can no longer stand the sight of each other. I throw in the towel; I have a flu that's not flu. It's a winter diabetic hangover like no other, that started out in autumn and it's time for my barely standing ass to leave the party. Clearly I am the one who has let friends down.

...

A friendship of mutual respect, admiration and alcohol; as amber blonde as any relationship; from the moment I step foot into *Flares 70's* bar looking for a job.

'Ah Paul, I? Joab interview? Somebody said you were commin in.'

'I.'

'Am Nathan, wit yeah drinkin? *Guinness*. Nice choice. So where dey ye drink? Wit dey ye day? No that it matters.'

'Just working up at the *GFT*; drink down at the *13th Note.*'

'You drink down the *Note!*'

'I. All the time.'

'Fuck, so am ah; me and ma brothers are doon there aww the time. Where de ye sit?'

'Upstairs.'

'Doonstairs!'

'Do ye know him? Do you know that? Cool as fuck, you've goat the joab; I'll tell Donnie, he's ma Manager, am just a Charge Hand. Donnie is cool as fuck. He is up the road the noo coverin fir that pub where the guy got shot in their toilet. Mad bastard, ad never even step foot in there. Glasgow man, always somebody gettin murdered. Do you know how tay make a cocktail?'

Nodding my head, no idea.

'It's cool, come in own Saturday at three o'clock and we'll train you, then you start at five. Here, I'll introduce you to everybody. Everybody Paul, Paul, meet everybody. That's John and Malky own the door,' waving over, 'And a'll sort your wig and flares oot when you get in fir yer first shift. Aw fuck, wit will I put doon on yer joab application sheet, "*Really nice guy*," here we go.'

Saturday at three o'clock.

'B52s, its layers get mixed up; you canny serve thame tay the public, yeh drink them roon the back. Line them up; a'll have somethin purple next. I any time ye need sugar or insulin, just stoap whit yeh we're doin and go into the back. Take what ye need, crisps and ginger and just make a note of it so I can keep the stock right. Do yeh smoke? It's the only way yeh can get more than wan break in here. By the wiy, you might need tay work the Millennium. It says here in the works' diary that a've broke ma foot, or twisted ma ankle and Donnie has hid tay take me to the hospital. Hey Hey!' – Someone's been working hard on that joke.

Five o'clock.

In the thick of it; the place is mental with queues going from the bar, ten deep, to the front doors and up the stairs to Bath St. Seventies' chart toppers are on full blast from some guy who is living the dream on his wheels of steel.

'Can someone show me how to pull a pint?' – Me

'You're meanin to tell me, that you stood there getting pissed learning to make fuckin fancy cocktails, and yeh don't know how to pour a pint?' – Donnie, six foot four, scowling and laughing at me at the same time.

'I.' – Me. Fuck, I was a bit more concerned about how to figure out when I'd be able to stop to have insulin and food to think.

'Someone show him, quick, how tay pour a pint.' – Donnie

Around half past eight.

Everyone has emptied out of the bar; it's down to skeleton staff as they head out the back door. 'Paul, go oot the back way thame.' – Donnie

Bit daft to let everyone have their break at the same time, I'm thinking as I squeeze past revellers to the side exit, where I find a Staff Room filled with *Wombles*. What the fuck's going on? Aww shit, and now I'm joining them, I'm a big fuzzy fucking *Womble*; going out the back past the bottle bins and up the alley to yells of, 'Hey, hey we're the *Wombles*,' by every drunk arsehole in Glasgow, then past the longest bar queue, where John and Malky wave us back in. The crowd inside are going wild on seeing us coming down the stairs through painted windows and I am not enjoying myself one bit. – I was a taking myself seriously Art Wank last week, all comfortable in the womb of *Wooh-hoos*; what have I done? The stage has been cleared and they are all dancing about mental to the '*Wombles of Wimbledon*' theme song; loving it. I'm practically still, taking comfort in the massive nose attached to my face that gradually bobs up and down on an elastic band, being large enough, kindly, to hide my face from sight. Get me off here please: the moment seems to last forever.

Ten thirty on a cigarette break, I'm approached by a more senior figure, 'I, his that you goat that diabetes, I? You need tay eat loads aye cakes don't yay? I, a know a guy thits goat it; he his tay eat cakes ow-aye the time; he gave me a pearl necklace,' – this thing begins to gesticulate wanking a cock till it cums all over her neck, 'so he did.' My new Boss is a fucking charmer.

Near midnight; laughing and exhausted with Nate. Already figured out to give rude girls half measures in their cocktails and polite people double shots in theirs; it all balances out in my head; as for rude men who drink lager tops. Well, they are already drinking lager tops so there's not much can be done for them.

Lighting a cigarette and passing it to me, 'How was your first night wee fella? Did everyone you have ever met in your whole-entire-life who yeh widny want to see you dressed in a pair awh flares an a wig come in tonight?'

'Only my brother in laws brother, everyone I have ever been to school with and some prick from school who thinks he's an Actor now. In with his parents, his mother shouting at me to pour her drinks like she owns me, and her son's so superior, and the rest of the place calling me Michael Jackson. I only wanted to be a barman because I thought it would be a good way to meet pretty girls. Then I only took this job because no other bar would hire me without bar work experience. I can't believe I was just up there on stage dressed as a *Womble.*'

'I ah don't like it either; yeh don't hiv tay day it if ye don't want.'

'You might have told me earlier, before I did. – Fuck.'

'Some people like it,' shrugging his shoulders and laughing, 'A've seen people cry because they don't get picked,' hands me another cigarette, 'Right, where we oftay the-night? *13ᵗʰ Note?*

'I don't get paid till next week, definitely do it then.'

'Don't worry aboot that wee fella, ave goat money here.'

...

Keeping my eye out of the tenement window three floors up; Nate's due round about now, as a taxi pulls in by the Swallow Café; that'll be him there I think, running off down the stairs. Quick brush over my pockets to feel for insulin and sugar test sticks; make sure it's all here; I don't want to have to come home early again or stay out sick. Hand waves from inside the taxi and the door pops open, 'Paul ma man. How you doin wee fella?' Hands are shaken. 'Got your twenty *Marlies* right here.' 'Got ma own twenty *Marlies* right here. Got your twenty *Club* right here!' 'Got ma own forty *Club* here as well.' 'All be smoking them, when ah run out of *Marlies* later.' 'Where we goin? Start at the toap of Suchiehall St?' and we're off.

Drinking crap bottled beer down what used to be *Speakers' Corner*, is now a student bar where pretty girls came for two weeks, then were so outnumbered by ugly boys trying to meet them that they vacated the building. 'Is your mate Daniel still abseiling down they stairs way his wee tiny legs?' A sense of humour so identical to my own, it's like laughing at my own jokes. 'Here, have you been here? Day yeh know there?' 'I; a got my first blow job round the back of there.' 'Ah, Sleazy

161

alley. Classic place to take a bird fir a first blow job.' 'Chinese Waiter kept coming out with the bins and apologising.' – We fall about laughing in the corner table. Over the road to some Edvard Munch bastardising student venue, 'Own fir a game of Pool wee fellow? Hold own and I'll take the table auf thame and we'll hiv it aw night.' 'Cool and the Gang; I'll get the beers in.' – Getting my arse whipped at Pool. 'That's four in a row wee fellow. Pot wan baw at least. Is your wee mate Jamie still crying because I beat him eight games in a row, and he was so sure he was the man?' 'I think he's almost over it, I need the toilet again.' Returning later, 'Jesus mate, you awright? You've been away fir ages.' 'Shittin blood again.' 'Fuck mate; have you been takin it up the arse?' 'No, have a fuck.' 'Paul, I don't mind if ye hiv. Why is it you think you are bleedin?' 'It's a kidney infection I think, keep getting it at the end of every cold. Feel better now,' and the talking shite for Scotland continues.

'How you doin?' 'How you doin?' 'HOW you doin?' in a terrible Bronx accent.

'She came up to me all excited, going, "No way, I was in *HMV*. Did you know there is a band called *Cool and the Gang?*" Aww mate, I knew I shouldn't have dated a seventeen year old.'

'Mate, ah jist don't see the attraction there at aw.'

'I know that I can't see her anymore, she looks like my grandad.'

'You the man.'

'No, you the man.'

'Who the man?'

'Mate, that scary bird way the ginger hair, if she'd a wanked you way

162

they big haunds, you'd a hid tay a held up a *Mars Bar* next tay it to remind you aye the scale.'

'Slanger!'

'Mate, she is just like every other burd. She thinks we never met her before.'

'Slange!'

'*Counting Crows* man? Ah listen tay Peter Green. Jodie Mitchell.' '*Pearl Jam* mate, ye canny beat a bit of *Pearl Jam.*' 'Northern Soul.' – We agree to loan each other some CD's.

'Slange-evar!'

'She started talking aboot when we went oot together. And ah said tay her, "Ah wis never goin oot with you. I only shagged you twice when ah wis drunk." And she said, "I you were Nathan." How mental is she?'

'Slangar!' 'Does anyone know how to pronounce that?'

'Right, come own then; *Nice N Sleazy.*' 'How come everyone in here takes themselves so seriously?' 'Ah don't know man, fuck it. Finish these and we'll go to *King Tut's.*' 'Bit of a scene in here in it?' 'Finish these then we're off to the *Variety Bar* to see Eadie.' 'It's crammed in here.' 'Ah know a place, almost know where it is; used to go there with Gina. Let's go there, I'll find it. Down these.' '*Bar-celona*? Shit name for a bar; let's go in here for one first.' 'It's cosa Glasgow City Council, they granted licenses to everyone who wanted wan, noo awh the bars are open but most nights you only get two customers in each wan. Sept the classics. Here am no drinkin *Corona.*' 'Shame they closed down the old *13th Note.*' 'A wis never in the old *13th Note.*' 'Mate it was my life. Here, before we go, back in the *It's a Scream Pub* to I get cash back that I won't have in my card till Friday.' Then ordering, 'A pint of *Guinness*, Pint or Lager, change for the cigarette machine and fifty pounds *cash back* please,' looking around confused, some pricks have turned off the music to pay attention to the screen projecting reality TV, 'Right, where is this place we're going next?'

'Fuck are we? This place is lovely. When did you find this?' 'Found it way Gina wan night,' and Nathan falls into a complete slump, 'A bit of life story and heartbreak.' 'I'm the same with Cherry mate.' Followed by his smile, and, 'Here Marc was talkin about you, and he says you're an amiable wee guy.' 'Aw what a nice thing to say.' 'Ah know, and Marc hates everybody. A've no told you aboot the time when ah caught Marc hivin a wank hiv ah?' I'm already belly laughing on my barstool. 'Came home fay school early and climbed o'er the balcony into the living room, instead aye usin the front door. Walked doon the hall past the door ay ma ma's and ma da's bedroom; done a double take, kept walkin; thought, haud own that's no right and reversed like wee guys day. He was sittin there own the end aye their bed, watchin himself in the mirror, WANKIN! HIVIN A WANK! WATCHIN HIMSELF IN THE FULL HEIGHT MIRROR. AN AH CAUGHT HIM at it and he spent the next six weeks tellin me, "That's what big boys day when they get older." HAhaHa.' 'You shouldn'y be tellin me this.' 'Honestly, it disney matter. He's no even embarrassed aboot it any mare, a've went oan about it to him so much. – Slanger!' 'Don't think I can drink anymore mate. *Garage?*

Ten pounds of Nathan's money left, I return from the bar with ten Vodka *Diet-Cokes*. 'Are you alright with *Diet-Coke* in yours?' 'HaHA. Mate a canny even drink any mare.' 'Well, we canny waste these.' Stumbling out the door; onto the chip shop, 'I need to eat something and take this.' – Standing outside in my brown leather jacket; needle through my jeans, now I'm trying to tuck all the insulin and all of the emergency sugar I've bought to carry with me, all into my pockets. 'Here, you need tay promise me no to tell anyone aboot this. Marc will kill me, a've been goin oan aboot bein a vegetarian since ah wis twelve,' says Nathan, opening a yellow *Styrofoam* container to reveal a massive battered black pudding. Picking it up and shovelling it into his mouth in one go, 'Awww mate, that wis lovely. Don't tell anybody. Please.' 'Secret's safe with me fella,' as we head toward the West End and *Café Insomnia*, stopping instead at a paper shop further up, 'My sister, and our mate James Duffy; when we lived in Gloucester, we used to put plastic toy money into these to get chewing gums and bouncy balls.' 'BOUNCY BALLS MAN! A'VE NOT HID WAN AYE THEM IN YEARS,' stuffing handfuls of change into the shin height red vending machine and turning the nozzle, 'Here ye go wee fella, that's wan fir you, wan fir me.' Slamming brightly coloured orange and green balls off the ground to make them bounce higher than we ever could manage as children and chasing them up and down the streets laughing till we run out of breath and need to stop for a cigarette. 'Bingo!' I point to an abandoned peach sofa left on the road in front of a blonde stone tenement; all her inhabitants, lights off, curled up in bed. We sit back and spark up a *Club* and then another, looking up at the stars.

'Thirsty?' I reveal and can of *Coke*. 'You're like a *Tardis* in that jasket. Here let me see it.' Nathan beckons for my syringe; taking off the cap. 'Toatey in it?' followed by a pause and I know exactly what he is about to do. 'Don't!' 'Paul man, I need to feel your pain,' and he sticks it into his thigh. It's sticking out and he is looking ahead then at me in shock. 'You're fucking nuts.' 'Pull it oot.' I withdraw the syringe; keenly aware it's fresh out of the bag, never been used. 'Mate, anyone seen that, they are going to think we are fuckin nuts. – Fuck it. I don't even think you've even had a good night unless you have embarrassed yourself anyway.' 'I just don't care whit anybody thinks, Ah never hiv. A'm gonna sit in the gutter and look up it the stars.' So we get off the couch and sit on the pavement over the drains. 'That's got to be the best saying every.' 'Puff another Club?' 'I go on then. That *Zippo* lighter stinks of paraffin; I don't know how you can like them.' 'That's ma *Zippo* man, had it fir years. Marc goat it for ma birthday, or ma Christmas wan year.'

Hours pass; it's getting bright.

'Why Who? Is that really her name?' 'I.'

'That lassie Tinker met; she kept him drunk in her flat fir three days. Just kept own topping him up way Vodka and shagging him. Big fat burd and he was mashed; he kept trying to sober up and she kept own trying to find his left testicle. He eventually went in fir a shower, after three days, and says he finally sobered up enough to escape oot a the windey.'

'Neighbour turns up it ma maws hoose, "A think this toaster I bought affa Gerr; might be stolen?" and ma maw is aww, "Uff, that's no stolen, Gerr's no a thief. Gerr's been oaffa the drugs fir ages; he widney day that. How dare you!" "It's still goat toast in it," she says.'

Taxi to mine, hugs in the kitchen, while cooking noodles, 'Hiv you no just hid that?' 'I need to have more so I can have these.' 'Ah get yeh,' – short pause, 'I pure miss Gina man.' 'I pure miss Cherry. Look at the state of us man.' 'Ah no man, and no one to talk to about it fir ever,' – still hugging. 'When did you last see Cherry?' 'Aw fuck, man I was totally getting over her. Then Daniel who goes abseiling to manage the stairs bumps into her at the *Cathouse*. She spends all night telling him she misses me and she is as heartbroken as I am, and I get back with her like an idiot. I just couldn't stop crying the whole time I was with her, from then on. And after two weeks, we woke up the day Diana died. All the TV's and neighbours radios were on. You know that way, when something *has happened* in the news?' 'I, its aww eerie.' 'I, and *Channel 5* had just started so we were as excited about having a fifth channel.' 'Canny afford *SKY* either.' 'And we both went, "Ah well, the English will be going on about that forever. Possibly more than winning the World Cup." Then she went home that afternoon and I never saw her again. Fuckin miss her man, I canny believe I still miss her. – Aww Diana come back.' 'HAHA.' 'Shhh gonna wake up my mum.' 'Gina moved down to London, I'm still petrified every time I walk into her sister in case Gina is with her.' 'Do you want her back?' 'More than anythin wee fellow, more than anythin. I canny believe am eatin noodles at haulf five in the mornin.' 'Ah canny believe you were living just up the road from me in Cranhill the whole time. I was so lonely up there.' 'Am still up there, it's horrible.' 'How many generations of the same family do you get in one building now? We had three and one on the way in ours.' 'See it aww the time; my wee brother Connor was seein a burd and bein all quiet aboot it; no like him, so I kept own askin him aboot her and it turns out she his aboot twelve kids to twelve different da's. I was like, "Fuck sake Connor, does she live in a shoe?" Haha, shhhhhh.' Dempsey walks into the kitchen, 'FUCKIN HELL, the size aye that cat!' as he stumbles back into a rack of dry dishes, 'CRASH,' and wakes up the street.

# Our Glasgow

Music sounds better; sounds warmer, means more to me when I am drunk. Thoughts go deeper and friendships mean more; they will last forever won't they? These friendships they will last forever. My emotional range opens; not so subjective, then reaches down further grasping toward memories: reliving them. I can taste her again, I can feel his support, I can stand-alone and make this city my own.

So cold and so crisp, trying to hold onto the warmth of *Nice N Sleazy* inside our coats, we run from pub to pub fleetingly from either side of Suchiehall St. This city she belongs to me: danger close and combustible energy in the air. The whole world, I make it my own. Searching out that perfect girl, that hysterical laugh, the camaraderie, the bond, the cheers, the slanger: the complete escape from worry that rests within all our hearts, trying to make life better. As usual I'm having more fun than everybody else; perhaps I've got more to run from than everyone else.

Stopping at *All Days* for another packet of cigarettes: served by All Dave who hates his Boss and gets sacked next week. Why pay six pounds for sixteen in a machine? Cold journey for an extra four cigarettes, but we go through these things like there is no tomorrow.

Flag down a taxi.

'Auright mate? Take us doon tay the *13th Note?* Cheers. Mind if a smoke?' – Marc

'NO SMOKING IN THE TAXI.' – The Taxi Driver

'I awright then mate, I'd a blowed it oota the windy.' – Marc

The din of the diesel engine as I count, 'Twelve Marc, count them, twelve non-smoking signs in the back of this taxi.' – Me

'Idiot!' – Nathan

As this black cab slips down Bath St, on past St Vincent St, on by *King Tut's* and the back streets leading to Hope St. It glides on by a dozen green and amber lights. A parade of nobodies, wanting to be anybodies, punching at passing cars, tooting their horns. Groups of giggling girl revellers traverse blackened sandstone blocks dating back to the eighteen hundreds. Look up to see our monuments and clock towers, our wisdom and our detail triumph over how we were; bronzed and copper solid reflecting the sun, bountiful against dreich sky sat lifting rich yellow and red; soaring spirits raising ours. All left to mourn over a lifeline of rusted pale green; rather scrape it back a shortened triumphant return: lifting our hearts to the possibility of sparkling prosperity. Look up to see who we could be, look down to see whom we are; at clusters of girls littered like rubbish on cobbles by bin alleys in a glow never reached by any church candle, Catholic or otherwise. Entrances of thick framed modern glass blocks reflecting withered veins hopefully dead to the cold. Short skirts and shammy mittens, asking strangers, 'Are you looking for business?' then whisked away in unidentifiable cars in order to feed a broken soul, and a child's stomach, she never comes back: poverty in this city replacing an old plague with new. My mother's cousin was one of them I think to myself, found dead round at the Exhibition Centre.

'Technically they are the ones looking for business.' – I ponder to Nathan.

Short queue, greetings at the door, everyone is happy to see everybody and the atmosphere is electric; soon to be back in the glow.

'Fuck you ah was in '*Trainspotting*',' – commands Eadie on the door to some thespian trying to skip straight through following a night at the *Tron*.

'Just go straight up lads,' – says Wee Ryan, instructing us past the pay booth.

All is good in the world from this club, just past midnight.

'I'll have the Catholic Guilt the morra.' – Marc

'It's the Heebie Jeebies Marc, everybody gets them.' – Me

'Fuck that, you never grew up in ma hoose, you never went to ma school: way ma good Catholic Mother.' – Marc

'Let's do another *Sambuca*.' – Me

'Oh Paul man, I canny believe you even shagged her, look at the size aye they haunds, they're massive; she makes that pint tumbler look like a thimble.' – Nathan falls about laughing.

'I didn't even shag her, I kissed her once.' – Me

'Even then we fella,' nodding his head, 'Look it the arse own Tracy, fucking hell and look it ma wee brother Connor trying tay chat her up; jammy we bastard, I wish ah had his balls.' – Nathan

'Is it balls though? Is it no just asking oot wey every lassie at the table? Look at him, wan at a time, knock back – knock back – knock back; he is unbelievable and he always gets the wan own the end – the desperate wan!' – Chimes Marc. Nathan's elder brother, in his jaw length curly brown hair and chubby smile looking like Eddie Vedder, 'That boy plays by a law ow averages.'

*Sambuca's* arrive and lighters out eagerly.

'There's no point in setting them on fire; it only burns away the alcohol. What a waste man. Look at you all grinning like loons, looking at the flames. I'll try not to set myself on fire.' – Me

Time for some random dog's abuse from Marc: coming in thick and fast.

'You canny even dance! How much did you pay fir they shoes anyway and they don't even hiv an air bubble?' – Marc

'Oh Marc shut up. Whose goat tabs? There you go we fella, a pint of *Guinness*,' handed to me in a pint tumbler made of plastic folding against my hand. 'I don't know how you can drink that stuff, it looks good but it tastes horrible.' – Nathan

Have a piss and another drink.

'You with your pint of *Guinness* and your *Red Marlies* and your wee spectacles. Ah hud *Guinness* when ah wus in Dublin wey Marc to see Joni Mitchell. It was much better o'er there.' *House of Pain* '*Jump Around*' comes on, 'Here haud ma pint, I need tay dance tay this,' slightest hesitation, 'Have you seen ma jacket? It's oh right Connor will have it somewhere, an that's where ma other snouts are, there in ma jacket sky rocket.' – All smiling eyes and more personality than I have even seen in any single person. This is the guy and these are the simple times those tour operators try so desperately to cultivate and sell to the Americans.

'Green bastard?' – Marc

'I.' – Nathan, back and all pleased with himself.

'What is in that?' – Me

'We've been drinking them since we were wee guys. It's a haulf pint o lager, haulf a cider, Vodka, something else, – make it up at the bar, and *Grenadine* for the colour. Tastes fuckin disgusting.' – Marc

'I'll just have a *Guinness*, watch you try and squeeze more than a pint into a pint tumbler.' – Me

Wee Ryan pops over to share an anecdote, 'In ma day joab, dealing way junkies, and this guy a know his turned up fir work, the first time in three weeks, he tells me, "I just hid a wee spot oh that diabetes. But it's better noo." A just laughed at him, ah said you've no goat diabetes...'

Northern Soul punctuated by Hip Hop and I want to dance but high sugar has my legs bound as stone.

Three a.m.

'Three! Nooo waaay is that three in the mornin, where we goin new? Up the road? Am no goin up the road, no fuck that.' – Marc.

Cooling off outside after a dozen, 'See ye laters,' and, 'Where you goin after this?'

'IF YE LIKE A LOT OF CHOCOLATE ON YOUR BISCUIT JOIN OUR CLUB, IF YE LIKE A LOT OF CHOCOLATE ON YOUR BISCUIT JOIN OUR CLUB,' jump up and down and repeat till fade by Marc, Joana and Ali as we stand outside, warming our noses and

172

freezing our balls off waiting on Nathan to find his jacket.

There goes Riley getting all the girls to show him the top of their pants.

'Do you aw wanna come back to mine and listen tay ma bands new demo tape?' – Joana.

'Nah mate, all you bands sound the same.' – Me.

'Where is he? Where did aww they gay blokes go? Ma wee brother Connor went wey them, he'll be oaf wey them the noo, does that aw the time, finds the best party and fucks off, tells no one. What's a matter wey you Marc? You goat snouts?' – Nathan

'It's him,' pointing at me, 'See you ya jammy we bastard, ave fancied her for years and you walk in snoggin the face auf her, you're shaggin ma bird. Ah pure love her, Tracy's goat the best arse though, and that we Sharon, aww she'd get it anaw, ah they we posh Jewish birds.' – Marc

'Sharon's goat a tash! I've goat snouts. Have you goat a light? Right where's Connor? An we're off.' – Nathan

'Where?' – Marc

'Where is Tinker, did he even come oot tonight?' – Nathan

'He fucked off with they gay guys.' – Marc

'Who Tinker did? Connor? I ah know that, he always fucks off tay the best party.' – Nathan

'Whit, are they having a party?' – Marc

'You know that they are hivin a party, it was you that telt me.' –

Nathan

She is out there, I tell myself, the girl of my dreams. – I look up
ahead into a clear winter black sky, over the heads of buildings across
the Clyde. All this built on the backs of tobacco and slavery – she
certainly isn't in there, gesturing my drunk conversational self at the
club doors.

Wee Ryan nods an understanding goodnight to me through the
warmer side of the glass. He has no idea that tomorrow he drags
himself back to these doors after being kicked half to death by a gang
of Neds. When we finally recognise him, it breaks all of our hearts.

'Come on, chips and cheese and fags.' – Me

'Are you goin up the road?' – Nathan

'No, I'm getting some food and get some fags, I need to eat, are you
going up the road?' – Me testing my sugar.

'I was watching this thing own the TV the other night: it says that
the quickest wiy to give you sugar if you fall into a coma is to pour a
can o *Coke* up your arsehole! I canny wait till the day that you
collapse in front of me,' – a Cheshire cat's grin beaming on Marc's
face.

'Fuck off! You're not getting anywhere near me, you'll get so excited
you'll forget to open the can.' – Me

'Is that you testin your sugar again? Every time you see a good
looking burd you day-yer-we blood sugar test thing, drip-aye-blood to
get attention.' – Nathan laughing with his arms as much as his
mouth.

'Fuck off.' – Me

'I ye day, ah the time.' – Nathan

'Ave seen ye anaw. Ye day and that's what gets you in. It's certainly no your personality; am better lookin than you and you canny dance.' – Marc

'An ye know fuck aw about football.' – Ali nodding his head with a wry disapproving smile.

Nathan stops sliding down a concrete path on his bum like a three year old and returns to the very cold fold.

'No, am a fuck goin up the road, am no goin anywhere. Whit times it?' pulls up his sleeve like some eighties throwback, 'Look at that watch, ah pure love that watch, ah pure love you we fella.' – Huge hug from Nathan. 'Aww we fella, if you were a bird ad shag you.' – Nathan

'Ah widney shag a guy, but I'd take a blow job.' – Concerts Ali.

'You're aw fucking frightening.' – Me

'Right come own then, *Insomnia.*' – Nathan

'*Insomnia* is shite.' – Marc

Everyone in unison, – 'Where else is there to go?'

'How are we gonna get a taxi? That we Swedish birds eyeing you up, an there he goes. Are you taking her with ye? We Connor was chattin her up aww night and then you come steamin in there, as soon as he's away, as soon as his back's turned you're gonna shag his bird anaw.' – Marc

Me in tears with laughter and before I can even deny anything, 'Don't you even go there, what you did to me, ave been in love way hur for years. Fuck ah miss Carole.' – Marc

'Right, enough you oan about Carole. Shaggin your school teacher.' – Nathan

Bin van pulls up to lights nearest the bridge. Three blokes in the front, quiet, puffing away on rollups.

'Here mate, how much for a lift up to the West End?' – Someone, no one is taking the blame for this.

'Twenty.' – Laugh the Bin Men.

'I'll gee ye ten, naw haud own a need money for fags, Paul is she comin? Seriously: in a bin lorry? Right how much has she goat, ave goat five, naw six pound.' – Marc

Bin Men are just laughing at us, 'Right fuck it, I'll take the money and drop you off.'

Five boys and a Swedish girl tucked up on a bench in the back of a bin lorry, doing the introductions and puffing away. We get dropped outside of *Café Insomnia* at four in the a.m. a queue still half way past the bus shelter with a peach couch sat on top looking in on a bathtub with *some* still swimming goldfish in and tables full of the most haggard clubbers in Glasgow paying well over the odds for coffee, humus and chocolate cakes. Falling over each other on way to the toilet as they wave to mates outside and eye up that girl they seen in the *Brunswick Cellars* seven hours ago before the world made sense.

'Why are we here anywiy? How much? For a fuckin cake? This toast is shite. Why is this the only twenty-four hour place in Glasgow? And where the fuck is Connor?' – Marc

'Did she just bin you for a Bin Man?' – Nathan

'Here Paul, did you no used to shag her?' – Marc pointing straight into a complete strangers face as she hears everything he just said.

'Who, what?' pretending that didn't happen, 'He's at that gay party down the South Side.' – Me

'What, wey ah they gay guys dancin down the *Note* wey no toaps own? What's he doin there? Ah bet that's some party, fuck it we're goin, where is it?' – Marc

Now in a taxi.

'Here mate, can you take us to a gay party down the South Side?' – Marc

'Ah don't know where, we'll find it.' – All of us in unison.

'Here mate, can ah smoke? Is it awright if we smoke?' – All of us in unison.

'Cheers mate.' – All of us in unison.

'Here mate, do you want wan yerself?' – all of us throwing fags through the talking vent.

'Ahh hate Taxi Drivers who don't let ye smoke.' – All of us in unison.

'Here mate, do you know where a party full of bald fat dancing gay men is?' – All of us garbling over the top of one another.

Music blaring out of a top floor window.

'Right that's us, that's goat tay be it here. Here mate just droap us aff here. Did she really bin you for a Bin Man?' – laughs Marc.

Were all dancing to *Moby 'Play'* with no tops on, pissing ourselves laughing and drinking cheap beer with Marc nodding his head disapprovingly.

'Look at the state of you, am embarrassed tay even know you.' – Marc

Nathan and I sneak off into the kitchen.

'Cheeky fuckers have hid the fridge. Ah bet it's in there. Here move that out of the way,' shifting a concealing white board, – 'Mind the door. Ahhh champagne and *Holsten Pils* in the fridge, ah knew It.' – Nathan

'*All the sugar turns to alcohol.*' – In unison.

'They must have known you were coming wee fella. Here watch the door, am gonna neck this (bottle of champagne in the one) glug glug glug.' – Nathan

'Right Connor, were goin; have you goat ma jacket? Come own Marc, we're off.' – Nathan

'I, wit aboot yer boyfriends?' – Marc

'Where's ma lighter? Its ma good *Zippo*. Connor where's ma lighter?' – Highly strung Nathan

I awake the next morning, cradling a can of *Holsten Pils* in my arms as if the most sacred thing in the world and my mum's standing in my doorway asking where I got the bottle of *Marks and Spencer* Sparkling Wine from: commenting that it's only three percent volume. 'Eh – they gave everyone a bottle,' I say all gingerly with flashbacks of sneaking down a stone stairwell in the early hours; giggling like an eejit with Nathan, carrying a bottle each and jacket pockets full of cans. 'That will do Angela then, she's not been able to drink since having Rebekah; only has sparkling wine now.' 'What's that in your pocket?' – as my mum picks my dirty jeans up off of the floor. 'Cool its Nathan's lighter.' Shit, I've turned us into a family of thieves.

Now to lay here balancing *Diet-Coke* to cure my hangover with full fat *Coke* and hauling the head off it to sedate myself through till evening.

# Blind girl

Blind girl in *Nice N Sleazy*; she holds her head with such dignity;
poised and beautiful; sits with her friend, discussing the menu.
Friend of a friend has seen her before, knows that she got it from
diabetes. 'God, how does she manage?' I'm holding onto the table just
looking at her. Still, she is so pretty, and I don't know where to look
or what to do, but I can't stop myself from looking over. How does she
remain so graceful? Bar staff begin to fuss, one young guy goes over
and says something about there being a no dogs allowed policy
because they serve food or something. 'It's a Guide Dog,' I can see her
friend confused, why she is even having to explain herself? His
ignorance on returning to his Manager, who herself has become so
fucking offensively rude, at being drawn into this; clear she is
backing him up. Clear she sent him over. Asked to leave. They cannot
be serious, no fucking way. If there is a law you would break then
this is it? We chose not to cause a scene; we do not want to risk
causing the girl any more stress. Once they have gone, we leave
immediately behind them.

# Far from it

Fallen in love, with a woman, not a girl; a painter of abstract landscapes, twenty-eight years of age, part-time curator of a private gallery (I thought she was a painter and decorator); she borrows paintings of oysters to hang on her walls. I love that about her. The product of all girls schooling with a disillusion for boys, frowns a little when speaking of us, an almost alien species. Carries a sadness in her person; the result of a childhood, where her parents never hugged her enough. 'You have a beautiful cock,' she says, 'Not mushrooming, not bendy over to one side, not too large as to be aggressive, foreskin fits and no unwieldy balls,' and I'm thinking to myself, she has seen a lot of unlucky penis. *Swallow*, 'You even taste nice and sweet,' standing up, to wipe the sides of her mouth with the cuff of her sleeve, and a smile; eye contact lasting; I invite her to see into my soul, and then back on to her obsession with being Jewish.

One of her Primary Teachers had been anti-Semitic, and the added contempt it laid with her; of how her father was unable to join a social club due to member's disdain of his faith. Speaking extensively of *nice Jewish boys*, how she has seen them only ever as *brothers*, or "Ya boys" who drove *Porsches*. Gives mention to the guys who call with broken hearts that she can, 'Do without.' I feel someone is destined to be with a nice Jewish boy.

I can afford to take her out for dinner, her preference, only one evening per week; and together while watching sparrows, bundle and circle then group to nest, we walk on through cobbled lanes of the Merchant City: glancing into restaurant interiors, assessing for comfort and romance, scanning through menus displayed on outer doors. Finally we settle at a secluded little spot down on the Trongate, when, somewhere between settling, and flagging down a waiter for a sugary *Coke*, she produces a book on the ill treatment of her people; the atrocities committed by butchers in concentration camps, and I ask if I can read it later. 'Will you tell me of how your own family escaped?' A very intimate question, I'm aware. Oh, they came in direct from Russia, to the Gorbals; working, as a people, to better themselves; working in retail and tailoring, selling kilts to the Scottish. – Genius; building up to move onto Newton Mearns, where this Artist was seeded.

Doing the chat, past boyfriends, ex-girlfriends, have you been here? Do you go there? And she begins to dwell on this guy she has fancied for a long, long time, never having the nerve to go over and talk to him directly. He seems happy to smile back from a distance; he works at the bar I mentioned. 'The Canadian guy, yeah I know him,' digging my fork into my leg, as a waiter stands over us, and we rush to pick from the menu. How lucky am I? I'm thinking, as I scan on this lady, my date, a fluff of fuzz on her arms, elegantly protruding nose and, '*Rosh Hashanah*,' finally onto more cheerful topics. Her best friend had kissed a skinhead then proclaimed, 'I'm a Jew,' just to see the look on his face; the same girl having stopped drinking her boyfriend's cum over concerns of weight gain and that girl's father had bought for her a huge flat in the South Side, far larger than what this poor painter had so far been granted, with only two bedrooms and one to be used as a studio. 'What is a pair of cheeseburgers from *McDonalds*?' – Must be too busy ingratiating herself with salmon, 'How disgusting,' and the bus, she has never been on a bus before, didn't particularly like watching them go by. Under so much pressure to have four paintings ready for the *Art Fair* in London; still coping with the trauma, of her less talented mother's jealousy at her ability, and successive scratching of the *Rolex* she received on her twenty-first birthday. No, these paintings are far too personal to show to me, but she has been having more of those recurring erotic dreams, about eating her own vagina.

Her other friend had married a boy who is not Jewish, and she was not happy. His career far exceeding hers, and I can find myself about to sing, *"I belong to Glasgow."* Would I like to go on a trip to Ireland with them next weekend, a couple's jaunt, only a short break over the weekend, 'It will be fun!' *'To be honest,* I'd love to, but I don't get paid again till the very end of the month.' 'It's only eighty pounds.' 'I still don't have it.' 'What?' sits back in her chair a little confused, am I just being difficult? 'You must have eighty pounds. It's only eighty pounds; you must be able to get only eighty pounds.' *'Really,* I can't.' and she goes on and on. I'm thinking to myself again; I should have known this could never work out, from the moment she never licked her *Sainsbury's Organic Strawberry Yoghurt* pot lid. And to be honest, I don't fancy looking her friend's husband straight in the eye, knowing fine well my mate Riley is taking his wife for shag lunches twice a week. 'Can I have the bill please?'

Weeks wash into months and on into six, on every word there hangs a sob story; now the Internet's being claimed as a suspected source of evil; *www* transliterated wrongly in Hebrew as *six-six-six*. So how does that leave me? Clearly out of favour, no more a *creative*. Devil Worshipper? I'm seeing myself as a bit of rough; she want's to hang out, she want's to go home. She want's to hang out; she want's me to go home, constantly being dropped off in her car, at the bus stop, 'I don't mind, it's okay. I love you.' Broken up with and gotten back together again, all in a moment's notice. On a whim bent over how her emotions are feeling today. And all I want; to be with this beautiful woman and her long black beautiful hair. I'd never been around anyone like her.

Saturday morning, I'd been invited to stay a lovely *last night*; she looks demure, and accuses, 'I need to be with someone who has integrity.' What does this even mean? As I'm pushed away farther than I can ever reach back from. My answer, 'You're not born with depth, you're buried in it,' and there has got to be more to me than you. It's going to hurt, and it does more than I imagine. I can't be doing this to myself any longer. I'd promised myself after Cherry, this would never happen again.

No chance of going back now anyway, chased by his drunken irreverent truth, Nathan later confesses to a flea in the ear of her friend. And I don't even get angry. I feel sorry for him, his golden personality bleached to alcoholism, two steps from becoming a roughly cut silhouette in family photographs. What must she? Harboured doubts in me through his *drunken malign*, I don't know if I ever want to know. But then I'm thinking on how I was only ever appointed her *boyfriend* in the first place, when we bumped into the married man she so wanted to be with her, for years previous. My love of her a genuine, unfair, surprise. Still, I'm the one left thinking of her for years to come, every time I hear a Scottish band singing a love song, and wondering if it is her they are sing about. And she is sorrow.

Flowers cosseted in a bowl of ice, she didn't get it, a second in Psychology that couldn't see past its own expectation. She never taught you anything, never encouraged you, never made you happy when you were down, and never blinked an eye when she left you with random *Habitat* furnishings. She never wanted you back you never wanted anything more. – Hold on, even I can see a pattern developing here. And you (speaking to myself) started dating six girls simultaneously, desperately seeking a seventh so you would have one for each night. My mobile phone is on fire, 'Fuck integrity. Fuck guilt, I only live once, isn't that right Friedrich / Ennis / *'Big Issue'* Guy?'

...

After eight years sitting in his bedroom smoking dope, Nolan fancies popping out for a beer. Expectation to be a nicer person, from the moment I stand outside the *Cathouse* doors on Union Street, disclosing with much eye contact, 'I'm diabetic and carry insulin and needles with me.' Needle a better choice of word than syringe. Syringe puts people on alert. Nightclub Bouncers are waving me on through, calling through to other bouncers further floors up stairs, 'HE'S CLEAR.' Doormen's etiquette and public safety guidelines informing I'm a safe bet, a clear pass every time. 'That just gets you straight in there? You could be carrying drugs or anything?' says a profoundly concerned Nolan. 'Assumption I'm a good guy because I'm diabetic. Hold on, are you insinuating I look like a drug dealer?' 'Na mate.' 'It's not like I look like I'm about to start a fight. Look at me; he'd snap me like a twig.' Marked out as different? I think to myself. Not really, more a convenient reality, my size and physical demeanour give away: highly unlikely to be carrying drugs or a knife. Finally up to the payment booth, those stairs go on forever. I now have the *medical* one on me, obviously been radioed ahead; she is sweet though, 'Straight on in to the left, let us know if you need any help taking your needle.' Unfortunate I won't, I think she would enjoy it. I'll spend half the night pissing instead, perhaps passing blood. –

Keeping that to myself.

'Why have you started introducing yourself as Steven instead of Nolan?' 'Here check this,' approaching a group of people standing by a black wall, 'How yees all doin? Hivin a good night?' 'I mate, we're pure lovin it; whits yer name?' 'Am Nolan.' 'Roland, it's nice to meet you Roland.' Turns to me laughing, 'Come own, back to the bar,' one pound fifty for a double *JD and Diet-Coke*, 'I can still barely stomach the stuff since trying to do push ups at your parent's house.' 'Are you commin up?' but the old diabetic ice legs have me nailed to the sticky floor, now Nolan is moshing his tits off to *Pantera*.

I'm doing my usual, drifting into thought. I'm annoyed with myself to be honest, perfectly fucked right off. Why am I always the one to confide in, taking other people's feelings on board, entrusted to their grief and a drunken shoulder to cry on? Treating friends like Gods, then coming to terms with them not believing in me. Fuck me; everything's getting to me all the time. Am I always taking things the wrong way? Am I being constantly overly sensitive? I don't think it's just me. Snide comments barely palpable, by people I naively believed cared, "No wonder my brother hates you. You only went out with her to make him jealous." It's just constant digs. I get it all the time, "My wife spends all the rent and doesn't shag me anymore. I miss my ex, she said I was bringing her down all the time," followed by, "What would I do without you to fall on wee fella?" then as soon as they have something better, "You're not invited, it's just the lads out tonight." Why do I base so much of myself, of my confidence, on what other people feel? On how other people treat me? Becoming clear they are only pub friends and not real friends. No point anymore, keeping pub friends everywhere I go in Glasgow.

'Check her out mate is that Katrina?' says Nolan. 'No fuckin way, it is as well.' 'She's lookin good; she used to be a horror.' 'Or are we just mangled?' 'Ah don't care; I'm goin over to say hello. Buy her a drink to see if I can get her sweaties off!' 'That's fucking disgusting,' we stand laughing.

Back to barflying, chain-smoking, thinking to myself; these girls I date, all sweet and ready to step over me at a moment's notice; at a single glance from the first sign of anything better, half not even realising they are doing it. Why do I put up with so much from young women who have wanted for nothing their entire lives; given everything and strive for nothing. Maybe some would stay forever, but I'm not staying here. I understand love is more about time than we give it credit for, early twenties and life is about paths, now I choose to walk away first. *"Paul the Bastard,"* two of my other friends are calling me, *miby's I, miby's no*, it touches a nerve. Though I'm not going to let *care* slow me. I'll show no hesitation in care, not passing on another opportunity of a cracking set of tits juggling about in my bed for a night, as I have done so a dozen times before; *out of care*, nor for the feelings of anyone who can *"do without me"* later. I haven't got anyone pregnant, I don't owe anything to anyone, and I'm not about to. The only compliment I ever received, that I was complicated; and all of them falling in between and all of them sorrow. Fuck, I'm getting drunk, time for a pish.

Back from filling the toilet with thick fresh jam red blood as I held up my jeans to escape floods of other people stench, laughing to myself at drunk boys by the sinks, shouting over the dryers having the same conversations as Nolan and I had back when we had long hair. I move over to sit in the corner seats beside Nolan who turns to me and whispers loud as fuck, more into her ear than mine, 'Mind she used to be stinkin? She looked aboot thirty when we were seventeen, mind?' 'I.' 'Now she looks aboot seventeen and we look thirty.' I'm looking at him, pissing myself laughing into my hands, and he gives me a long hug, 'Awwh here mate, always good tay see you,' then he is back in her ear, 'Here, Katrina, mind when ah met you and you looked like you were about thirty?...' I'm stuck chatting with her friend; I don't think with this pair there is an ugly one. Only this one is around eight months pregnant and chain-smoking *Red Marlies* like there is no tomorrow, 'I, yeah see him?' pointing to a bouncer, at least seven foot tall, 'He's the dah and want's nothing to day with it. So am smoking to try and make the baby wee'er cos it's gonna be huge.' That's the saddest thing I've ever heard in my life, I'm back thinking to myself.

Christ, I mark myself out. I'm so sick of feeling weaker than everyone else. And what happens when it kicks off? As in Glasgow, it inevitably will. My head kicked in as adrenalin and insulin become irrelevant to my consciousness imploding like a dying star. Nervous when queuing at taxi ranks at four in the a.m. scared of walking around town after closing time. Had enough of fucking junkie *'Big Issue'* sellers, sniffing me out a mile away, intimidating as they *instruct*, "BUY THE 'BIG ISSUE".' Growly faces, *always* their last copy and they want to hold onto it. Glad to have the nerve to look them dead in the eye and say, 'No,' rather than, 'Sorry.' In no doubt, I'm being singled out because I look the victim.

Do I want to be a Barman forever? Do I want to be working the same pony jobs, long pony hours for the same pony money? Surrounded by you fucks making me feel out of place for wanting more from life? Arrogant because I won't drink in the same dens my whole life, I don't feel the world owes me a favour and I'm not content with my lot. Far from overjoyed with your own, "You look sluggish. I don't know why you don't like her." "Hold on, I never said I didn't like anyone." Not content to be miserable, wanting to bring everyone else down with you. I won't allow myself to become one of these people I'm surrounded by, refusing to see the bigger picture, living in each other's pockets, blaming the world together, pissing their lives away. Happy to be hard done by; confiding in jealous sneers, "That's no good enough for you, is it?" I'm perfectly prepared to strive as best I can to get as far out as I can, 'I'M GOING TO BARcelona,' lifting my head as I say it out loud, awakening myself from my inner drunken conversation. 'I, you ready to go up the road?' smiles Nolan. Yet, why do I need their company so much more than anyone else? The camaraderie doesn't cut it anymore. I'm turning off all emotion, before I take the chance to be hurt anymore.

Understanding nothing, underestimating everything; not so cool to have ambition in my social circles, goes with my explanations of, "To be fair, if I have to wait to meet a girl who none of you fall in love with from a distance, then I'm going to be waiting forever. And what of dating girls you have been chatting up for months, why bark when your dog can do it?" 'How much have you hid tay drink, come own Paul. Have you checked your sugar? Goat your insulin?' loves Nolan.

Fuck the cold is sobering me up as we near the door. No fear of Neds tonight in this weather. Too cold for scumbags in their trackie bottoms; ascends the subconscious of Glasgow. And I'm with Nolan tonight; the real deal. I have never heard this man say a bad word about anyone, and we are indestructible tonight on *Jack Daniel's and Diet-Cokes*. 'Paul, c'moan. You're hammered mate, fuck, am hammered. Right mate, see that shoape ower there that charged me fifty pence fir usin ma *Switch Card* earlier? We're going in there; am stealin a bar of chocolate to get ma money back.' Filling our sleeves with *Mint Aeros* and *Dairy Milks* as I purchase another packet of smokes, falling about with laughter outside, and near slipping over on ice, it's so bone numbing cold. Night buses have been cancelled and I'm nipping around a corner to find a spot for a piss, as a girl as fat as could humanly, possibly, fit in that dress, pulls up her tights as she stands from her crouch behind two wheelie bins and pronouncing in one swept motion, 'If you never smoked, a'd find you attractive.' '*Silence*,' falls form my lips, as I step away backwards onto Hope Street.

'FUCK other people's opinions Steven, and anything holding me back. Fuck love, fuck religion, and while I'm at it, fuck animal rights. If it wasn't for experimenting on pigs we wouldn't have me in the first place. – Insulin delivered by pigs in the first place, an ah would be deed.' 'Ah know mate that frightens me. See how skinny ma da is noo he his goat the diabetes, type two a think his is?' 'I but he should feel better for it.' 'Experimenting for beauty products? That's horrible.' 'Well, that's different, sure, but you're only going to kick the dog if you get shampoo in your eyes and it stings,' I continue my own line of conversation, as I appreciate and hate where I am at the same time.

'Fuck em Steven.' 'Fuck who this time, who we fuckin?' 'Fuck my own family who left me to rot in this hellhole, the ruin of my diseased father. My mother got us out from under, and has managed to buy a home. What's stopping me from here?' 'Nothing mate.' Not so cool to have ambition in my social circles, 'Fuck all these miserable bastards Nolan, I believe in me.'

'Here, remember when we were sixteen and you told me to put salt water in ma hair?' 'An put a glass ah water beside the bed, so your hair would crawl to it when it goat thirsty, HAHA. Did you day it?' 'Here, remember your dad used to come into your bedroom all the time and say,' both of us in unison, 'CHRIST, STEVEN, OPEN THAT WINDAY!' 'Aww mate that room was a cloud aye dope, I couldn'y breathe in there.' 'He used to drive me mental coming in to talk awh the time, "DAAH GET OOT MA ROOM" did ma nut in.' 'He loves you though; he always wanted to come in and hang out with you. I'd love to have had a Dad like yours Steven.' 'I know man,' Steven burst out crying, 'I pure love ma da,' and now he is laughing and crying, wiping away his streaming eyes.

'Come own?' both of us pointing, 'TAXI,' at an abandoned shopping trolley. 'Perfectly good condition mate,' as he pulls it back from the drain lid its backwards wheel's been stuck on, 'Hop in!' 'Rattle rattle,' up and down pavements, jumping off kerbs and my back is in bits, all the way from the *Odeon* to George Square; pulling up to anyone standing at late night bus shelters, 'HERE, YOU LOOKIN FOR A TAXI? Jump in.' 'Art's the connection between the consciousness and the soul; proving very little yet believing in almost everything. You Nolan, as a Painter and Decorator are the balance of Glasgow between the Neds and the Art Wanks.' 'What are you talkin aboot?' – Actually interested, 'Get back in that shopping trolley!' Shouting over at people, 'Happy Christmas! Happy Christmas! Happy Birthday! Hahaha. Look PROSTITUTES!' A meat wagon pulls up at the lights, and the Officer just nodding his head at us, as we chuckle and head our way home. 'Can't believe I never got ma hole tonight. But I'd rather be on a night out with you than with some girl who won't give a fuck about me tomorrow.' 'I, keep in touch way yourself,' huge grin when Steven walks the rest of the way home.

One more cigarette at the foot of my mum's block, 'And fuck you Bar Guy, standing behind me at the bar, mouthing the words, "So neeeegative," Fuck you Glasgow,' this city she hates herself.

# Career development

I should be doing my dissertation; I should be doing lots of things. I am reading on-line reports of an Internet bubble going burst. I'm little surprised, as it's falling into the same pattern as photography; I'm a little relieved as it should hopefully wash away every idiot who can save an image as a *.jpg calling themselves a Web Designer. I'm a little bit, *the carpet has been pulled away from under my feet*, because I'm yet to complete my *Hons* year and the World Wide Web still in its infancy has raked in shareholder confidence and pissed it against the wall.

All summer long, on completion of my *BSc*, I have hunted around the Internet, emailing off CVs, trying to get my foot in the door, "How much experience do you have? Minimum of one year required. Sorry." Knack all is my only answer, along with every other student studying in the same field, and the four years advanced bookings for the next batch lined up behind me, not to mention the aforementioned *Web Designers* capable of saving a *Word Document* as a *.html.

Knowledge of the Print Industry stands me in good stead; a basis for conventional print-to-web design, and now in more ways than one; a little podgy chappy I used to print t-shirts for not so long ago, standing in front of me now at the bar of this snooker club where I find myself working. This guy knows all the buzzwords and is looking up at me, dead chuffed with himself, 'The Web. I the Internet,' nodding his head up and down, up and down, as do those little plastic dogs you find in the backs of passing cars, 'I know it aww. E-commerce, that's the future; that *Java* script; that HTML they Hyperlinks!' Smile and jig of the shoulders, almost bursting from his barstool because he can talk the shit, '*Dreamweaver, Apple Macs,*' rounding off a one-man game of bullshit bingo, 'I we've goat aw oh thame. Expanded so we hiv, doon at the *St Enoch Centre* noo; apparel decoration and aw aye that. Look it ma logo?' Hands me a business card, it's the *Gap* logo with his company name on it instead, 'Created it maself. Day it aww wee day.' 'That's brilliant.' I'm sure I wanted to shag his blonde wife at one point, I'm thinking as I'm nodding, while he is getting off on mock admiration as I would if my Pamela Anderson and Claudia Schiffer calendars came to life. Then his tall skinny brother walks in, 'Here day ye remember him?' pointing at my head, like I'm his dog, 'Think aye that face way long hair, mind? Always countin the stones own the grun when printin thame *Baby Chaos* t-shirts fur us. Mind?' My face has gone red for all the wrong reasons. His brother's head jumps up in surprise like a Jack in the Box, now I'm a long lost relative when the bullshit offensive kicks in, 'Is that right? Is that you? No way! That's amazin! Fuck me. No way. Yer jokin? I? No way! Yer Jokin? Seriously, is that you?' How high can the pitch of this guy's voice go? Now the tag team comes into full effect, 'Get this. Tell him whit you've been dayin?' Nice, I'm being instructed already, 'Web Design at uni.' 'Noooo way? Yer jokin?' the short fat one is grinning on his barstool, gleeful bright red face: arms crossed almost making it over the width of his chest but not quite. I just know that at the other side of this bar he is trying as hard as he can for his feet to find the floor. – Dramatic pause and they look at each other, 'Ye want tay come and work fir us?' said in such practiced unison; it's *meant to be* bullshit. Not exactly how I envisaged my future out of uni, but anything beats working in a bike shop begging them to let me build their web-shite and I need my one year's experience from somewhere. 'I alright then.' 'Come in an see us the morra,' hands me the third business card of the conversation, then his brother the fourth; but he has to be the one with final word, 'Am a businessman noo; It's aw aboot lifestyle; I'll teach ye everythin ye nee tay know aboot the world.'

...

High ceilings; great views over Alexandra Park and a toilet, 'I'll take it.' In the fridge, I have *Diet-Coke* for everyday use; two litres of normal *Coke* for *heavy hypos* – I'm taking no chances in case something bad happens when I'm on my own in the middle of the night; a *Snickers bar*; tons of insulin; four for a pound *Muller Corners* and some butter. Making use of said butter, I have on the table two plates on rotation and twice as many in cutlery, two family sized bags of crisps, mixed flavours, and a loaf for making crisp sandwiches. *Heinz Soup*, six tins, random flavours because I like a surprise; two Beef *Super Noodles*, two *Sweet and Sour*; a *classic* selection of *Pot Noodles*, that means *Beef and Tomato* or *Chicken and Mushroom*, nothing fancy; twenty-five pence each or five for a pound non-English speaking noodles: I keep twenty packs still in their carrier bags to stay tidy, all chicken, and I'm still not sure if these microwave sausages go in the fridge.

To the hallway, a large cupboard, empty since I found Big *Ragu* asleep in it last week and leading nicely onto the connecting bathroom; capturing breath-taking sunlight in through a sash window, draped by half a yellow curtain. – I don't care if anyone sees me naked. Furnished in toilet roll, Ketone sticks for pissing on, some bleach, some *haute couture* towels that won't get me dry, just make me fluffy

194

and a *Habitat* bath rug that all the little woollen nubs fall from, trailing through everywhere else, as bad as my used blood sugar test strips.

Spacious double bedroom, couple of poly bags fresh from my mum's, containing two pairs of *Diesel Jeans*, thirty-two inch waist thirty-two inch leg, kept on rotation, and a pair of scruffy ones for emergencies; half a dozen or so t-shirts, the same number of long sleeve tops, a smart jumper and a scarf should I go somewhere particularly nice; all cooked at forty degrees on a full spin. Loitering beside these are two pairs of trainers and no shoes, you don't need fancy shoes when you can get away with a good haircut and a chiseled jaw. In fact, you get away with murder with a good haircut and a chiseled jaw; girls just want to take you home and look after you, hence the *Habitat* furnishings and stack of condoms holding up the pillows.

I sit under a *Habitat* lampshade, in no way a ubiquitous sphere with a spiral of wire holding tissue in shape through which I can see the bulb, but a canvas cylinder clearly defined by someone who can't say hello without sneezing, '*Bauhaus.*' On a King's diet of *Beef Hoola Hoops*, Instant Mash and gravy, mixed in a bowl for dinner served almost every night; It's brilliant how they mix together, but not on a chemical level, a can of *Irn-Bru* always kicking around beside half a crisp sandwich, for chance at hand hypos. Convenient access to a Chip Shop for when I can't be bothered cooking, and a corner shop with long opening hours in case I fancy some microwave affair. TV set for nights in, *Calor Gas Canister* for warm nights in. Two towels and a HiFi that only comes on at four in the a.m. but that's OK as the old woman upstairs is tone-deaf and I'm now shagging a Goth from directly downstairs, when she pops up, when her boyfriend pops out.

Comfy sofa because I'm not quite settled enough to sleep in the other room on my own, and some random friends I have not seen in ages pop over for a cuppa, when I bump into them on Duke Street; one taking a hand gun out of his pocket, placing it down on the table like it's a book so he can get comfy. Girl from downstairs has popped in, door's always open, her dog shits on the floor boards, I think it speaks for the both of us.

...

'That's very kind of you; I'm a very kind man,' potential opportunity arising at his mutterings on every opening door; desperately trying to find a fellow member of the *Masonic Lodge* to do the funny "*wink wink, nudge nudge*" with. 'I only speak to decision makers. I know the guy,' and so it goes on; my computer monitor brought in from home, attached to his desktop with a sticker of a cow on it and crammed with pirated software.

Three pay cheques in with three different company headings; addressing to me a breakdown of thirteen thousand pounds per annum rather than the agreed fifteen thousand and I'm thinking of making a run. But I'll keep my trap shut; see if I can see this through to the six months experience mark. 'If you hid tay take the word of a great philosopher, or the word of yer ma, whose *word* would you take?' Maybe he has a point there somewhere. 'Ah Don't subscribe tay it, "*Just tell us where and when,*" that's whit ma pals *Gun* said when they goat the opportunity tay tour way the *Rollin Stones*; that's whit ye say when ye get offered an opportunity. Don't fuck it away by making demands. Give me a hundred grand and I'll make you a million. Give me a thousand and I'll go away. Canny argue way that.' This is his actual business case: the little podgy shit, self-empowered authority on living. – Only three months to go. I could have completed and handed in my dissertation by now, been on track for an *Hons*, but I'm too happy to get angry and for once wearing designer clothes.

'But what is it we actually do as a company? That I can build a website and E-commerce around?' 'I'm a genius, that's whit I day. Everyone who meets me says it. I'm a businessman, that's whit it'll say on ma tombstone, "Businessman." I only talk tay decision makers, I know the guy.' – Two months three weeks to go. I've designed and built a website based on the t-shirt printing side of the company, 'We can expand it with different channels to encompass other services later on,' trying to do something with nothing my expression hangs. 'His it goat awh the bells nd whistles own? Sell the sizzle not the sausage.' – Two months, two weeks and four days to go.

'I was the last man in Glasgow tay develop *Rickets*.' 'How did you get that? You have got to be *ages with my mum* and she got the *Rickets* vaccine when she was a kid.' He falls quiet on that one, and now they are debating, between three brothers and some guy who mooches around, 'Who day yeh think hid it toughest when growing up?' The skinny one now almost in tears, 'You sent me oaf tay be in a Foster Home! Ah wiz a Nurse before you made me come here and work fir you, ahh wiz happy.' 'It's all aboot *lifestyle*. Whose comin fir a bevy?' – Two months to go.

'Sports merchandising. Apparel decoration. Am tellin yea, this is war. We're goin to break into this on-line in a big wiy. *Pub Grubs 'nd Tubs* (or some crap).COM. We're buildin it noo, the Venture Capitalists are comin in next Friday. You've hid your tainin, get buildin the WYSIWAG. When ah stand up people listen. Am tellin ye, am a genius.' Two pizzas of explanation later, 'So it's the same as what '*The List'* magazine are doing with bar and restaurant reviews?' I enquire, in a tone of are you serious? 'This is war. None of these people know wit ah know.' I better shut up and get building; I'll go for a diabetic

197

shit first, the kind that wakes me up when I have started digesting again. And sure enough the following Friday a bunch of Savile Row tailored, bespoke shoes and haircuts with neatly trimmed sideburns that spelt these men were the shit and could VC your ass from zero to hero have entered the room. A step forward having last week laid off half of their on-line business because the Internet bubble has well and truly burst, and are now looking over my shoulder.

'Is that right? Now way! That's amazin. Here Brother, did you hear aboot?' 'I, he was just siyin,' shaking his head all over the place in faux disbelief, 'That's amazin!' Full grown gentry taken in by this pish; it can only last so long; flattery and platitudes bestowed in admiration sure to break down any social hurdle: here comes the technical bit, 'That's the latest WOP technology fir they mad phones.' Flinching at my Bosses sales monologue, 'It's built fir they WOP phones.' The room falls dead, my grin nearly licking my keyboard. Non crease water proof suited desperation on my right; deft silence, cheque books closed behind me to my left. 'That's a nice website,' one states as he taps my shoulder on leaving, to unabashed cries of, 'But its pure magic!' I already sent him my CV last week so I'm delighted he liked it. I'm also delighted to in that same afternoon receive an invite to a job interview the Artist who recently dumped me found in the '*The List*' whilst doing research. – Five months well spent.

...

'Diabetes! You might only die. I have IBS. I might shit myself!' calls *the big M*, my Edinburgh HQ based Director delivered in a golden Irish accent. I don't mind telling people what my insulin is for, if anything it has become a nice way to break the ice. I do notice however that I have to pee a lot more than everyone else and concede to feel a tad embarrassed, every time, having to walk past the same people to go to the toilet rather a lot more than seems humanly feasible; in fact, I have to be peeing out more than I'm taking in. Made worse now working from this trendy building on Bath St; all stained glass stairwells, polished metal surface floors and unisex toilets. Nothing worse than going for a poo in a cubicle when the woman you fancy from the recruitment company in the office adjacent is applying too much makeup by the sinks.

A rush of adrenaline going into work in the mornings; facing the world, believing myself to be indestructible, knowing I can stare down the sun. I never take a day off, thriving on coffee mocha from the copper token swallowing vending machine. Martie announcing himself at around a quarter to ten; glides in, handing me over a bacon roll with brown sauce on, 'What do you think today *Sparkey*, good Cop or bad Cop?' before wasting hours on the telephone losing arguments to Car Insurers and Banks. Popping out for lunch, *Greggs the Bakers* no more, instead, its three pounds and fourty-five pence for a (*how middle class*) *Pret A Manger*, Brie and Saumurer Baguette. 'Tastes okay, but what is actually in it?' 'That's cheese and pickle Sparkey, thank God you never got beef and mustard, we could have been here all night.'

Eight p.m. and I'm loving it; beavering away on *Showreels Direct*: a proof of concept allowing clients to open a modestly secure on-line account; select, preview and order from a library of commercials, to be recorded onto *Digibeta* Tape by the VT Department in Soho, London, and then delivered via Runner direct to their office. Figuring it out as I'm going along to be honest, but it's all coming together as it should and I'm taking so much pleasure in both boffing a Fashion Student over Martie's desk and topping myself up with countless mochas; working into the twilight hours night after night, developing an idea that will make tomorrow a better day. Right, project complete, I better get out of here before I'm the only one left in the building; left trying to figure out how to operate the alarm, and get myself over to the Social Worker girl's house for my night-time insulin and run a few more tests through the world's slowest Internet connection. 'I know you are a vegetarian, but you do have to take the bacon out of the plastic before you put it under the grill.'

...

A trip to Amsterdam, all I do is dump for days. All that coffee and stress I didn't know I had. I think my body has finally relaxed from all the long working hours and brews. Smoking pot just makes me feel sleepy but I love the fresh omelettes each morning. Ripped off for a Euro or two at every opportunity; men staring at my girlfriend, assuming she is on the game, and staring them down with all the Cranhill training I thought I would never need. Day five before we make it to the *Van Gogh Museum*, and on the way there we stop by a canal so I can take my insulin. Locals are looking at us funny, people on barges are pointing over, when it occurs to me: they presume I am *hitting up* in public. Okay, twenty more bells ring at us to get out of their way, and we are looking dead straight into the connection between the consciousness and the soul.

Then the worst happens. September eleventh and the *Twin Towers* fall to the horror of the world. Kids along canals are chanting, 'USA, USA.' Stuck in Europe, watching their world fall down; they didn't know what else to do.

...

I'm terrified for the world; I love the Artist girl and I'm with the wrong one; I am a terrible person. Stuck at the airport for the return journey home, *easyJet* staff just up and disappear, our plane delivered to someone else. I'm sorry but it's now five in the a.m. and there is nowhere for me to buy sensible food. The crew arriving an hour later as if nothing has happened, descending into near interest when I explain, 'People need to eat. I'm diabetic. I can't survive on vending machines while you disappear off to your hotels.' Panic, 'Your medication is in your luggage?' 'No, I have my insulin.' Panic over, no danger of suing them after all: handing me seventeen pounds worth of vouchers for the now opening stalls, this is turn causing a near stampede of angry Glaswegians shouting, 'Where's ma vouchers? How come am no gettin vouchers and he does?'

...

Stuck at opposing desks with Internet Radio Stations streaming all genres of American Rock from the puny speakers of Martie's designer *Vaio* Laptop, 'These page dimensions irney right Sparkey. Am hivin tay scroll doon to see haulf this Home Page.' 'It's not the height of the home page; it's the non-standard resolution of your monitor. We can't build for four hundred pixels high to suit that thing when everyone else in the world has a minimum screen height of seven six eight.' 'But it needs to look good own here fir demonstrations.' 'Then it'll look half arsed when they get back to their offices and look it up on their own computers. It'll only fill half their screen. I'm not changing it.' Laughing because he knows I'm right, 'I'm yer Boss and I'm thirty-four years old. Day what ah tell yeh; aww fuck, now a've only gone and depressed myself that I'm thirty-four.' Phone goes, 'Ahh it's they London wankers. Work work work... I yeh might earn twice as much as ah day, but remember your hoose costs three times as much so a've still goat mare money. It's Martie, not Martin.' I'm rolling on my desk, listening in. 'Listen to this. He just told me that they have convinced the idiot Marketing lassie down there that there is a fifteen-minute time delay between Scotland and London. That's frightening!'

Smell of piss wafting in from the air conditioning unit wakes us like smelling salts. 'So what made you pick me over the four people who interviewed for the job?' 'You really want to know the answer? Bearing in mind you don't know what cheese and pickle is?' 'Go on.' 'Well of the four; one didn't show up, one turned up looking like he woke up in a skip and the other was wearing half his big brothers suit and the other half I think was his dad's. I knew we would be locked in this small office together because the *BBC* won't let us webcast from their offices, and you seemed like the only one I'd be able to hiv a half decent conversation with. Although I don't know how that's going.' 'Thanks.' 'Is that you, ye happy. And your portfolio CD didn't even open either? By the way now is a good time to tell you, we won't be making any bonus this quarter.' 'Ha ha, the news just keeps getting better and better. Come on, we've been listening to that for ages, log into my radio station for once and we can even use my desktop speakers.'

Lunchtime passes, 'What's that you're having for lunch?' 'Ahhh ma pet hate. Hate it when people look at ma dinner and comment before I get to eat it. Go away; you wouldn't understand, its no made of crisps or haudin doon yer jacket pockets way cans of emergency *Irn-Bru.*'

More conversation to run out of, more random questions, 'So how intelligent would you consider yourself to be?' 'Me, well a lot of my friends actually consider me to be somewhat of an intellectual.' 'You serious?' 'I. What aboot you?' 'Well in my past jobs I've been called Smudge and Peachy, and now you call me Sparkey, and at the end of the day I get to design websites for a living; getting paid to do what I love; can't get better than that. And I shag for Scotland and I earn more in an hour than I can drink in an hour. So I might not be majorly bright, but I'm doing okay.' 'Good answer Sparkey.'

I pick Martie up a case of *Becks* for his birthday and a ticket to see the *Stone Temple Pilots*, for letting me text him on his work mobile last night, saying, *"I'm having a great night out and would it be okay if I go to a club and come in late tomorrow?"* I love it here.

# London, notions of wealth

'It's Martie, not Martin. I said Martie. My name's Martie no Martin. I said Martie.' – Martie completely cocks up a job for a major client concern, the Private Investment Bank, *Dresdner Kleinwort*, and his business case has been flagged up as being written on the back of a fag packet. His pronouncement that DVD would soon become a latter technology, ill-fated in the hands of Video on Demand, more ill-fated in the hands of those who earn twice as much but their houses costing three times more. These copper coffee tokens and my flights to attend meetings in London costing more than my salary; plenty more than we are bringing in. But the Directors can see promise in my work, in my ability to modify video for transport over any network type and package this in a *client-friendly* web interface viewable on any device. This means the absolute world to me. 'Would you like to move down to London and develop what you have been working on?' 'Absolutely Moses, and absolutely *Nick the Hatchet*, I would.' Seven thousand pounds added to my salary, plus four grand in bonus paid over the year and a thousand pounds *petty cash* to accommodate the expense of my *flitting*. Not to mention a company mobile phone and a laptop, 'Just tell me when and where.'

...

Wee Ryan has warned me, not to come back a homosexual. My

mother, not to come back voting Conservative, and Victor, not to let celebration of the Queen put me off a good party. I kiss Dempsey on the head as I depart.

Five thirty in the a.m. on a November morning and I've not slept a wink with nerves; last night I cried my eyes out in fear of what lies ahead. Quick wash, slug of coffee, phone goes one ring and the taxi is waiting outside. Grab my bag; beautiful tanned leather given to me by Victor, he had travelled with it his whole life and it had stood him well in Elephant and Castle. Now jam-packed with jeans, trainers, t-shirts and insulin. A few good tops from *Frazer's* hide my travel money, bankcards and a first month's rent: between this and the cash they gave me to relocate plus the hundreds I have borrowed from my mum, it is more than enough to live on till my first big payday. Making more now than my mum has ever earned in her life and I've only been working a year.

Dempsey walking around the hallway, looking up and wondering what all the fuss is about at this time in the morning; he is old and frail now; I pick him up and kiss him again on the head. Quick nod to my mum as she nods past in her housecoat, to get at my coffee; half asleep, definitely going to burst into tears the moment she closes the door behind me. 'You be careful down there son, I know you're going to love it and have a great time, but be careful and you can always come home if you don't, the door is always open.' Huge hug and now I'm humphing my bag through the narrow, half-open, landing doors and down the stairwell; can see my trainers poking through the side as it's banging off my calf as I jostle with the ensuing pins and needles down my hands. I just know it's pissing with rain outside and sure enough I can hear it clatter on the plastic security glass. Unhook the clasp on the storm door; swings in towards me and there goes my shin; rain's lashing down and the sky's that black you can only see it

205

through the orange glow of street lamps and passing *Cleaners'* buses.

'Awright mate?' as I pull the door shut behind me and shuffle along using my bag as a foot stool. I'm not letting this out of my sight I know there are loads of thieving bastards down there.

'Off to the station Son?'

'I.'

'Where you ofta?'

'London.'

'Have ye goat a joab doon there?'

'I'

'Fucking brilliant son, that's the game, I've lived doon there – oooh must u've been twinty-five, twinty-eight, thirty years, thirty-two years ago... ma sons doon there the noo, he loves it, you'll have a cracking time.'

'I, my grandad used to live down there, he says it's great, just no to let people celebrating about the Queen to put you off.'

'I, you'll meet people from everywhere in the world. It's no cheap mind; there we go that's three pound twinty son.' as I'm reaching back in for my bag, 'Where is it in London?'

'Soho.'

'SOHO! Ya dirty bastard, you take care son.'

Laugh, 'Cheers mate.'

Quick splash through some puddles, lights on from the *Blue Lagoon* chip shop; I was out here drunk only as many hours ago, trying to get chips and a taxi. I'm looking up at the big clock; it took all of four minutes and I gave it thirty-five just in case. I'm not risking fucking this up: quick check, bag's still here, no one's been near it and the studs are keeping it safe from whatever that mark is on the soon to be shined clean by the man in his little sweeping buggy floor. Quick pop into *WH Smith* for some fags and magazines; one headphone in, the other around my neck; girl behind the counter is Crowe's girlfriend; he's a lucky wee fucker. Time for another paranoid check and organise my bags before getting on the train. How much sugar could I possibly need and I've a year's supply of insulin.

Looking over at the glass elevator, that was our meeting point for a while when I was a Grunger. I got Nolan and I a bottle of *Mad Dog 20/20* there on my birthday one year, his was blue and I had it in orange, he was so drunk before he hit the bottom of the bottle and I had drunk myself sober, or so I thought until I came out of the toilets and swayed like a sailor before attempting to smoke Glammy Tear's joint lit up the wrong way around, just puffing out clouds of dust as all around me fell about laughing. Happy days.

Comfy on the train, snug beside the window, bag on the table; I'm not leaving it up there in the cargo hold. Fuck have I got my insulin and my money? How could I not, I've checked it a hundred times already, but I am incredibly fucked if I lose my insulin. Watching the man and woman struggle on board with the coffee and snacks cart, I look forward to that later, have enough crisps here to last a life time and how many hypos could I possibly have on a seven hour train journey with all this chocolate and *Cola*. Stick the headphones in; they're still clattering that cart everywhere but on the train. That must be an awful job going up and down on trains all day. Whistle blows and we're off, '*Radio 1*' are playing '*It's been a while*' by *Stained*; I watch the rain fall over a dawning Clyde, all blues and forgiveness, looking down and back at the *13<sup>th</sup> Note*; aww man.

In Edinburgh Waverly now and it's still lashing it down, half of Motherwell getting off and I'm paranoid checking for the umpteenth time whether this train is indeed direct to King's Cross or do I have to change? Newcastle and it's still raining; I'll give Daniel a call, see how he is, and hope he wonders how I am, we have not been getting on too well recently and I'm pining for old friends. He studied around here; in Sunderland he learnt the craft of glass blowing, then he got to go out to Slovakia and study under the Artist whose work had inspired him in the first place: so magical. He also had constant run-ins here with guys in his Student Union, about him being from Scotland, to which one-day they lit a match and asked, 'Do you have fire up in Scotland?' and he replied 'You should know; we burnt down half your country on the way to London.' I hope not to have such run-ins and seriously dread any anti-Scottish sentiment. York and it's sunny, in fact it's roasting and the countryside is so pretty. Coffee trolley has finally turned up; just give me twenty minutes to find my money now fallen deeply down the side of my bag and into my shoe. London King's Cross, and this is clearly the biggest step I have ever made in my life, wish I never wore all these clothes. I'll jump a taxi, make it easy on myself; nice bloke, usual chat, five minutes, five more for traffic, 'That's twenty seven pounds please?' still I have to walk half way down half of Great Marlborough St and Noel St because, 'It's a one way system mate! Ain't nothink I can do, bloody Council.'

...

I enter my new place of work, the *Digital Media Facility* (DMF) of *Megalopolis-Transmission*, Soho, London. 'Oh there he is, you cunt,' delivered with a big grin, 'Oi everyone, look at him, fresh down *frim Glasgey*. Look Gary it's Paul the code warrior. Did you bring your hammer and chisel down with you? Streets are paved with gold you know. You cunt, you're going to love it down here. Here Matt, that's Paul, down faye Glasgey.' 'Yeah we spoke on the phone mate,' gives a wry smile. 'Awright Paul, I'm Bill. Oi Garry, take those fucking headphones off and meet Paul.' Gary looks up from his chair in the corner; fastidiously staring, nose up against the glass; he has not moved a muscle since my last visit down two months ago. Big smile, 'Alright mate, are you down today? Is that you just *doon*? Do you know Nigel, yeah, Nigel Regatta, he just got completely fucked.' Everyone laughs.

'What happened to Regatta?' – Me.

'He went to start his new dream job doing DVD's for a snowboarding resort and they went bust before he even got there; tried asking for his job back here but they won't take him, what a cock.' – Everyone laughs.

'Here, Matt takes a smoke,' calls out Rich, 'Paul, go out onto the balcony with him. Matt, are you skinning one up? Do you take a smoke mate? You're going to need to in my house.' Nigel walks in and stands there in the corner like a tart. 'Did Martie tell you I was going to treat you like I'm Dennis Nilsen? You already know Regatta don't you? Look at you two northerners; nah mate you're going to love it down here, it's pukka. Here, let's all go for an omley. Hey everyone, Paul's staying over at my house for a month, what a pukka Boss am I? You're going to love working for me mate; I'm a top Boss. I'm pukka aren't I Nigel? Ahh you don't work for me anymore, you got yourself a dream job. Ha ha. I could buy and sell you mate.' – Everyone laughs; everyone's standing out on the fire escape shivering

209

to death and I'm standing in my t-shirt smoking on my comforting *Marlies.*

Up Oxford St and into Tottenham Court Road station; across the road from the yellow glow of *Virgin Records* flagship store; I've never seen so many people, all Christmas shopping. I'm following Richard like a puppy and he stops at every turn, every ticket barrier and every escalator to find me and allow me time to catch up, 'Here do you recognise this? It's the train station from *'American Werewolf in London,'* pukka init? I love Jenny Agutter, loved her for years mate.' Down further tunnels, he knows a short cut and we're onto the platform heading west, at the tracks crushed in a wave of businessmen, tourists and people just trying to get home. There are mice under tracks and I am barged through the doors before the last few people have even got off. 'There you go mate, a seat for you and your heavy bag; a long way from *hame.* HA, my dad is Scottish, I told you didn't I? He's from up north; proper Scotland, not Glasgow.' – What did that even mean? I'm just laughing at everything, half in hysterics and half nerves. 'Did you bring your *Pearl Jam*? *Your Nine Inch Nails*? Dark Green likes *NIN*, you will like Dark Green, he's a top bloke, doing some programming you ....train rumbles to a halt at St Paul's and twice as many people get on as got off, how can this thing even move.... yeah you will get on, he is doing a web build for a bloke he knows, you two might be able to help each other.'

Carriage rocks from side to side, Richard falls silent, I can see the day's exhaustion draining from his skin, and he is worryingly thin and dressed like a Glasgow football casual from the eighties. 'Do you like that mate? *Sergio Tacchini,'* pinching on the logo, 'Original mate, classic, don't make them anymore, and me *Stan Smiths*; I got six pairs in case they stop making them, don't want ever to run out.' The train passes into a tunnel near Stratford and he nods and grins as my ears pop then we're out into open air. As we pass a graveyard he quickly blesses himself with his hand pausing slightly at his lips; not for him you could tell, for others, maybe someone he knew. I could tell already he was a seriously good bloke and we get off at South Woodford. 'This is all Essex mate, well it used to be before they expanded the boundary of London. You can see it on all the old signs, see it?' pointing to the old brickwork above the *Railway Bell* pub with Essex imprinted, 'I was born in Colchester mate, Essex through and through; here look at me dagger key ring, that's the lick init? Still go to see them play with me old man, me brother Simon comes sometimes too but he's all married up now, she's nice though, lovely girl and me sister got married to a Doctor when she was younger, they got a *TR7*, remember them?' I'm laughing and nodding, trying to take it all in as we walk up a pretty, little quiet town High Street. 'Just round here mate, behind *Sainsbury's.*' *J Sainsbury* no less, very posh, we go through the car park, up and around some broken brick stairs, 'You will meet Dark Green, I've known Paul for years, we've been mates since we were kids. Paul's his real name. He's not left the house in three months,' as he pushes open the door, 'Dark Green?' knocking on an internal ground floor door: the place has not seen sunlight in years, is lit by the dimmest bulbs illuminating an ever present waft of cannabis cloud. This perfectly normal and nice bloke steps out – Ah thank fuck for that. 'Paul meet Paul; got a bit of work on at the moment you might be able to help.'

The three of us in the kitchen, Richard is rolling his first of the evening.

'Can I put my insulin in your fridge to keep it fresh?' – Me

'Yeah, put it on the tray where the eggs go; I'll do us a nice Thai green curry tomorrow, made with carrots.' – Richard

'How is web bird, did you meet her?' – Richard

'No, I just kept my head in and drove slowly past when I saw her.' – Dark Green

Richard offering Dark Green first dibs, 'No, I've got one going; I need to be getting back on with this.' – Retires slowly back into a green haze.

'Yeah, Paul's a code warrior; he might be able to help you.' – Richard

'Yeah?' – Dark Green, popping his small, cropped head out.

'Yeah if I can mate.' – Me

He disappears behind closed door and I can hear the faint din of broody techno.

'Yeah Dark Green likes *NIN*, you'll bond with him over music.' – Richard

'Has he really not left the house?' – Me

'Yeah. But he did meet a bird on the Internet.' – Richard

'How much are you a month in rent Rich?' – Me

'This place, it's nine hundred a month, pretty big place, got loads of rooms; I used to live in a squat. Dark Green's got the biggest room.' – Richard

I hand him some notes, 'What's this for?' – Richard

'Three hundred; my third of the rent for the month.' – Me

'Pukka mate; are you sure, you've not even seen your room yet? I've been using it to dry my washing.' – Richard

'I'm sure it will be fine mate.' – Me

Rich unwraps one hundred and fifty, 'Here, Dark Green,' a head on a stretched out neck motions back around the door, almost surprised we're here, there you are mate, Paul's rent, we're his Landlords now Ha ha. Remember Dennis Nilsen?'

'Oh cheers mate, I'm well skint.' – Dark Green

'That's your room there mate, will that do you for a month? Your birds coming down int she? I'm just in the room across the hall; chap the door if you get frightened; I'll leave the toilet light on for you, careful you don't fall down the stairs, I nearly did once, Dark Green's done it a couple of times, I think he has, has he? I don't flush the toilet neither, keeps the water for the fishes and the trees. Fancy a joint? Come in and see all my records.' – Richard

Boxed room, nested in LP's with a bunk in the corner.

'You've got thousands.' – Me

'Yeah mate, there is only a few there, the rest are at my maws and paws; been collecting them all my life. Vinyl mate, vinyl. Talk to me about techno, always got time for techno mate. I still get Royalty Cheques through the door; yeah, when they release some of my old music in Eastern Europe or somewhere like that.' – Richard

'Do you still make music?' – Me

'Yeah mate all the time. Into me Pedal Steel now I am. Do you know *Gram Parsons*? Better than that *Radiohead* shit you lot listen to.' – Richard

Puff.

'Do you know if *McDonald's* stopped killing livestock they would free

213

up enough fields to lay grain to feed the rest of the world?' – Richard

'What do you mean you don't have a TV?' – Me

'Com'ere and tell your Uncle Ricky!'

And countless stories, starting with life as a drama student, in the middle somewhere something about living in squats and broadcasting illegal images on late night German music television, then he starts doing a dance they all did in some nightclub, *back in the day*, using only the motions of going skiing without the poles. Everything else is a blur and I awake the next day.

...

I'm short. That's the first thing I notice. *Oyster Cards* and *iPods*; everyone is reading the same book as everyone else on the underground train: no one is sharing. Ethnicities and features on flip down chairs, the perfect game of *'Guess Who'* waiting to happen. The art of, 'Excuse me,' lost to taking old people's ribs out with laptop bags. "Stand to the right of the escalator." 'You can't sit there; those four empty seats are taken.' 'I'll have the post-modern lemonade please.' 'Cheers love.' 'You're alright darlin?' 'Oi Oi.' 'Yeah, *laters!*' Cafés with no toilets; paintings hung on bar *gallery* walls; works you would have to be drunk to appreciate and an expensive way to impress a *"snooty cow."* Everyone is a cheeky cockney. Aspirational: 'How much was your house? I've got a mate who pays more than that to live out in the rain; right hand side of a small shrub in Islington. Likes it though, it's very Bo-ho.' Spatial awareness gone, push you out in front of a bus in the blink of an eye, then coming to a complete halt in the middle of Oxford St and pretend like it's everyone else's fault as they tut and trip over. It's so anonymous that nobody cares, let alone takes offence. It's a free for all, make it your own, fresh start in life; no matter if you're an Italian Goth from some small village, where your family would hate you for dressing like that, an English Bank Manager, or a Brazilian Tranny; everyone gets treated with the same *contemptible* lack of respect, everyone is equal.

...

Social Worker, moves down and moves in; one of the few, the true and the good. I can't stand to be in her company; downing red wine like *Guinness* to listen to her moan, smoke by the sincerity, never going to win the, 'I've just had a shit day at work,' conversation. Tell her of my childhood, she enquires if I am sure: my pain for all the children under her wing. Social butterfly, she likes all the music I like, likes all the friends I have, but in London I have few and for her Barcelona is never a possibility: London is to be our meeting point in the middle. I'm fucked if in ten weeks, never mind ten years, I'm going to be stuck in a room with a girl whose breathing makes me want to scream, thinking on how I wished I had fled to Spain when I had the chance. She takes the *Xbox* as her two hundred pound shortfall in the deposit, because her anger won't wait a week. Returning to Glasgow, and she is sorrow I can long do without. Take it with you, take it all; and as soon as she is gone, a diet of crisp sandwiches, canned soup and banoffee (banana milkshake replacing milk in my coffee).

...

'I met her on the Internet,' wild eyes and cunning smile, this old boy Les is giving us twenty-something's a run for our money, 'Just out the hospital; was in there for months; thought she couldn't have sex again. But she could!' Found the right spot, found the Czech Bar on West End Lane, West Hampstead; opened for Czechoslovak Soldiers after the Second World War so they would have somewhere to go; frequented now by Czech and Slovak Au-pairs, sent here by their

Agencies so they will have somewhere to drink; contrasting nicely, the mid-fifties building merchants baked in Duty Free *Marlboro Lights*, *Budweiser* and *Slivovitz*.

...

On the surface of this city, no one wants to talk, no one wants to make friends, and it is all about making money; scratch a little deeper and you are surrounded by the warmest, loveliest people you could ever hope to meet, from every region of the world. I never knew Glasgow to be so small till I arrived here; Theatre at the Strand, Open-Air picnic concerts at *Kenwood House*, drug dealers every five dusty steps I tread in Camden. It's busier in Soho on a Friday night and the atmosphere more electric, than Hogmanay back home. Feeling as though I am holidaying all of the time, and the women, my God, are like angels. I never knew back home to be so small till I went back to visit *friends* who had all slated me to every girl I had ever dated. I'm settled in after six weeks, this city is my home now; I live here.

...

West Hampstead flat; tap water that tastes like its been through eleven other people first; I'll just move onto only drinking *Diet-Coke*; a clothes rack that doesn't seem to have permission to be out of the shop, a bedside cabinet for socks and it only takes four seconds to walk from the back wall of the bedroom, past the toilet door in the hall to the front living room wall. It always seems to be dusk in the summer time. Scaffolding outside used as a private balcony on balmy nights; Jehovah Witness neighbours upstairs can't stand the sight of me, Muslim family downstairs bring me some cake on *Eid*, having heard me sneezing through thin floors. Lights come on around the back and my bedroom illuminates; cars drive by out front and the living room falls into the path of passing headlights as Film Noir. I find this to be so comforting, and who cares that I can barely cover the cost of rent?

Conkers falling down from the trees as I stand one morning on West End Lane, over from my new Doctors, waiting on the bus to take me to work; held back on *Abbey Road* as tourists write their names on the iconic white wall, – often confusing *The Beatles* with *The Stones* and the studios with neighbouring buildings. I am able to walk home in the evenings, all the way home from Oxford St and never get so much as a dirty look. That smell, when moisture from raindrops falls upon the summer's dust is here and no longer have I to worry about bumping into her in the street. I need to admit to myself that as much as being here is great for my career, it is as much about getting out of heartbreak's reach from her.

# Megalopolis

Meeting with Miles and Giles by the lift, day one, I simply must be in London. Seven years working for *Megalopolis-Transmission*; rich for the first weekend of every month; client lunches to stave off starvation by day twenty-eight; change from expenses pocketed till payback on the Friday to cover travelling expenses. Stock Exchange; pharmaceuticals; entertainment; tobacco; defence; global comms and alcohol; a client list reading as a zeitgeist; *GSK* Patient Insight events and my life's expectancy decline by five years every time. The staff are in awe of their own aptitude, shareholders are marvelling over stock prices, umming and ahhing over whether or not to purchase *Boots*, and I'm thinking, 'What the fuck, it was only down by ten years last time, and I thought I was beating Sister Shepherd, now it's back up to fifteen, what happens next week?' – Sitting on JP's desk all day whilst testing web casting equipment; a looping corporate promo, timed in our minds to perfection, to look up at the moment the smiling woman with big boobs jumps to head a beach ball: eating Mr Garnier's biscuits would not be helping my tiredness matters any, but these are amazingly buttery biscuits.

Fascinating to listen as, this man discusses how it costs billions in any currency to develop new medicines and how *no* governments contribute to fund in their research and development of new drugs;

costs instead being met by profits made from the sale of domestic brand name produce such as *Lucozade,* and *Sensodyne*: leaving all Pharmaceutical Industries in the tricky situation of not being able to give away medicine for free, or even at a price affordable by the financial standards of most developing nations. Cost price per pill often more than a week's wages of the average citizen; should *GSK* give into media pressure and give drugs away for free, they would simply go bust, no more cures in the pipeline. And further demands on exclusivity, with patent portfolio times being reduced by *"independent governments,"* resulting in less time to sell more drugs to recoup these costs. Vicious circle or downward spiral? Who gets the surplus cash, those suits aren't cheap?

...

Annual appraisal, one year, two months and twenty minutes late; to be honest, they could have informed me as and when it was happening, not wait fourteen months till they had a detailed little dossier to scold me. There is nothing like being told, 'Half the building find you aggressive, unapproachable and basically an arsehole.' My back is broad enough, and I go down to the Marketing Dept to tell the lady I am sorry I had caused her any offence; certainly none was intended, and then up to the Bookings floor, calling out a few of them for a moments interrupted attention from busy phone lines and forms to fill in. Again I explain, I had never meant to be rude to them, nor would I ever feel any urge to, nor ever even have reason to. I do this with a lump in my throat; genuinely unaware I had behaved in any way approaching the unapproachable. Certainly not aggressive; cultural differences, that I was from Glasgow, and to them a little rough around the edges, taken more as hurtful and not reason enough, though given by a close confidante as reassuring comfort. But when that bitch thought to question, 'I expect it's got something to do with your upbringing?' realising she may have crossed the line and looking down at her desk; amateur psychologist, gone too fucking far by me. 'Where do I see myself ten years from now? Well, I'll have my own company. Working here allows me to practice and learn how to run my own business, using your money.' Slap back in the face, put that in your notes. Anger almost pulling up tears. Still, clearly my diabetes isn't upsetting just me anymore. – Going into work feels a bit shitty for a long time after this..

Fucking Bookings floor, where fat sweaty and acorn peckered, skinny mockney telephone operators fall head over heels in love with bad teeth girls, but that's a terrible thing to say. This whole group and the Receptionists are the real heart of media, the ones who like to brag and boast in bars of how they, 'Work in media darling.' But aren't they just answering phone calls and booking things in? Seems it's uncouth to say that out loud. On the other hand, just get back to fucking work you bunch of whimpering bell ends. Wanting to stand around chatting all day, being *luvvies*, waiting to be *discovered*. And everyone is making a movie and everyone is writing a script. At least they talk the talk and that's what they like to talk about. – High blood sugar my arse, these people are fucking morons.

Head back in the game, back to building up a client list by doing four Video on Demand jobs, three quotes; sending invoices downstairs to Accounting so they know I'm still alive; co-ordinating three live events, pitching them three more; never mind the technical support required with half my kit broken, being sent via internal mail. 'Foe Mark init?' pronounced by a Receptionist in a *thick* South London accent, shrugging off her shoulders. 'No, For Attention of Mark in I.T.' Diabetic Mark sitting there chewing his way through half a packet of *naughties*. At least I can bribe him with the odd *Sugar Free Turkish*

*Delight.*

I have moved home four times in under two years; the stress of moving house so frequently like being on a witness protection scheme; I've called back to Glasgow and every time; my cat is dead; GT is a heavy drug addict; my gran is in hospital and now I'm shitting blood again. I hear Cairnsey has been murdered back in Cranhill: beaten to death then stabbed with the broken end of a golf club outside the grounds of my old school. Fuck you my blood sugar is high, leave me alone. I wasn't that bad was I...? Oh God, and then there was the phone call with Billy.

...

Had better pick things up at the gym for my own sake; eating *Twix* bars as I work out four nights a week to the disdain of just about everyone. *Snickers* bar on the way home trying to keep my sugar up. Early night's drawing in along with hooded tops trying to pry my mobile from clutched hand. Boiled eggs and tuna fish for protein when I get in, with plenty of mayonnaise to make it edible, and a big plate of pasta in tomato and pesto to see me through the night. Kept passing blood anyway, the Doc gives it its medical name, as did the last one and assures me, 'As long as it's of fresh blood,' that it is of no real concern; so I start taking tins of soup in with me for breakfast to help heat me through and count those slices of toast with melted butter as two units in each.

...

Time off from work becoming increasingly frequent; complications from diabetes ranging from flu virus, which would not let go and burning stomach pains, to forgetting my night-time insulin and having to turn around at the bus stop, to go home for a couple of

221

hours to sleep it off as insulin kicks in. A trip to another new *Diabetes Clinic* held within the *Royal Free Hospital*, Hampstead. 'Are you still on this?' surprised and concerned about the world outside her Specialist Diabetes Unit, this bashful woman. 'This is out of fashion, must be four years now. Twenty-four hour insulin you see, this one only lasts sixteen to eighteen. Let's try you on this instead, should notice the difference as it lasts twenty-two to twenty-four hours and it means you can skip breakfast and sleep in if you want to.' – Fashion? I garner profound concerns over this term *fashion* being used in conjecture with medicine. My life changes for the better, in a moment, in a sentence. The following week, and she twitches when I say, 'Thank you,' a job without applause apparently? No one gives me a hard time about it though, '*Rinsulin*,' becoming the term: rinsing a few more early afternoons off work to attend the *Diabetes Clinic*, at the rate Gary is off having tailors amend his trousers. Colleagues more concerned with convincing the Receptionist as she arranged the cutting of new business cards, that I was not a Web Developer, but in fact a Web Arachnid. Never a concern with the higher ups either, we are owned by *WPP* and as such have a fairly secure Human Resource criteria, able to verify a long term employee over long term performance; besides there were another two or three diabetics over in SE1 and I don't think I am the worst.

...

I stand at the side of my colleagues on the seventh of July, and feel a London changed. I weep on the bus the following morning as Johnny Vaughan pays tribute through the radio on my headphones to the people of London for not letting it hold us back, paying particular respects to the ones who could not be with us today. My world went numb as for one day the people of London did not jostle each other, but walked in silence.

I called the Artist girl when it happened, I didn't know why, for something. I got an answering machine and I said, 'Something.' I had a date lined up with a *web bird* that same evening, we both felt it wasn't a night to be spent alone; both of us had to talk with someone. I had plenty of wine in my fridge, she was able to get a bus here, skirting around the cordoned off Zone One. She turns up with one leg shorter than the other. I mean for fuck's sake.

# Philly Cheese Steak

'Welcome aboard Sir, Diabetes, yes that's fine and if there is anything we can do to help,' before further reassuring, 'We have plenty of *Diet-Coke* on board sir, for all that complimentary vody soon to be in your body Sir.' – A gentlemen's understanding I feel.

Someone has just pulled a hand grenade at the airport, and it's all over the news, "As it happens, on the scene, no fucking about." Someone has just, "Fired shots downtown." I'm not even leaving this hotel room. I'm climbing back under my duvet, beside a half-eaten room service cheeseburger. "Prime time, in the day time," the TV is barking away; flashing lights and logos; they have *'Buffy'* on at this hour? What time is it? When did I last have insulin? Freaking nine hours' time delay: I'm jet lagged all over the place and hung-over as hell. Heady blue sky revealed beneath orange blackout curtains, I see the *'Rocky'* steps through the eye of a massive *GSK* crest; world perception framed in brighter orange logo haze. Slide back curtains, hiding in a flickering half glow. "The hand grenade was a fake, but everyone else is dangerous and has a gun," they loop on local news channels. I've got a cheeseburger instead of a gun. Is this why they put us up in the *Wyndham*? So no one ever need leave the hotel, just straddle the secure corridor, past the branded golf merchandise and straight into *GSK* HQ?

'*KNOCK KNOCK!* Is it breakfast time? 'This is REAL *Starbucks Coffee.*' That was my last conversation; not impressed, did he really expect a tip for *Starbucks*? 'Yeah whatever mate.' How does this tipping process work anyhow, and where are my shoes? Who? What's this leaflet for strippers and steaks? Is it nine hours or four hours? The clocks changed, so am I behind or in front, three hours or ten hours? How do I adjust my insulin to this, and is it at all worthwhile when I'll be heading back to London in four days? If insulin is $x$ and time is $n$, fuck, I'd need to be a Quant to figure this one out. *"Free entry into, Delilah's, The Gentlemen's Club and Steakhouse, for guest of the Wyndham; just present your room key."* Where the fuck am I? I'm supposed to be working?

Steak and strippers; can't get it off my mind; not yet, I'm off down in the elevator to get a fresh cheeseburger with fries, and a BIG icy *Diet-Coke*; maybe a litre of water and borrow a lighter. Woman in the lift with the thickest New York accent, amazing; black hair with a big nose, billion floors down of us going, 'What? Where? New York? Glasgow? No Way! I love your accent, just visiting yeah,' eye contact with *the smile* at the end, 'Sorry to hear about your Diana.' 'Don't worry about it.' I certainly hope to bump into her in the hotel bar later. And now I see her with her son and they are pointing over to wave, he has got to be the same age as me. This is never going to happen. She was being genuinely nice; I hate it when that happens.

'*Philly Cheese Steak?*' smile and nod of friendly presumption. 'What is a Philly Cheese Steak?' I'm kind of guessing, steak and cheese. Aww man, that was a Philly Cheese Steak, served to me on a platter, by the same dainty lady in her late thirties; two kids, twice as many jobs, and limping from the glass cut out her foot from her hairdressing job the day before. 'Sorry about your Diana.' Amazing how quickly you pick up some peoples life stories. Her Bartender colleague all camp and hair: doing fuck all and dreaming of becoming an Actor, 'When you are in the Barbershop, who do you pick to cut your hair? And when you are in a Strip Club, who do you...' 'Just finish your joke and fuck off mate,' my hung-over head almost banging off the bar is saying to him. It's easy to see who makes the tips and who takes home half of the tips in here. I'm going back to bed. I can't sleep. I'm up again, in the hotel foyer, 'Shops over there have cigarettes,' says the same waitress lady. I didn't even have to speak. I must look like crap.

Stocking up on smokes, and my God that is one hell of a selection of pornography, and *diet* absolutely everything, 'I'll have one of sugar free everything please?' Porn mags on the top shelf for the travelling salesmen, don't they have the Internet in their room? 'Proof of ID?' 'I'm twenty-eight mate, thanks for the compliment though. Can't be looking so bad. Now a few puffs as I stand outside, still arms-reach of the hotel's entrance in case someone pulls out a gun; watching my breath chill to fog under the safety and absolution emanating from the glow of *GSK* orange above. It seems to me an unintentional piss take of '*Christ of Saint John of the Cross*'by Salvador Dali.

Morning comes, well I think it's morning, my phone is, 'Prrping,' and 'Thrrumming,' on the floor somewhere. It's my client in the UK, he isn't flying out till tomorrow, 'Fuck off you wanker, it's four in the a.m.' I wish I could say out loud. Kick my feet under cool sheets for a while, 'knock knock.' Ahhh breakfast in bed, 'This is some fine ass, *Starbucks Coffee!*' Really, better than last time? I'll skip to chasing the dragon with freshly squeezed orange; each gulp intensifying that instant hit of refresh all good diabetics *live by* on a vocational calling, deep to the last sip where I know my sugar will now be high; empty glass so cold against my cheek, my jaw and ridge of my neck, clunk of ice always watering it down all too fast. Hotel showers and I could

226

stay in here forever, dragging a layer of skin off my back like a hot girl's nails. Out of the shower and a little Asian woman is folding away my clothes, 'Yes please take away that terrible coffee. Sorry about the mess,' cans and packets of last night's, salt tasting, can't leave them alone, cheese and chive crisps, with raspberry, chocolate and lime zero carb melts: cast aside as a bulimic frenzy. I feel like *Sting*, and the conversion rate is two-to-one, so give her twenty dollars and hope she plants a tree. She reminds me of my gran, all cleaners remind me of my gran. – It's like the time when Holly gave me a hand job in a photo booth, and I had to stop because I didn't want some poor old woman like my gran clearing up after. I'll need to make sure the place is spotless before I leave.

"Prime time in the day time," here we go again, I'll just settle down with this gallon of vitamin enriched, bright orange, zero juice and large bag of low-carb crunchies; technically the combined equivalent of one regular bag. And the good news continues on discovering in the fridge, a carton of toffee-chocolate-milk, with no added sugar! Four units should cover everything, and I'm in diabetic heaven. "Crime in Philadelphia," flashing all over the screen, triple bold and double American. Is this really the same place I am visiting, because the people in the hotel are lovely? "Hand grenade was a dud," they are still going on about that, don't they report further than ten blocks? Quick look out to the world without the squinting headache; what am I on the three-hundredth floor? Looks like some sort of festival is going on down by the '*Rocky*' steps; I think it might be an art gallery. How ignorant am I?

Time to skip outside, my first time really outside since I got here, on my final day before work begins tomorrow. *Pretty kind of them to allow me near three days to adjust to jetlag, and enjoy the city in advance,* I muse, wondering around the foyer, half lost, inhaling heavily conditioned air. And on my second pass of the escalators by a man dressed masterfully as Tiger Woods, surrounded by vampires, I'm wondering how a blind person is ever going to find the braille on those inch square lift buttons. Waitress lady waves over, back on already, pulling long shifts; serving Pharma salesmen perched upon high stools cramming for todays' exams: discussing amongst themselves and to anyone who will listen, techniques on selling to Doctors Vs. selling *direct* to the patient who in turn will persuade the Doctor to purchase their brand of medication; chewing on *Zantac* and fries, looking like exhausted crap. I bet those laptop bags are full of *razz mags*.

I'll go for a walk around the block, puff a few and take in the magnificence. Scale without shadows, details carved in smoother stone, effortless skyscrapers. Clean lines and polished surfaces alight history with sophistication. – I'm not here long enough to understand the textures. Look up to bluer sky, down to newsstands stacking comic books, just how I dreamed of as a kid. I can't even believe I'm here, all the way from Cranhill. *"LOVE"* I have seen this statue in design magazines. What a cool sign to put anywhere, but here it sits perfect, all makes sense. Who wants to be an asshole around a sign marked love? And everyone is feeding off of it. That reminds me, I'm hungry, what time is it? Am I due insulin? I'm still all over the place, better get something. *Starbucks*, fucking *Starbucks* is on the corner, I'm being haunted by *Starbucks*. I'll have a *Starbucks*. – Ahh they got me. Do I tip in here? I think so. This is nice I hate to admit it. Gone in balls deep with the double whip caramel everything, balance out all the insulin, think I probably had too much with the diet food earlier. Better get something substantial though. *Subway*, how cheap is this compared to back home? How much can the team of four of them fit into a baguette? No I'm not supposed to tip? Yeah laugh at the Scottish guy; you're the ones who just said no to money and would suffer a seventy-five percent redundancy rate under common sense: come the recession Billiam the American Network Consultant is expecting because every time he goes abroad his dollars are worth less than the fake fiver a London cabbie palmed him off with.

Walking along towards the '*Rocky*' steps, circumnavigating the widest road, my life in my hands; these cars are larger than my flat; this city is not designed for the pedestrian, nor the man just knocked clear off his bike in front of me. This city is designed for Goliath. All of these little makeshift wooden cabins full of slogan t-shirts, what do they say on them? I need to get up a lot closer to see. It's *Diabetes Aware Day*? No way. I'll get some Diabetes Aware drinks here I'm sure, *whey-hey*, more diabetes aware crisps, no way, and they won't let me pay because I'm diabetic! How cool is that: *almost as if it was supposed to happen*. Underneath the bright orange bunting and face paint they all seem a big bit moody though.

Up and up crushing steps to the *Philadelphia Museum of Art*, kids reaching for the sky with the theme tune to '*Rocky*' blasting from their stereos, "*Rocky tune in the background*," I've done it I've conquered America!

Brrrp, vibration, in my pocket; on the phone again, 'Hi, yeah, yes,' not this guy again, I'm trying to enjoy myself. 'What do you mean, I can't wear jeans? – Cords or a suit, smart casual. Are you joking? It's bloody America, they invented jeans. I thought they would be proud?' 'Bla bla bla, angry because his daughter is always shagging on his literal doorstep and his wife left him, but taking it out on me.' 'Right then, I get it, I'm off to the mall to get some cords.' Now at the mall: shit they only sell clothes for people twenty times larger than I, who dress up as *Cypress Hill*. Could someone please show me how to use these phone cards? I need to dial how many numbers? Oh dear Lord

229

no, as I glance into a store on my left; found my cords; I'm wishing I hadn't; dreaming, seriously considering, almost tempted to pretend I haven't. Gravy is the only description worth attempting. I could get stabbed for wearing these in Cranhill. Balls to it, chess club chic it is, it's the new look. I'll tell Nathan and they will all be wearing them. Thirty-four inch waist? They must make them small over here. I'm thirty-two, thirty-two back home, always have been; I pride myself in being, perfect square, model size.

Back in my hotel room, I'm parched, anymore of that *Starbucks*? 'So what's this leaflet I picked up anyway?' I enquire with the concierge, 'Is it safe?' '*Delilah's Steak and Strippers*, they will take care of you, just present your room key. Tell them the *Wyndham* sent you,' in a chocolate brown voice, as he ushers me off into a cab knowing I need ask no further questions. Out of the taxi; walk on in through the gun scanner unannounced, insulin, who gives a shit, and onto drinks and private dances. 'Do you want to come in the Champagne Room?' 'Well hell yeah I do, but I've spent two hundred dollars in twenty minutes so I think I'd better take it easy.' There is no way of mistaking whom to tip in here.

Taxicab back and the exhaust pouring fumes into the passenger seat like a bit from a faulty washing machine. Driver pulls up under a bridge with no lights and no distinguishing signs; sits quiet. Either he has forgotten me or he is a serial killer, and I'm being slowly choked to death. Couple of moments later, 'Here mate, want tay get us back tay the hotel?' I say through plastic shield glass, with my strongest Glaswegian safety accent; he accelerates completely unfazed and moments later I'm drinking *Samuel Adams* at the bar, thinking to myself, what the hell?

Following morning: everyone has Christian names for surnames and

I'm bored rigid by the corporate speak of *Velcro* suits, trying to *outflank* and *outmanoeuvre* next year's department, – this could go on for days. 'Meeting of the global giants: just got off the phone with the President, and Bill Gates. Whose fault is everything? How do we obtain the credit for this? It's good for CAPEX; good to go; ducks in a row; *buying loyalty*; culture of blame. Is this a robust road map going forward? Let's take this one offline. Who has the most *Air Miles?*' and dramatic pauses punctuating the end of prepared sentence; straight from the book of middle management training on, *how to make people sit up and take notice.* Pathetic; only beaten by my own, days late Senior Colleague asking a waitress to meet him in the toilets, and my gasping like a schoolgirl seeing a penis, when noticing an Undercover Cop's gun as he leant forward at an ATM.

Get me out of these open plan facilities, get me off down the two separate lifts, past the coffee and the diet confectionery vending machines, let me back with the real people of Philadelphia; the rude girl *I still had to tip*, serving up flat beer in an Irish themed pub, who sighed because I requested an urgent *Cola*; the long day workers driving home through snow to their loved ones: smiling warmly in sports bars, feeding on an array of light, diet, zero, low carb, low cal, no sugar, high volume, mass variety, multi pack, everywhere on every shelf and in every fridge everything. A diabetic's dream and I'm sad to be catching the plane back home to *Diet-Coke* land. Equally sad I can't manage three buttons of my jeans or the last four holes in my belt. How the hell did this happen on a diet of *diet food?* I'll need to rock the chess club chic; one button left hung open; ride it all the way back home to London. – And I still haven't tried *Taco Bell*.

# New York, and I'm never

# going home

Its not their smiling faces that annoy me, nor their glossy beauty; I am happy for them. It is their infuriating levels of energy. Never let up, always on the go, oblivious to the privilege of being awake; taking for granted the joys of non-lethargy, unappreciative. Their get up and go hasn't fucked off and left, leaving them wanting to sit down with a coffee. I put down the '*GQ*,' and pay the man at the newsstand. Steam pouring up through drain covers like something from '*Teenage Mutant Ninja Turtles*;' two blocks down from Park Avenue, South. I stand on the set of '*NYPD Blue*,' '*Hill Street Blues*,' all the blue shows before they moved them onto Chicago for tax incentives. Walking around Manhattan, and the intimidation continues; watching the executive class in suits, working fourteen hour days, six days a week, a wife, an ex-wife, two kids, a new kid, a dog, goldfish, mistress; nights out, jet lagged, working holidays, positively buzzing. Retire? Never. – Bastards. Where is that coffee shop? I still haven't tried *Wendy's*.

Over here attending another *meeting of the global giants*; paying us what I would consider a small fortune for advice on global communication strategy; for them it's a pittance to further brand outreach and connect with some unrealistic definition of the man on the street. Self-assuredness, that's what all these fuckers have, in completely unnatural levels; self-motivated on pillars of self-esteem, building to a crescendo of pish and greed. One decides over a technical term and flattery that I should do his bidding; he doesn't know what I do. – What is this kid from Cranhill doing here, advising and constantly surprising? But selling sand to the Arabs is so, last generation bastard, for these guys it's delegate responsibility and wash your hands time, proper Judas style. Clearly this man is unaware of my *halfJesus* esteemed qualification from high school.

I'd better start paying attention; just glad I didn't lose my Doctors note this time; oh he is addressing me again, 'Words, vernacular, deceit, smiles, I do this, I do that, he gets someone else to do something else. Good to go.' 'Now the reason that's not going to work is this,' hate to be the bearer of bad news but sometimes with these pricks you have to, 'I have never heard of them, so we won't be using them. We run this project. We are only considering subbing out elements of the project to you for reasons of logistics. Stop right there and do what you are told.' No one is smiling anymore; my new CEO, sitting to my right has written his company wide business plan on a napkin: here purely on this week's fashionable parental company term *synergistic*, though all he can smell is domination, so he is staying mute. That other guy on our team who calls himself a Senior Colleague; well he came home from working on a similar deal last winter, to an empty home; wife had taken his kid, his newborn and their furnishings; her Solicitor demanding the rest via the home of her high school sweetheart whom she rekindled with on a Social Network. I wouldn't know how to describe him, other than fucked.

Okay, I'm going to be sick, 'Jet lag; point me to the toilets.' Spinning,

233

wish I could vomit; grey cubicle, all toilet cubicles make me think of Goon these days. 'Arrhhhhuuu,' and there it goes; Vodka, *Diet-Coke* from *Heathrow* to *JFK*, whilst chatting up someone's gorgeous PA on the way, she was kissing my neck by the time we landed. Three, four, five in the a.m. GMT, seven in the p.m. NAE? Time for insulin? Of course I don't know. I need to learn international time keeping; I have a meeting with a voice on the phone client/colleague/partner Randy, in one hour's time. Taxi and a, *'Wahoo,'* I'm on a famous bridge; don't know what it's called but I've driven over it in a *Ferrari* on the *XBOX*; maybe she is out here somewhere. *W Hotel*, Union Square and already it's apparent my Senior Colleague is still living on his company credit card, because we can't get booked in. 'At least this time my flight was paid for,' I smile to the Finance Director; have no idea why she is here either, then off into the lounge to get Randy.

Pleasure to meet someone who rocks up with a deserved sense of confidence, laughs at how *tipsy* I am then proves to catch up fast. I'm yawning but he wakes me up, 'You know Paul, I'm a little surprised you're not homosexual.' 'What?' 'Didn't you know this hotel is the gay capital of NY? You had no idea right. This is the *'Queer Eye for a Straight Guy'* domain.' 'No way, Ha ha.' 'Don't sweat it man, everyone comes here.' My esteemed colleagues have things sorted out at last, joining us, and the usual introductions: client/partner meet astronomical midlife crisis and jollies. Randy raves about me into my CEO's ear, while I try to remedy who I've been billing these drinks to.

Well that couldn't have gone better, plenty of future work secured over cocktails, and I'm taking in the coldest *fall* night with a cigarette in my mouth. He told me there is work here for me if I want it. I'm twenty-nine with the world at my feet; I portray the deserved confidence and I'm respectful enough to go so much farther than I would ever have dreamed: leading the life of the proverbial cliché has its merits. I see no downfall; what I'm lacking in exuberance I acquire in dig-deep Glasgow, nothing can stop me, and I'm plain too frightened to go back. I manage the occasional twenty-four hour shift with the rest of them. I'm going to live till one hundred. New York and I need another century on this earth just to appreciate this city.

This crazy smoking ban is working, how much longer can I stand outside puffing in the cold air before I give in? I don't know, maybe sometimes we need a Government to make the big decisions for us?

# Bursting

'Frequent urination,' *they* just check a box, 'Yes and dry mouth, it's very common in diabetes.' Thanks for the understanding.

Trying to go to sleep and I need to go again; fuck I'm so tired I really need to get a good night's rest. My tongue's dry like sand paper, driving me mad, like people lost at sea glugging salt water. I need to pee, here we go again; no, don't pee into your mouth, that's no solution no matter how much you don't care to get out of bed. Two minutes later, up again, tap full of water and I'll be peeing that out within the hour. What the fuck? I haven't even left the bathroom, and I need to pee again. Maybe if I tiptoe to bed my body will forget. Eight in the a.m. I've been up seven or twelve times already. Feel like I haven't slept. Up and dressed and twice more, now just one last time before I get the tube; I must wash my hands more times than someone with checkers disease.

Wee Ryan in the *13ᵗʰ Note* Club, 'Paul. Am assumin that's you in there. Whit is it this time, yer ma's lasagna?' and a lengthy, familiar, anecdote through the door. 'In ma day joab, dealin way junkies. And this guy a know, hisney turned up fir work in two weeks. He says tay me, "I've hid a wee touch aye that diabetes." Shockin in it? Tellin yeah mate, these fuckin scabby junkies I need to deal way everyday. Wanaye thame talkin aboot no bein able to come owf the needle. Says he went own it because, get this, he's dug died. I said tay him, "A've goat a best mate who is diabetic and he's goat nay choice but tay inject." These fuckin people don't get it at all day they?' A moment before a guy who must have been holding in ten pints starts spinning around with his pants down, lashing everyone, impersonating a garden hose. 'YA DIRTY BASTARD!' I hear Wee Ryan scream, as I stand safely behind cubicle doors, hearing the man being dragged out of the building with his pants still round his ankles. One up for the everyday diabetic I tell myself.

*GFT* and I find the non-monetary contents of a woman's bag strewn everywhere, whilst going for my fifth work break lash. 'No I won't mop up the mess from blocked pipes while I'm in here. I disagree it comes under odds and sods in my contract. Written warning? You don't have to; I'll just give you my notice. What is it two weeks? Here you go.'

Getting up from my desk every ten to fifteen minutes becomes embarrassing. When colleagues answer my direct line to inform the Boss, 'He's in the toilet *again*,' no matter how humorous and no offence meant; it's embarrassing.

Getting up three times during a ninety-minute flight, to use a cubicle beside the woman who looks at me funny every time I draw back the blue curtain; spend the rest of my flight awaiting the light to inform me its *free*, with the accompanying, 'Bing bong,' to consent I can get out of my seat; embarrassing, uncomfortable and annoying.

Three cups of black coffee and this café has no facilities. Public urinals and you know the feeling when people are looking? One on either side peeking down before I emerge to Nigel Regatta's Geordie glee, 'Haven't you heard of *cottaging*?' 'Jesus Christ Nigel, that is horrible.' 'It's the norm in London mate.' *McDonald's* on Oxford St, the

237

guy actually said, *"Fuck you,"* to my face when asking to use the bogs. *BK* on Piccadilly Circus, I'm not a Russian Bear; I don't need to be caged in.

On the *Guinness* and I'm finally level with the three-for-one, broken the seal, cheap lager drinkers, as Maz manages table service and Irish John throws me the keys to the wheelchair accessible; packed high with Sunday newspapers; could be a lock in.

Toilets in the *Odeon Cinema*, after holding it in half the film, eventually giving in to push past the grouchers; what are these children eating that their shits smell so bad? Don't their mothers teach them to wipe the seat? I knew I shouldn't have had that hot dog. And now Natasha won't believe me, that I've seen Slash from *GnR* in the foyer. Annual General Meetings, and the more wealthy the client the more filthy the toilets; a lifetime of Nannies, Swedish Au-pairs and cleaners wiping their arses for them has caught up in manhood.

Pretend posh bars with some poor bastard making more money than I do, on tips for a stick of chewing gum, something weightier for a splash of aftershave in the eye; don't even think about asking for a *Chupa-Chup* lolly pop; and always a dirty look for the diabetic fed up greeting him like a Banshee. Hope not to wake up dead tomorrow with a comb in my hair. God bless the *Savoy*, I could sleep like Goon in here.

Pausing every DVD over and over, being tutted at by the disabled for using their *special* facilities, it's not like I pulled on the red cord. Causing confusion, leaving my coffee on the far end counter at *Starbucks*, having quickly ordered a Venti Black Americano, paid, and run straight by into the cubicle. Buying three *Diet-Cokes* I don't want just to use the toilets in knees-up pubs throughout London on a general shopping spree. Being instructed by Police just to piss in the street corner at four in the a.m. because it's not *strictly* safe to pee in public urinals at this time.

Rock concerts and waiting in the second slow *poo queue*, whilst everyone else *leaks and goes*; these toilets don't even have a hook on the door for coats; they are strictly, *get in and get the fuck back out,* again toilets. All I can hear in the background is *Pearl Jam* singing 'Even Flow,' the song I so desperately wanted to see playing live, echoing off white tiles each time someone opens the swinging entrance doorway. Frustrating; at least I can sit down now and enjoy the next twenty minutes of the show, relax properly, get some beer on the way back, may as well.

*Bitches and Homies Store*, they don't even have a working bulb in the cubicle. Last time I was in a *BHS* toilet; well I got done fast then I got bored waiting on my mother and sister. I then found myself distracted by a cracked fire alarm. Needless to say the bells rang, customers ran for their lives, thieves removed racks of clothing and a hand over my mouth told me to hush in no uncertain terms as I tried to say, 'I think that was me.'

Trying to concentrate on writing this book and I need to go again. My sugar only "5.2" this is driving me nuts. It's frustrating and it's uncomfortable. How long till it turns into peeing myself? Becoming a pissy old man stinking of piss and biscuits, making people boak and their eyes water, whilst trying to be polite not causing a scene in *Sainsbury's*. Man I just refuse to even let this bother me anymore and chalk it down to just one of those things. Scratch that, three days of good sugar, excess sugar and insulin removed from my system, I have the water retention of a camel.

# Paul Vs. Boots

I remember Doctors being like Gods when I was a child, as teachers were esteemed genii; I mean, how hard can it be to prescribe a repeat prescription? Local GP has just tried to fob me off with a single bag of syringes to last six weeks! 'There is a numeral two on here with a red line through it. I'm pretty sure these shouldn't be used more than once,' I explain on a frequent return visit, as he flicks piss all over himself from almost obsessively doing my urine test. 'Well you should know better than me. You are the diabetic,' he continues the fob. 'No I'm sorry; you are the Doctor, you should be able to prescribe for me accurately. I have brought you in my medication; you have given me it before.' 'But they change it, don't they? It is for you to keep up?' Third time coming back with the wrong prescription, having also been turned away from the pharmacy because they don't even make half this stuff anymore: would it really be so hard for him to just look it up on his damn computer? 'I only took the syringes in an emergency because the last insulin vials you prescribed did not fit the pen,' I plead, 'I need you to get this right. If they have changed it, then it must be on your computer. How am I going to find out?' 'Well it says on my computer that your Hba1c came back from the hospital as "9.2" that is disappointing.' 'Well yes I expected it to be high, I had a flu for three weeks, and it always sends my sugar rocketing.' 'Then why did you have it done if you knew it would be high?' He is all

240

angst, but I know the answer to this one. 'Well, I don't think I should be hiding it. Is this because my blood sugar statistics impact on your *performance indicators*, as they said on the news?' Now he is in a real tiz, as he bangs down the lid on his printer and looks at me dead in the eye, 'I have one man who comes in here already trying to sue me for losing his foot, claiming he was not properly looked after.' Hold on; is this about my health care or the perception of his practice? Ah ha, a prescription finally handed over to me with a grudge.

A procession of General Practitioners over the years; conclusion, all local Doctors are the equivalent of that guy the Letting Agent sends over to do repairs; never actually qualified to do anything, but having a loose affiliation with the people who do, and maybe one day he will get it right, but in the meantime nothing works as it should and you end up meeting over and over until your confidence rusts and you finally convince them to put you onto an exceedingly long waiting list in the hope of getting someone who does know what they are doing. – No it won't get better on its own.

Finally found *Dextrose Tabs* behind the carb control drugs, what on earth is going on there? Do these people even think before allowing their Marketing Team to stockpile shelves? Think on it later when I've got some of this in my system. 'No, you need to queue at the other side,' says the girl with the hairy arms. 'I'm having a diabetic hypo; I need to buy these now.' 'Just a minute sir, I'm explaining to this customer what the three-for-two special offer is,' as she nods her head at him; she is teaching him the rules of *three for two* and I'm the arsehole? I'm such a fucking inconvenience. Now Security man is looking over at me funny as I open a packet of orange flavoured *Dextrose* before I've paid. – The size of his belly, he will know all about it soon.

241

'It's only one hundred on here,' take it or leave it in her eyes, 'You will just have to take the same amount of as everybody else.' – Hold on a minute, I don't think she is qualified to amend my prescription, she is a check out girl; she's not even the Pharmacist.

I can stand happily in any queue in the world except for the Chemist's, 'Your prescription is being made up for you now if you would like to come back in fifteen minutes?' Twenty minutes later. 'Your prescription is almost ready; be with you in five minutes, the Pharmacist just needs to check it first.' Ten minutes later. 'We only have five percent of what you ordered; take this slip with you and come back and wait around again tomorrow.'

'How can you not have enough insulin in store? That's like a bakery running out of bread. I don't want to go away with a ticket and come back another time. Don't you read the news? There are thirty-two million of us in Europe alone, three hundred and fifty million scattered around the planet; if we all jumped up and down at the same time, caused by the same huff no doubt you have put us in, the Earth would implode and that's a threat! Just order in some more. Do you want to see my, *prescription not paying* card or not? Stop being so random about it; the clue is in the prescribed medicine, only used by diabetics who in the UK don't pay for prescriptions; it's not *Nectar Points*. What do you mean you don't know what cold and flu remedies I can have? Jesus you must have something sugar free? Yeah I expect us diabetics are a miserable bunch to deal with, as per the half terrified look on your face,' I feel bad now.

Assumption by a member of staff behind the prescription counter at *Boots* on Oxford St, London that I was a drug addict; given the corresponding treatment because I tried to purchase syringes over the counter. He walks back a few steps, opens a random drawer, pretends to look inside and says, 'We don't have any in stock.' 'I am diabetic; I have somehow managed to leave my screw top needles behind at home and have insulin vials in my bag. I need to take my insulin now, I'm getting ill; look, you can even check my blood sugar.' 'We won't sell insulin syringes; you will need a prescription from your Doctor.' 'That's completely hopeless.' My reaction based on if I were a drug addict, then he just sent me away to spread HIV. I kicked up shit. They got on their knees and I doubt that clown still has a job.

Catching myself being all grumpy and not giving the Pharmacist a reasonable chance to make a general human error, I stop myself, apologise and ask, 'Are a lot of diabetic customers really grumpy?' to which he replies, hesitantly, 'Tend to be a little bit yeah,' poor guy having to put up with us.

'This blood sugar test monitor; it stopped working; I don't have the receipt, but I did buy it here, and if you look me up on your computer you will see that I get all of my blood sugar prescription test sticks from here.' 'Well,' shrugged shoulders in my face, 'What about it?' 'It doesn't work; I need you to replace it.' 'I'll have to ask my Manager.' 'Very well,' I stand for ten minutes as she points over at me to indicate to a girl chewing on a pen that I am being a pain in the arse; then she traverses the cylindrical spinning medicine cabinet, under begrudging instruction, 'Yeah, we will swap it, but shouldn't really without a receipt.' Well thank you for making me feel so fucking great about myself. Actually no, that chewing of the pen has really pissed me off, so on the way out of the door I ask a lady stacking shelves, 'Could I speak with a Manager please? I need to make a complaint.' 'Yes certainly, if you want to stay right there I'll pop upstairs and get someone down. Won't be too long.' Few moments pass, 'This is the gentleman here, wants to make a complaint,' shop floor whispers. 'Actually, this is the Manager I want to make a complaint about,'

243

looking at old chewy, 'Could you please go and get your Manager?' Yeah that will cheer you up, try taking that pen out of your mouth. Big Manager comes over, 'So you do agree that through me you do make a fortune on distributing blood sugar test sticks. The ones I claim on the *NHS*, which I prepay for in Tax and National Insurance. I don't mind if you can't change my broken monitor because I don't have the receipt; I mind that you employ people who choose to stand far back at the other side of the counter and nod their head while they chew their pen at me. Yes I agree, perhaps they do need more training.'

*Boots* on a Saturday and my tail between my legs, 'I've run low on sugar test strips, and I'm late in requesting a prescription from the Doctors'. Could you possibly advance me some?' 'Yes that shouldn't be a problem.'

This guy on the bus who sat and watched me do a blood sugar test then inject insulin before making up his mind to be disgusted and avert his young son's eyes as he takes him away to protect him. What is this, diabetic apartheid? Then there was the Indian man who told me on the underground when doing the same, 'You are very strong.' Jesus; blew me away having someone reach out to me in such a caring, respectful light.

# Self-satisfied

Billy has drawn a penis on the carpet by spraying bottled water; Gary is hiding in a box, jumping out and frightening the life out of Bookings Floor staff when they come upstairs; the technician bod who smells of milk and, 'Cooes,' like a Dove has high-fived Richard, himself shouting out to anyone who will listen, '*Talk to me about techno mate; if its not techno, I don't want to know,*' passing on the stairs. Hannah is yet again heart broken and Wesley is trying to get home early on his first day back because he has another gig, while some tit has even bought himself a snowboarding jacket with built in *iPod* controls. Happy New Year is on everyone's lips; grateful to see one another, high spirits are all around.

I'm gearing up for the year ahead; no I'm not, I only put down my last and final bottle of *Peroni* seven hours ago; I was only pleading with Nolan, 'Shut up and go to sleep, please. I've got work in the morning,' not so long ago, on answering the building's main door, three sleepy floors down, to be greeted by a verse of, '*YOUNG MAN!*' The first two words of '*YMCA*' sang with strange actions, repeatedly, every flight of stairs because he only knows the first two words. And brought with him, one more friend from Glasgow he will be travelling back with round about now, and two of my other friends who they get on far too well with Hailey and Jean from South London. Seemingly no one else needs sleep at all; but they do need to be fed as they unwind together on the couch at the foot of my bed in my, 'Pure Baltic in here!' studio flat on Abbey Road. 'When ah canny get the sound or anything to work on ma TV, ah just swap ah the wires oot and put thame back in again.' Pretending to be asleep knowing Nolan is screwing my surround sound system, 'Paul, gonna make us something tay eat? Am pure hungry, we're your guests remember?' Cheeky bastard Janice; now I'm up in the kitchen, oven heating my last slices of pitta bread with melted cheese on and sprinklings of pepper for the gannets now pilfering my cupboards. Five weeks to go till payday, I don't stand a chance.

The phone goes at my desk; Reception admonish, 'Hi Paul, it's for you.' 'Hi Paul speaking.' 'Is this Paul Cathcart, previously of Dynham Road, West Hampstead?' 'Yes. Who is this?' 'Hi Paul, it's James from *Black Katz* Letting Agent. I have some pretty difficult news to tell you.' 'What is it?' (Those fucking people from upstairs who bought the place downstairs and hated me in the middle still complaining and I don't even live there?) 'The current tenant of the property had received a very important looking envelope through the door addressed to you so he thought he'd better open it. I'm sorry to tell you, it says that it's from your Uncle Samuel Cathcart; it's about your father, he has throat cancer, and he says, "If you are ever going to make peace then you need to do it now." I'm sorry.' 'Jesus. Fuck. Shit. Mate, thanks for letting me know; aww fuck. Listen don't worry about it. The guy is a complete wife beating alcoholic fuck amongst other things. Cheers for letting me know though. Is there a number on there for Sam?'

I haven't even managed to get as far as leaving the building; telling people who need to know that I have to go home. In some or total shock I don't know but I have never felt this angry inside. Walking in the cold from the corner of Regent Street onto Oxford Street; January Sales windows all lit up and slush on the sidewalks; so angry, bursting with rage and strength and hurt and betrayal; I call Nolan, unsure if he will even be off the train. I need to talk, I need to tell someone and there would be no point talking to my family now. 'I, how do you feel about that then?' Nolan, I love you, but fucking useless.

Don't know if I should be continuing to sit around the house or going out for a drink. I share his name, I see him in the mirror, I more than see him I feel his presence within me. The bullshit confidence smile, at least he was good looking. The guilt I feel, the responsibility bleeding me for what he has done. This man responsible for me being here, I can't take that away from him. – How can I be mourning losing you? As many reasons given why he never wanted me, but I never understood any. What comfort did he find in being drunk that he didn't feel in his own family? 'Your da; truly evil through and through,' I had been told so many times from a young age. Why has he left me with this scar that does not heal?

My creator; conversation with him over safe distance of a phone call and he tells me he spends his days walking on the beach, laughs in my mum's name and refers to Angela as my little sister. Poison; as an adult so apparent; I love him with everything I am, but I hate him. My creator: an early afternoon, on any given day, I don't know much about it. My mother and father found a dead boy on the road, newly broken, where a car had struck his form. My father removed his own jacket and placed it over the boy's head. The only thing I have ever been proud of him for. This man who got so drunk when I was born, he almost missed the signing deadline for registering my Birth Certificate. This man who caused such embarrassment, I had to be christened in a kitchen sink in the hands of my mother with no witnesses. Christened Paul after my mum's favourite *Beatle* not William as he requested. The time my mum and him got lost somewhere in Belfast, 'I'll be murdered, you'll be raped.' This man who made my sister hold his cigarettes, while he beat our mother, and what of the girl from Ayr?

He is my father and I can't change that, and I don't know if I would. I'm in the shower and I'm crying, I'm screaming, I call him once more from a scrap of yellow *Post-it,* his number scribbled on in blue ballpoint, given to me by Sam with some *too familiar* reassurance that he wasn't on the drink. 'Alright stranger?' is his response. 'Why do I cry when I'm in the shower? I hate you. I fucking hate you. JUST DIE, DIE, JUST FUCKING DIE,' the line goes dead; he hung up.

I call my big sister in bits and she offers to pay for me to go up and see her. Tells me I'm okay, reassures me it's over. Conversation with his hospital Nurse; timid when informing me in sympathetic voice, she did not expect he would be around for much longer. She did not suspect what would come next; 'He's not worth being concerned about,' informing her of a few home truths. I wonder how that revelation assists in his care, for those Nurses are better people than I; it's as testing angels.

My father, my creator, I love you because I am your son and genetically I am programmed to do so. Just die and do the world a favour. See an end to all the guilt I feel for what you have done. Stop me from feeling like some kind of monster. – No one in his family will call me back, no response given to restore with peace of mind he has ended. I discover when writing this, he clung on in a hospice for two more years. 'The Devil looks after his own,' my family always said.

...

Blood sugar completely out of control for so long now; mild panic and pain; neuropathy in my legs as I awaken during the night; going all quiet one minute, raising my voice the next; well, actually screaming, 'CUNT!' in an auditorium whilst setting up equipment. Some leave from work, some official complaint to HR, some meetings I still attend for major opportunities because I can't let my life come to a standstill. But I do need to talk to someone and I can't wait two to four months for an appointment with the Diabetes Clinic at the *Royal Free*, well aware of falling into diabetic no man's land. My breathing is short, my hands are shaking, my calf's cramped to make me limp and I'm near to spitting sand. I need help now. I need to get on top of this now before it takes me over.

'Look!' Showing a young male Triage Nurse a blood sugar test reading of, "18.0" and clicking back to recent reading display of, "13.0" in dismay, 'And I haven't even eaten anything. It's going up on its own.' 'No one is going to be available. We can't just admit you into see anybody from the Diabetes Clinic from here. You will have to go back to your GP and they will make a request to put you in the diary.' 'But my blood sugar is prolonged at eighteen.' 'You may be testing too frequently.' I am sent home from A&E under instruction this is the wrong time to be giving up smoking and drinking, that I should go for a pint and allow myself to settle down. I'm onto five injections a day because no amount of insulin will bring me down and I fear a seizure of some kind.

...

Shot of insulin, shot of some girl I met last night. Everything seems pretty real today, no abstraction or perception, drifting into and out of sadness. Have a neighbour who owns a gallery in Knightsbridge, where he frames works by Matisse and the like. Have a suspicion he borrows them to hang on his own walls, by the way he answers the door ajar, only by sticking out his eccentric mop.

*Megalopolis-Group* holding onto my share options for the benefit of major stakeholders, maybe if I hadn't taken so many sick days I wouldn't have been on the redundancy list in the first place. Staying home watching *Film 4*, with half the audio still out of sync like old Kung Foo movies. Thanks Steven, I raise a smile; between girlfriends I pick up my old sketchpad: tucked away in my flat I find happiness, the true meaning of being alone, squirrelling away on my '*Moco*' storyboard. Someday I'll get this finished. Find green calm within copious cups of black coffee well into the wee small hours, and if I awaken with even sugar in the morrow I will have a good day.

More time spent taking care of myself; Glasgow Soul Food, stovies, mince and tatties, beef lasagne and extra beefy bolognese. Gym twice a day, fresh orange and diet lemonade. Blood sugar at least eleven before I'll clamour into bed to advocate the risk of waking, tripping over with glass leg the small plinth leading from my bed. Eyes feel they have gravel in and I can no longer wear contact lenses, whilst inking onto pages. Waking with level sugar always feels like good luck.

...

Nolan makes me Godfather to his firstborn, reaffirming my belief that this world is a good place and I have a deserved place in it. He even gets around to starting a band.

Talk with my mother eventually, she is skeptical to take it in; so many hard feelings she does not trust him to die. She will not be relieved, but she has other news having bumped into a relation on the bus, and been informed that her father too was dead; 'The

250

bastards are dead, we have outlived the bastards,' I say with my hand over my mouth.

# Behind every man is a good woman, and plenty of bad ones

I make acquaintance with an old man; older than his years, dying through some medication or another. 'What is he doing over there, speaking with him?' The aspirational lifestyle looking over; they all have better things to do tomorrow, people to see, loved ones to nurture. Cold pale room. Impossibly tidy. Absence of anything, I am so alone. Shortest distance to the warmth of love?

Four thirty in the a.m. on Baker Street, frost sparkling on the road ahead; she must be out there somewhere. I walk home alone from Soho; feels as though the world, she belongs to me. Should be feeling pretty good about myself right now; a kiss on the cheek goodnight as I send her off home in a black taxi; if it weren't for the sliding scale of quality as realisation to how I've been burning the candle at both ends.

Seventy pounds for a bottle of wine, when did that happen? Media exec; denim skirt, *fuck me boots* and black woollen tights covering thunder thighs. Brazilian girl with an incredible chest but if she doesn't remove that blackhead from her forehead the next time she visits the bathroom I'm out of here, and French girl; big old unit, surely the warmest of winter's nights, though doesn't give me a card on my thirtieth birthday. She gives me a balloon left over from her friend's birthday party, and we chat over a bottle of wine about past indiscretion; her having slept with a previous boyfriend, then popped upstairs and shagged his mate. How free spirited! Broken up with her in my head midway through her sentence.

They are all rolling into one. Intended Glamour Model; best of luck with that one love, bit presumptive to assume I'd want a second date. Jewish Solicitor on a break from her *soon to be* husband, takes one look at my foreskin and jumps back three feet as if it's a snake. Woman who spends the night and then sends a text the following afternoon saying she didn't fancy me. Girl undressing and I'm already wishing her home. Two Nordic girls, one short, curvy, brunette, all smooth; one taller, blonde, skinny and full bush; both happy for me to buy their drinks all evening, they don't live up to their reputation at all. To be fair I never went all the way so not a total slut.

Curves in all the right places light brown girl I met in a gay bar, texting repeatedly to say she is stuck at work and on her way; I'm good thanks. Don't bother. I'm already walking home in the rain. Kiwi girls; one giving it, 'But what about your girlfriend?' well pronounced considering her tongue resting in my mouth; the other, inquisitive, 'How are you? But how are you really? How do you really feel inside?' before informing me of the most savagely intimate personal details of her closest friends. *Pimm's* girl, eating the contents of her drink like a salad, I go over to the bar and get her a fork. Spanish hedonist, 'Would I like to do a three way with you and another guy? Bye.' A girl who works her day job in *Selfridges*, got a taxi home from my place around two in the a.m. my phone goes at around two thirty, has she forgotten something? No, she has run off without paying her cab fare, would I care to cover the charge? Left a wrap of cocaine on my coffee table, a tip from her clothes off evening job; flush. Some woman, allegedly Italian, supposedly standing outside the front door of my building the following night; calling, texting, pressing my buzzer over and over, kicking my car, 'But I don't have a car and my bell's not ringing so I don't know whose house you're standing outside you maniac.' A girl with a body like *Baywatch* and a face like a Flumpet, 'I was really drunk. Please stop texting every Saturday.' Crazy LA girl I met on my way home buying cigarettes has started turning up on my doorstep at all hours, when I couldn't less have wanted someone. High sugar, I don't wake up very well, 'What do you want? No this isn't spontaneous, this is annoying.'

Amazing how dating a black chick briefly qualifies to be smiled at by the staff of *Blockbuster* and *Sainsbury's* on the Kilburn High Road. Takes her wig off and leaves it on my ironing board; I almost leap through the ceiling. Schoolteacher with nothing to say, at all, ever, not even particularly bland; just here for a couple of weeks, turning up, going home, texting and turning up again. Marilyn, met her at the gym's Christmas do, the only one also drinking so we head downstairs to the attached *Maida Vale, Marriott Hotel*, stroking her back and she is stroking my inner thigh under the table. Flowing blonde locks over her Adam's apple, and her name is Marilyn, need I say anymore? I roar with laughter all the way home.

Interrupting any chance the blonde glow of a fuck has of turning to love, I stop for a blood sugar test, a glass of *Coke* and a *Mars Bar*. In fact, I'd bet the only thing any of those women would find memorable about me, is my refusal to share my *Coca-Cola* and *Mars Bar* with them.

The last time I can even remember caring for someone; a waitress just turned eighteen with ambition to become a Lawyer; no way I'm keeping up sexually; I can't put her through what I am going through emotionally and I'm only going to hold her back in life. All I want is a cigarette and a blowjob, preferably at the same time. And before her; Black Rum and *Diet-Coke* to get through it with the Czech girl; red hair and Glaswegian tinge to her English; ran out of personal things to complain of one day, went on to begin telling me of the woes of her family's friends.

...

Lactating during her period and something didn't sit right. Suddenly in an Observation Room, Head of Department and his junior, could cut the tension with a knife. 'Have you been suffering headaches? When did you last have a headache? You're not having a headache now? Are you on any headache medication?' an interrogation behind closed doors and all four of us have become terrified. Had I seen sign of breast milk before? 'No, and I would have noticed.' They explain her symptoms as being the sign of a brain haemorrhage, and now I'm hoping this girl I realise I have always felt so sorry for is pregnant.

Breast examination taken by junior overseen by his superior, pushed along, 'Take samples of fluid from each mammary separately.' He uncovers her breasts one at a time from under a Mary blue sheet, looking to me for approval. 'It's medical, please do what you have to do,' we plead with him; she is so frightened, staring up at the ceiling. Junior squeezes milk from one nipple onto a stick and presses toward the tip of a sample bottle, flicking contents over into the air and landing in his Boss's ear. Bent over with a paper towel, picking it out and feigning professionalism, his mouth wide open in anger and disgust, we the four of us give in and roll around laughing. The sample is clear, pregnancy negative and lactating confirmed as *just one of those things* by a woman on the Maternity Ward who knew what she was talking about. We go home arm in arm a new lease of life together.

Drunken hysteria when surrounded by people enjoying themselves, a handful of pills at her worst when requiring attention. Walk to the hospital at one in the a.m. no money left for a taxi. Doctors and Nurses staring at me into the early hours, believing by default it must be my fault. Back loitering in my flat for month after month chain-smoking in tracksuit bottoms, crying when I broach the subject on what she wants to do; till her country becomes part of the European Union and she gets a job in her old position: arriving home finger fucked by a Surgeon's Apprentice. – (me me me me me.)

Wrecked my flat on taking her belongings; I meet her at a bar months later; she wants to say, 'Goodbye,' for some kind of closure. Immediately find myself feeling sorry for her, the draw of repressed comfort. Quick think of something, 'Actually I have started taking lots of heroin since you've been gone.' The look of disgusted horror, and finally she leaves forever, and she is sorrow. And all the ones that fell in between, all of them sorrow.

...

It has come to pass; hacket women and alcohol; I blow chain-smoke through chill air from a cold room, trying not to care. A bottle of *Baileys* in case of hypos; I have become a bastard, I am sorrow and I am so fucking alone. Listening on repeat to the songs that make up excuses for how I feel. Thinking on the women who cannot remember me.

Why do I feel grateful to you? His fault my health through childhood stress. He made my childhood nightmares, he did his best to ruin our fucking lives. Not permissible to love him. God I'm definitely not as hard as my family back home whom I offend by merely being upset, unentitled to speak his name. 'I don't understand why you even care Paul.' Perhaps overly sensitive to things outside of my control; perhaps only the genetic link between father and son. How dare I care; what a disappointment to my real family and what they have gone through. But I remember her telling me it was okay still to love him and miss him when I was young.

If I could drink and smoke without ever getting ill, would I even need anyone? Shit to be around and wasting my life; all the ones that fell in between, blaming everything on everyone else. I have become sorrow. Galvanised by high blood sugar knitting with a genetic trait to blame everyone else. I have become a bastard and I am sorrow.

...

Back home, two thirty in the a.m. having safely returned an old woman to her *stations of the cross*, I piggyback onto a neighbour's Wi-Fi, then sit down to watch some porn. A MILF enters a college dorm wearing only her apron to cover a massive inflated boob job, and carrying a prop wooden spoon, "Hi – giggle, I've come over to bake you boys some cookies." Cut to next scene, she has baked said cookies and is straddling the kitchen island; removing her apron to reveal enormous tits over a tray of freshly baked choc chip. Hold on, those don't look warm. Surely the best bit about home baked cookies is when they are piping hot. In fact there are no flour marks or crumbs anywhere to be seen. Those cookies are clearly out of a jar. Wish she would move those fat collagen lips and cellulite hips out of the way. I

257

want to take a closer look at those cookies.

...

Washing my clothes with dishwasher tablets. A need to be out there almost every night, because she might be out there somewhere. Stood at the bar, light on the eye with legs that go on forever, her arm around me the next day walking down Willesden Green; when I met Natasha it was as all emotional piano wire attached to ex-girlfriends had been severed and I do nothing but sleep on her shoulder for two straight days. I take Natasha for her first ever *McDonalds* and she eats all my fries then hides hers down the side of the sofa, and I know I love her.

Moving in together, it's all, 'Oh we have the same *Tracy Chapman* album. – I haven't gotten around to listening to it all of the way through either. Why doesn't she just sell that *fast car* and put the deposit down on a nice wee flat? Check her dad into rehab and cheer up a bit? I love the *Counting Crows* too, *The Spin Doctors*? No way, I thought I was the only one left. You were in Philadelphia at the same time as me? You were in NY the same time I was. You were actually in my local club a few years ago and I tried to buy you a drink one night but you were too drunk to remember.' And then you hear, 'Hey, what's happened to my *iTunes* library? I can't find all my songs. Why is all your music on my *iPod*? I don't even like the *Nine Inch Nails*.' 'Hold on, *The Best of School Disco, Hootie and the Blowfish, Shanks and Big Foot,* who are you? What do you mean I'm only the second best looking guy you have ever kissed?'

# Love

You see the difficulty in being diabetic only starts with high sugar, diet and insulin. It only ends for many in death *due to complications with diabetes:* but the difficulty in *being diabetic* is in the living and how blood sugar changes you.

*Cheekbones and back along the ridge of my brow furrow, skin pale, eyes narrow and divisive. A piercing fault as I usher aside-clouding thought: that knot which resides buried deep within my forehead.*

*I'm trying to concentrate on what you are saying but instead I become frustrated. I look hacked off but I'm trying to pay you the attention you deserve. I'm shaking my hands and I'm trying to follow and focus on to realise what it is that you have to say; then sharp of tongue, 'WHAT?' 'What is it that you are trying to say?' but not because I want to snap at you: not because what you are saying has little substance or I'm disinterested, 'What?' because I can't think, because I'm trying to understand. I'm trying to relate to you, to empathise with you although I'm clearly not coming across this way.*

*I am like this because my head is clouded and agitated and buzzing and I'm trying to communicate with you at the same time and it's smothering me. I want to be there for you, I am there for you: I am here for you always. And I'm not ill tempered, especially not ill tempered towards you. But what should be clear; clear and simple open and just us becomes for me disagreement;*

*disagreement repetition and frustration. Sharp of tongue and tense in tone, impending by pushy, wallowing then withdrawn and it's horrible. You shouldn't even have to try to understand.*

*I want to be a better person for you and I'm only four points of sugar away. My life is run by this simple biological block of not being able to cope with glucose on its own. I won't let it continue to hurt me and I won't continue to hurt you. I won't allow it to stop me from becoming a great Husband and a great Father.*

*I know now why I'm writing this. I'm writing this book because I'm ready to settle down and I can't be living or behaving like this anymore.*

*My love.*

*My love.*

*My love.*

# Fifteen years and changing:

# diabetic solstice

Diabetic Vs. Time; I'd forgotten all about the fifteen-year milestone. I never paid any notice to the anniversary; things have just started going wrong and getting worse. A fumble of footfall, something is not right. Independence giving way to dependency: shameful burden I have become opening into a financial black hole with diabetes creeping into every corner of my life.

Hypo and my eyes go all fuzzy like a broken TV set. Salt levels changing, causing brief spells of confusion; I get up and start changing the track on the CD player and mumble on about it sounding like something else instead of eating the *Dextrose* tablets in my hand. Bed sheets always drenched in sweat during the night; I awake freezing cold, my sleepwear on the floor. Death warmed up and my GP's solution is to prescribe anti-depressants? Which, I reject. Sitting in on client meetings, completely useless I'm sure they will agree; trying to keep myself from falling asleep, can't be very flattering for anyone in the room; their own fault for being cheap-ass and not supplying coffee. Stomach balloons to three times its size. GP now prescribes six boxes of *Fibogel* on diagnosis of constipation, which in turn bloats further, to the point where it's making it hard for me to breath, bringing on panic attacks, and I'm back in hospital being told, 'You're fine: it's not ketoacidosis. Go home.'

When did I become a weak person? – Round about now. Requesting to see a *Diabetes Expert* at the A&E of the University College Hospital, London (*UCH*) because my body could not take it anymore and being sent away without even a future appointment. Losing track of even more important Diabetes Clinic appointments and turning up for ones cancelled without notification: an automated appointments system keeps changing dates every time a Consultant takes a holiday. Support requirements taking leverage over everything I had worked so hard for. Neuropathy in my legs, mood swings getting worse; I'm a living storm cloud.

Manage to turn up to an, actually happening, appointment. This one has not been cancelled, or postponed; I'm in! Diabetes Nurse at the *UCH*, looking at me in complete terror, 'We need to get on top of this neuropathy because long term this is what can lead to amputation.' This dainty Asian Nurse lady further asks with genuine concern, 'Why do you think you are like this? What do you think is making you this ill?' I attempt to surmise, 'I'm struggling to deal with work, to even get into work. I can't take more time off. I'm struggling to look after my sick girlfriend.' Injecting me now with more quick-acting insulin and instructing me to start taking my night-time insulin in the day to help prevent the very dangerous hypos in my sleep. Hypos so bad I now leave a *Gluco Syringe* at the side of my pillow with clear instruction for Natasha. I'm really worried now that I'm going to fall into a coma. The Nurse even gives her mobile number for Natasha to call in emergencies; her support holding me up she also manages to push me onto the Consultant's list.

And finally I get to see a Diabetes Expert Consultant, none too pleased to be seeing me. First he has the lovely Nurse run me up the usual; scales, height and blood pressure. I go in thinking I'm five foot eleven and my usual ten and a half stone; turns out to be, that I'm five foot nine and a half and a chicken wing away from obesity. Natasha is on the floor crying with laughter, 'I mean, how could you possibly be five-eleven, when I'm six-one and you only come up to my shoulder?' Then we get some one-on-one time with the man. The Consultant Expert, dressed in respectability: has barely asked me a question; grumpily enlightens, 'You must lose some weight. You are very overweight! I have lost lots of weight and I feel great. In the meantime, have some more insulin to cope with your additional weight gain. You are clearly not having enough insulin to cope with your mass.'

'Cheeky bastard,' I'm dismayed to Natasha, as soon as we're *puffed* out of his office, back in the holding area, watching him leave his office again, approaching the Nurse's Station and onto his next patient. 'I no longer have to lose weight. I have lost lots of weight and I feel great!' impersonations on repeat and back out toward the lifts. Well great news for him, but what about me? Is that it?

Second opinion GP, on getting an up to date prescription for my buckets of insulin, finds a lump in my stomach and declares out loud, 'I can feel a lump.' Well thanks but can you do anything about it?' 'I don't know, you should maybe see a Specialist, I can ask reception to put you on a list.'

Human Resources are in a huff and they are pulling me in for *the talk*. Why am I ill? When will I be ill again? It's very busy, they need me to understand; I can't be swanning off to the hospital all of the time.

Nine hundred pounds borrowed for a CT scan, paying to go private to get back to work ASAP. I inform HR, now showing full Cheerleader support, 'Really appreciate the efforts you're making Paul. If there is anything we can do?'

New Governmental legislation coming into place at the end of the month; demanding financial institutions clearly identify and disclose key shareholder information on Investor Relations web pages. We are providing these at a loss in a grab for market share: I'm banging out seven a week, through variable legal definitions. Sundays on-line with India, Monday's, I'm having panic attacks before my jacket settles on my chair. 'I'm sorry but I have to go home.'

Acute allergic reaction to Iodine, but they can't keep me in for observation because I'm only paying for the one procedure and not covered by Private Health Care Insurance. So they send me home with a packet of *Piriton*, instructing Natasha to call an ambulance if my throat swells back up.

CT scan couldn't find anything other than guilt and an impending moral crush, so spit roasted by a joint Endoscopy and Colonoscopy; found nothing more than a small hernia, some tiny ulcers and hard poo blockage caused by poor diet. 'Perhaps it's to do with diabetes hindering your body's ability to digest due to nerve damage caused by high blood sugar? You should ask your Diabetes Clinic about it.' 'Yeah I would if I could get the miserable bugger's attention during appointments when he is busily daydreaming out of the window, wishing it were Friday.'

Sacked from my job at *Acronym Indecipherable & FFS* anyway for missing so many days from work. On terminating my contract over the phone she says, 'If there is anything we can do?' – It hurts and ruins you most when people don't believe you are ill.

...

HR always having this habit of leaving the distinct impression that I am wasting their time, staring at the phone during meetings and talking more about the next meeting they have lined up, to get to, as I get shoved out of the door. Obviously hard pressed dealing with more important matters, unless of course you happen to have some gossip they can share with the I.T Department, whilst flirting across the office landing; one by the filter coffee machine the other by the photocopier, purring at each other and fantasising in innuendo.

At first it's all, 'Welcome aboard,' and, 'Give us your bank details: we want to make sure you get paid ASAP. We certainly don't want you to miss the three-to-five day payment window depending on whom you hold your account with.' 'Hmm, will that be the last day of the month? Last Friday of the month? Twenty-eighth of each? Or just plain late because Doris messed up the *BACS* payroll system again?' Just before they scowl back into their little hidden screen and research on *Facebook*. Be sure to get around to checking references and screwing up my rate of tax later.

Grown accustomed to a Media Industry, still immature in their perspective that they can bring in rolls of employees for projects the Sales Team have recently won; binning them again as soon as profits dip. As a diabetic my coat rests on a shaky nail. I was hoping in this instance, their boasts of having David Cameron; soon to be Prime Minister on the Advisory Board would temper rash decision and stand me in good stead. Now David is in charge of the Country; implementing changes as he sees fit in health care reform plans; shaking down employees' rights to attest. I have Grave concerns and near one thousand pounds in bonus *made* for beating all work related

265

targets.

...

Six injections a day; insurance declined, 'If you had diabetes before you took out Payment Protection Insurance on your loan and credit card then it is a pre-existing condition.' Transliterated as, 'We've taken you for all you had. Your health is of only your own concern and our perfect exit plan. We say we record calls for training purposes. I assure you, we don't record promises made by our Sales Team that the obvious terms of your insurance policy would fully cover for instances of poor health caused by diabetes, which you certainly discussed in some detail as you're not a complete idiot and we're a bunch of sly bastards. Next caller please?'

Waiting for someone to at least tell me I'm ill and give permission to sit down and recover. I have become a dependency; all I feel now is guilt. Considering moving back home to Glasgow: giving up entirely and writing myself off. A life begins of waiting for someone to tell me I'm going to be OK.

# The blind leading the blind (struggling to support a loved one)

What they wanted from her she could no longer give, what they expected from her in return for their lack of enthusiasm and scant consent could no longer be granted. 'Some fresh air? It will do you good, and a glass of wine, it will cheer you up. It's good to get out Natasha.' Hysterical screams, falling apart was there anything left? Her legs gone out from under her in the bathroom, water spilling from cold taps barely holding her conscious as she drifts in and out: sick all over her nightshirt, trying to change her into underwear, cover her as best we can manage in time for the ambulance to arrive.

Glandular fever, only fluid supplied, 'Your temperature has come down, you need to go and see your GP; she should never have prescribed you *Penicillin* in the first place,' even the graveyard shift Doctor furious at her GP's neglect.

How can you rest when your mind boils and all they can say is, 'It can take up to a year to get over, go and have some more blood tests. Maybe you should speak to someone? Can you go private? And while you are here can you start swallowing these non-specific, non-targeted anti-depressants, they can't do any harm.'

How can you watch the person you love more than anything else in the world fall into depression, the emotional equivalent of a severe car crash and watching it all happen in slow motion? She can see no light at the end of the tunnel; our calls further echo and confuse; quickly her physical form gives way as she is left for months on end heaped in a ball, defenceless on the sofa, collapsing in the hallway, weeping throughout the night. Contact with friends drops to a bare minimum. Natasha sees only through frustration a shadow of herself, but at least she is finally resting: soon I pray she will ask for help.

'Are you not better yet? Are you feeling better now? You're looking good Natasha, will you be returning to work soon?' Her husk bears it for as long as they stay, cries out when they leave, though not enough to extol guilt from their sentiment, which sighs with her as she lowers her posture to surrender into the gloom. While final clasps at a time barely six months ago when she was the belle of the ball and a kick ass career girl are let go.

Finally she sees someone, just when you think there is nothing left, back in her brain is some reserve, her backbone and character have peered out to identify and exclude the medically incompetent; qualifying herself with past confidence all but forgotten, she knows she needs to seek out some real help.

Dr Davidson, a small balding man whose simple expression, demeanour and mannerisms make you want to open up and fall apart, even when you are only there to hold the patient's hand.

Glandular fever is what she had, chronic fatigue is what paralyses her now, and I'm sorry but the stress of trying to look after her is hurting me. I'm so sorry. And in a way it is made worse because in a way I am jealous because I know that for her this is temporary and for me it is forever. – I do not at this stage comprehend for a moment how bad this will become for Natasha.

...

Spending my nights in *Liberty City*, we have inadvertently cut ourselves off from the world. Sleeping through crisp winter's sun, awaken by four in the p.m. eating by six, thoughts at seven, *Love Film* till late, with dreams to follow as light scratches at window panes. Cairnsey would have been getting up to steal milk around now.

Awake only in the dark, we see only each other and the pizza boy. Barely keeping time with bars and walking in the smallest of hours: Oxford St, Piccadilly Circus, and London Bridge, shop light and moonlight. The bustle removed we lose touch with normality. We need to get back in the sun, eat fresh food and partake of conversation. Eight in the a.m. and I can't keep my eyes open, two a.m. and we can't sleep. We are depressed and when we do we sleep deep, we love each other. 'God who was that? I can't believe someone called at four in the afternoon, how rude and selfish is that? Oh it was a Recruitment Agent. I've only gone and got a bloody job.'

One year anniversary together and we know we have been through a lot, we know we want to survive together and we know our honeymoon period has to be out there somewhere waiting for us. 'Natasha, will you marry me?' I ask her in the private grounds of Park Crescent. 'Yes.' 'I love you so much, thank you for staying with me,' we both say, hugging under a new moon. And followed up by an equal request on New Year's Eve, sipping Champagne from *Becks* tumblers; we will never let each other go.

# Fifteen years and changing,

# and the damage is done

Blood Gas drained directly from an artery in my wrist for the umpteenth occasion. It has become as simple as step two following on from sugar high panic attacks. 'If it's not ketoacidosis then you're not considered at any imminent risk,' they tell me, leaving Natasha and I cold as I pull back on my jacket, 'Please let me stay? Please help me long enough just to get my sugar level. You are sending me home and it's fourteen, I can't get it down any further. Please.' I'm crying and my body has long since buckled. Mouth so dry I'm slurring my words and legs barely hold gait still. 'Please let me stay?' They send me home. I say goodbye to the man, built like a brick shithouse, who woke up strapped to a wheelchair after collapsing into a diabetic coma earlier this afternoon. I have about enough time remaining to rest before getting up for work.

I can't hold my eyes open during the night with rocketing high sugar trying to comfort you. I can't manage to pull together this new position when I'm so worried about you I can't think. I put down the phone to you at lunchtime knowing fine well you are on the floor in

271

tears: twenty minutes away and I can't help you. My stress of loving you and FUCK I am so sorry, I can't cope. I cannot manage. I am unable to be there to make you take your medication and try to establish myself here. I am buckling under pressure; this is killing me.

The Concierge of our building is looking after me, outside is Regent's Park in the summer's morning and birds are flying together as silhouettes against clearer blue sky, while Natasha calls my Boss to get details on what exactly has happened, but instead is told not to be so demanding. I remember being dizzy getting into work and dizzy asking my Head of Department to call a taxi to revert me home. She paid no mind when I couldn't fully remember exactly where I lived and was back through tinted revolving doors before I'd closed the cab door behind a street that was too bright for any time of day. I'd found myself on Great Portland St, stranded and lost, following streets that look familiar, eventually making my way to my building where I didn't fully recognise my own Fiancée. An ambulance takes me to the UCH where more Blood Gas is painfully extracted from a tight artery, in my left wrist this time. I'm beginning to get used to this like I did blood sugar tests; people should never get used to this. A drip is fed, and two hours later an all clear for ketoacidosis. Begging again for them to take me seriously and let me stay in overnight, 'Please fix my sugar?' They finally let me stay. 'Bloody easier to get into a manger.' hisses Natasha.

Sitting in the ward listening to a Lithuanian man without an interpreter clearly begging for help, couldn't feel more sorry for him. And now a Nigerian Nurse comes over and tuts through her teeth in my direction; informs me the reason for my sugar being high is, 'The bottle of *Cola* by your bedside,' as she tries to remove it. 'I need that for hypos!' I say, in a tone reserved for speaking with mad cows.

Hospital menu, fuck that life is bad enough. Tash does a run to my favourite Italian joint; down the street for Carpaccio and Lasagna before a young male Nurse is back over looking at my sheet on the board, hanging at the foot of my bed. Can't tell what time it is and not hard pressed to ask. 'Says here your sugar is only seventeen and your ketoacidosis came back clear. You shouldn't even be here.' 'Do I look well enough to go home?' 'Well it's not that,' taking my sugar count, looking at it and wanting to forget, he certainly doesn't share, 'It's what it says on the sheet, and it says you are fine.' Later night drawing in, how does a fluorescent bulb lit room seem darker? But it does. And we sit surrounded by distress and languished pleads, 'Hush now,' to calm. Ward Sister insulted that I won't risk her inducing a massive hypo, and I don't accept an understanding, '*They have plenty of sugar* when you have a hypo,' to be sufficient over a basic knowledge, the insulin I had only two hours ago has yet fully to kick in, and as such an extra injection at this early stage, even to mitigate sugar of nineteen, could prove hazardous or work the other way and induce my body to create loads more sugar. I do however want to have more insulin in three hours' time, when she and all of her staff would be unavailable. Her protest of, 'My parents are both diabetics, I look after them just fine,' only filling me with more dread on behalf of those poor old sods. 'It must be like '*Misery*',' says Natasha, holding onto my hand and refusing to leave until I feel safe, 'If I wanted to become a murderer, I'd become a Diabetes Nurse. In fact they should change their uniform to a black cloak with a fucking scythe.'

I survive till morning; test my sugar of fourteen and hand over yet another cardboard cup of urine to a bereft; we get the picture response of, 'We won't be needing anymore of these.' Well you requested them; I think to myself, do you only want them when showing pleasant results? Surely you should be morbidly concerned

273

this stuff is acutely orange. Tash is here.

Meeting with the Head Consultant of Diabetes Medicine at my bedside; yawning and arrogant; that's new; grin on his face as he scans my chart, his team of trainee Nurses getting wet on his every word. I explain what has been going on with my blood sugar levels throughout the past months and he informs, 'Have some more insulin,' prescribing me Quinine tablets for cramps and smiling to the team, 'It's what they use to flavour Gin,' all very dashing in his delivery. 'No that's Juniper Berries, Quinine flavours the Tonic,' Natasha is savagely hissing to herself. Discharged within the hour to barely a sideward glance other than, 'Is he gone yet?' Blood sugar has not come down below fourteen but clearly I am safer on my own and the whole world can go fuck itself as long as she understands.

...

Phone rings at two in the a.m. to remind me that my taxi has been booked; two forty five to inform it's been dispatched. I can hear the fucks holding in the giggles before they start sending text reminders and I know the game is to wake customers as many times as possible before their early morning pickup to the airport, because I'd be doing the exact same in their position; so my frustration is one mixed with humour. Not too bad a way to start the day.

Buzzer goes, taxi is outside somewhere; I walk half of Park Crescent before I hear the din of a diesel engine and he switches on fog lights to highlight noir rain. 'No conversation,' not a whisper I want to hear from this man, there is the best part of an hour's snug sleep to be had in here if I put my mind to it. But to be polite, 'How are you mate?' 'Yawn, bigger yawn,' hand held over his mouth, 'Gasp for air,' exhale yawn – dramatic pause to gather his thoughts, 'Move to the other side please?' 'Why?' – This guy, he doesn't like people sitting behind him, but he has parked up the road to stand outside his cab smoking a cigarette when he should have been parked outside my building opening the car door for me. I'm thinking to myself; he can fuck off. On the other hand, as I gather my laptop bag to suggest swapping places, 'Mind if I smoke?' Clearly he does, it's a forest of pine fresheners in here, 'Okay, but you must move over my friend.' Things must be tough in Nigeria to become a paranoid London cabbie. 'Long shift?' 'Seventy-two hours, you are my last fare, then I will go home.' Fuck, why did I have to ask? As he taps the Sat-Nav for *"collect,"* answering his mobile phone to a permanent fixture of ancestors back home: I hope his wife and her mother are enough to keep him awake. I'm certainly not drifting anywhere. Puff.

Marylebone Road, Baker Street, sun ebbing over the heads of buildings spectacular; to imagine their stature when newly built: stone walls and marble surfaces shining bright, "Rule Britannia," a stage set for horse drawn carriage. How many Victorians lost their lives building these monuments to who we could be, never to be repeated? Stopping at traffic lights for no one, streets are practically dead. Some movement over by phone boxes, a small figure in muted tones and nondescript rucksack tearing down cards, to replace with those of his masters. London; legal to operate a brothel with up to two slave girls, perfectly legal to attend, participate, to pay to bruise; straight to prison if he is caught advertising them. Death, taxes and marketing reminding us who we are; never more than six feet away from a rat, a slave girl; brutally, repeatedly, raped for fear of her Eastern European captors hurting her family and a *Coca-Cola* in this city. Besides, I doubt the girls kept in box rooms of modern plague are half as hot as the photographs displayed on cards with phone numbers and postcodes underneath, as do images of cheeseburgers on bus shelters.

275

Edgware Road, past the *Hilton Hotel* on our way out to a motorway junction somewhere; a fox crosses our path; nature stops society in her tracks, with eye contact tracking: light reflecting in her pupils dilated, dawn on her coat; we are on her terms and I feel nothing but charm to be living in a city commendable by its inhabitants who love this vermin. In her own time she shutters off and we move along; calm, now I can rest.

Airport.

'Did you pack this bag yourself?' 'Yes, and it does contain sharps. I am diabetic; I carry insulin and needles with me.' 'I need to see a Doctor's note.' 'Thought you might. Here you go.' 'Right, is that all of them? You can't carry this bottle of *Coke* with you.' 'That's the sugar I carry with me for...' 'No you can't take that through when you can buy another one inside.' Okay; and they wonder who profits from terrorism, I'm thinking oh so deeply into myself. 'Is that everything? All your sharps in this bag and you packed this all yourself?' 'Yes,' trying to get past a banshee here. 'The rest of the bag is needles free?' 'Yes, as far as I can tell. I emptied it before I.' 'YAWWWWWOOWWW!' What was that? Fuck what is it? It can't be? She withdraws her hand and gives me such a deservedly filthy look, handing me over my brown leather satchel and I withdraw a loose syringe with bent needle tip, missing orange cap. 'Fortunately it's not broken the skin.' My heart is in my mouth, 'I am so sorry.'

Meet up with colleagues and silence; surprised not to be in a holding cell.

St James Gate Dublin; guy in a pineapple shirt, instruction and I'm sure he would argue I was paraphrasing here; on how to sneak through the ambiguities of legislation to sell as much poison addiction under susceptibility of social acceptance, whilst keeping under the radar of bad press; God forbid, no press and price increase caused by undue accountability. Punctuated only by his colleague's assertion, 'Only once you have passed the exam will you be allowed to sell the dream. And if you fuck it up we have the power to ensure your employer fires you. Have a nice day and thanks for attending our media training camp.'

Well plenty to dwell on there as I stare out from a museum dedicated to the notion, history is written by the victor. Repetition of logos and caricatures magnified, reflecting an epoch cast so dark as to think there is someone behind you. A pint of the black stuff in my right hand; still getting over the shock of this morning; I take a sip thinking on Nathan and it tastes exactly the same here as it does anywhere else. Blood all over the back of my mobile in the other hand – every time I reach into my blood sugar test sticks pouch it makes me smile inside; makes me think of Victor reaching into his *Shag Tobacco* pouch for the contents of a *rollie* and that little ritual. Those buildings over there look too familiar and I think it's them; it is where Angela and I went to visit with the Duffy family when we were children, to find a week's escape from my father, where we listened to ghost stories about Banshees and witnessed a shooting star... this is the last thing I ever expected to see.

...

Nothing like poor art to make me contemplate my existence; where am I in life? Again considering writing myself off and returning to Glasgow. Can't get my blood sugar below sixteen; all pissed off and miserable, making everyone else's life around me miserable. I bring the storm cloud into the room just like my father did. I don't want to be that guy. Can I see the end of me? I don't know, though I've begun to walk home again in the evenings to capture and make the most of these last summer nights; glances at the way life should be. The question, which always niggles at me; should I have been brought up in different circumstance, would I have been healthier? Would I have achieved more? Would I have been happy? Would I trade in my past, which would mean trading in my family for a shot at health? No way, not a moment without these people I love, and their lives, which got me where I am today, even if it is fading, fast.

# Brighton

We came down here a few months ago, we came down for a day and a night so Natasha could get some fresh sea air; maybe switch off. We stayed for three weeks, moving from hotel to hotel throughout, avoiding staggeringly high weekend rates and achieve the best view of storms pounding the shoreline. – Starlings in their hundreds and thousands, climbing and tumbling as silhouettes against the coastal sky, then falling into place under shelter of the Marina by sunset. I hold her still, 'Natasha, look at me please. You have to stop. You have to rest completely or you're never going to get better. You can't keep putting yourself through this cycle of putting off work for a few days so you can try and heal, then putting it off again for another few days, you are putting yourself under too much pressure to return. You need to stop and rest fully, not be thinking about going back in, you're not allowing yourself time to switch off. No, you are not letting anybody down; those people would replace you the following day if you got hit by falling debris; they are not important, you are. FOR FUCK SAKE WILL YOU LISTEN TO ME? You are recovering from being seriously ill. Only you know how hard this is, you are the one going through it. Please take a break from work for at least a few months or you are going to get worse. Please fucking listen to me. Stop. Just stop. You need time to heal. That's the only thing I know, I'm not a professional care worker. I don't know how else to look after you. I only know from what Dr Davidson has said, you need to remove yourself fully from stress to fully heal. You need to take a step back or I'm scared you're going to fall into something so deep I won't be able to help pull you out of...' We hug for a long time, side stepping around scaffolding above. Natasha snuffles and giggles into her tears, a little coy a little bit impish, 'Shall we move here?' 'Here? With the seagulls tearing at bin bags worse than foxes and living off of fish and chips?' 'Yes?' 'Yes. I love you.' – A hug that lasts forever, 'Sorry for swearing at you.' Knew it was the right decision when arriving at the station overlooking a blue horizon.

Lugging myself to the station in the black of morning, standing outside shivering, taking comfort in a cigarette or two; listening to *Pearl Jam* through headphones, waiting on a train to arrive at the platform. A blanket of cold sweat and shock layer between my skin and a *'PAC-MAN'* t-shirt hidden under my favourite shirt: a laptop weighing more than a desktop swaying off my hip; dragging it along with me, at the exit platform it repays the pleasure tugging me down greasy stairs. Cigarettes, cold air, hands in my pockets; my phone is in here somewhere, *"Hi Pooh Bear, I love you,"* send.

Victoria Station; get on the bus, give my seat to a pregnant lady. Fuck knows what my blood sugar is but I definitely need a pee, then I look over at the War Memorial standing poised in the cold brittle sun as I chudder along. *'Metro'* newspapers everywhere; celebrities are being shagged and the poor shot all over London, "Gun crime in the day time." Off the bus, cigarette, heavy tinted glass revolving door. Account Managers look so bleeding bucky in open plan hell, I'm getting ready to roll over and die as I unchoke myself of this digital appendage. Finally I get to pee with just enough time left over to plug in this damn thing, arrange planning documentation and grab a cuppa before the team meeting.

You need thick skin dealing with these people and mine is translucent. Cup of tea reaching up the back of my throat, running out of *Monday's* team meeting to be sick again down the toilet. Head sweating suggesting it's time to head home, back home early again. Disillusionment lurks around the table, already agreed *he is* letting everyone else down. Even if *he is* telling the truth, I doubt it. Jacket still warm, 'Remember we have a breakfast planning meeting tomorrow pre eight a.m. Try to be here.' 'Yeah, but I'm fucked if I'm carrying that with me,' I make as mental note to myself.

...

Walk into town to trade some video games for food. Last night Nathan texted me his card details so I could order in a pizza, total lifesaver, and a mountain of insulin to digest, 'Get whitever yeh want mate, whitever it is. Are you okay? Are you sure you're awright?' I don't know that I'm coping at all. I'm pretending to be. I will send him up a copy of '*THE WIRE,*' season one, box set when I get paid on Friday to say thanks, knowing he will be chuffed. Would have asked my mum for help but I want to scream on hearing the voice of anyone who loves me and we have barely spoken for months. I don't have it left in me to explain how I am and they have enough on their mind; so easier to assume that I'm happier being arrogant.

Sure I ate plenty before I came out but already shaking like a leaf on Upper St. James's Street, "2.4" and falling. I can feel my legs going away under me, my head is too bright and such with worry; this is going to happen. Ambulance coming towards me, what a relief in a washed out at sea kind of way, hold on, is it just me or don't they seem to want to stop? Have my arm out waving for them; half way onto my knees trying to stay upright I can't be any clearer. That's a

281

bit of a dirty look from the passenger seat. What the hell, at least they have chosen to stop. 'What's going on?' 'I've run out of sugar and I am type one diabetic.' Total turnaround in their demeanour; I'm being lifted onto a bench, like clock-work one is passing over the equipment, the other testing my sugar, the other now trying to find that last tube of *Glucogel*, 'Should be around here somewhere. Can't have run out?' I don't want my last thought to be a sarcastic, *"Brilliant!"* 'Got it,' here we go and down the hatch in one. In the back of the ambulance, how did I get in here? Blood pressure being taken, personal details, contact info, concussive chat, have I banged my head? Occupation? 'I'm a Senior Project Manager for a media ad agency, when I'm well enough to get into work.' despise how real that sounded when said out loud. 'Tell you the truth mate, we were nearly tempted to drive by, we thought you were a junkie looking for attention.' As I come to it becomes apparent the other one is in a bit of a state, his colleague explains they have just got back from a particularly abusive callout, 'If anything, seeing you has helped to ground our day.' My sugar reading "5.0," 'Can't give you any more sugar when it's above five.' But the understanding is that it may fall well below four again on my way back; so they let me walk a tube home. Cheeky fuckers, assuming I was a junkie. I don't care how bad their last call out was. I must need a shave or something; looking in the mirror, fuck all I can see is a very fat fourteen and a half stone, bearded duck.

...

Mum asks If I will be a Pallbearer, I can't. It's not only physical strength which does not exist, though she could not remain more than five or six stone, but mental strength retired. Her closed casket before me, near arms reach and clasped shut. I want to open it. I will never have the strength to look inside. I wish someone would make

282

me. I want to see her one last time. My niece, my god daughter eleven years old, Rebekah sitting behind me so strong. I am so proud of her. To my right Natasha holds my hand.

The Priest, shares his spiel, he seems quite decent at first; I mean he isn't Jesus or anything. He is not very respectful; everyone lets it go. I don't think he had met her more than a handful of times the way he refers to her, if he had met her at all. If he was blessed with the love of God he would not speak of her in such a way, 'Hearing about Katie, she liked to, "Tap a fag." There will be no tapping fags in heaven.' Fuck him; in her absence she bears a million times the humanity he ever will.

Catherine was her Sunday name. Friends and family called her Kate, Katie or Cathy, depending on when they met, followed by Munley, McEnroe, McGarvie, Lindsay or Waugh. Perfect skin, and we seen the first indication of her going down hill on my birthday, a card delivered with a picture of a Jester on the cover, inscribed, *"If you're looking to fool around on your twenty-first birthday, then I'm your fool!"* She did not presume respect, she did not stand between adoration, praying on the purse of the poor. She met *Odd Job* from *'James Bond,'* she went to stay in a hotel in London, only to be turned away at the door because it turned out to be a brothel. Condensed orange juice and cod-liver oil; distributed to defend children against *Rickets*, and just to be sure she procured a second dose for my mother each month from a neighbouring parent. She believed in cleanliness as currency and her proudest moment; receiving a personal letter, *signed* from the *Pope* himself: instructing her she was forgiven; not for marrying an evil man who tore out her hair, not for divorcing to escape or even given permission to marry again, but forgiving her for marrying a Protestant in the first place. She ignored this letter and went onto re-marry, to my Protestant, grandad, Victor, the best move she ever

283

made. She was proud of Victor for being a cook in the army. They helped my mother drag us out from hell.

Couple of days later, at the *Cottage Bar* on Shettleston Road visiting Victor. This proper old man's drinking den; a half and a half: whisky and a beer; we the contents of the bar stand outside nestled in from the rain, bundled into the doorway rolling *Shag Tobacco* from little pouches, large drops of rain falling down the napes of our necks. Pouring back in one after the other, Victor already keeping Natasha company, 'Yeeh alright, Bigyin?' she looks a little out of place, all tall and elegant with her own teeth. A sinister old bastard approaches from behind, I was at secondary school with one of his kin, he too was a terrifying little fucker. He limps up from behind Natasha and whispers into her ear, 'Alright … sex.' The snare from Victor, the scald, the dead eyes. So fierce I have never seen anything like this from him. The old chancer melts, 'Right, that's me, am goin up that road, a hiv tay hiv ma jab, av goat that diabetes,' he says, this McGarvie man. What he was trying to say, 'Alright sexy?' all humour lost in a high sugar mouth strained with *Grouse*. He had after all been present at my gran's funeral, where he sat quietly on a far back pew dressed fully in black. This McGarvie man.

…

Train on the way back; my nerves so wrecked I have almost convinced myself I have MS because I keep dropping everything. I have these lumps forming under my armpit and my thigh. I haven't received a call back from work till this time, this very point in time their number displays on my mobile and I answer, 'All shitty and scathing waiting for me to bite,' no background noise, she must be in the *War Room* for this call. Her hand is shaking on the other end and mine finally calm. I have waited for this moment since they cut access to my *Common Theory, Abbreviation and Dwiddle* email account. 'Something about being fired, not only for attending my gran's funeral, not for the audacity of taking time to be upset in the first place, but for asking them on the morning after I found out she was dying to stop calling over-and-over with meaningless questions. Some salt into the wound; shouldn't really have been upset anyway, as a Grandparent she did not qualify the HR requirement of a direct relative. Now something about me having to come in and sign some papers to confirm I have been fired.' 'Yeah, that's going to happen,' squeeze of Natasha's hand, 'I fucking hated that place anyway.'

...

Starlings in their hundreds and thousands, climbing and tumbling as silhouettes against the coastal sky, then falling into place under shelter of the Marina by sunset; walks on the beach holding hands, Natasha's health returns slowly but steadily and at last she is able to return to the world. Thank God for the Banking system meltdown; the man from downstairs has finally stopped trying to take Natasha into his employ; though fortunate, and in perfect time, an old colleague Andrew has been listening out for her revival and opens the doors wide for this protégé. Looking into the sea and it's so impressive; we all seem so insignificant: putting everything in perspective. Making the thought of becoming a Lemming and walking off into waves entirely conceivable, perhaps time to move out to the countryside.

# The talk (human resource)

HR bring me in for *the talk*, to see how I am doing. Offering their support, 'Is there *anything* we can do to help? Adjust your working hours? Just let us know. We are here to offer you all the help and support we can. The door is always open.'

HR bring me in for *the talk*, 'Will you ever be ill again? If so, do you know when and for exactly how long? It's affecting the team; they are managing to arrange cover for now but it's getting a bit much for them to be fair and anything you can do to let them know in advance will be great. In the meantime we are extending your three month probationary period; already two months in during which you received an amazing first month's review; by another three months.'

This guy should have a placard on the wall behind his desk, reading, *"You don't have to be a spineless, conniving cunt to work here, but it helps!"*

HR bring me in for *the talk*, I've been ill again and it's really letting them down. My Boss has come along to make this an all the more formal affair with no warning to me whatsoever. I'm not feeling so supported now. No one is happy when I request still to be paid for the pre-arranged working from home I did whilst ill. I am informed, 'This will no longer be an acceptable procedure.' I inform them of the Bank Charges they owe me resulting from delayed payment.

HR bring me in for *the talk*, 'Lilly here – the head of Resource Management – suffers from migraines and she really understands what you're going through. Would you like us to put a bed in an empty office for you and Lilly?' I'm trying not to fall off my chair at the ineptitude of this man's statement. 'That will make you better. If not, would you like to take a few months off to get better, completely unpaid of course and we can get someone in to cover for you in the meantime, it's no problem honest – smiles.' I won't agree.

HR bring me in for *the talk*, sending me to see the company Private Doctor to get to the bottom of this. Someone reported back they had seen me drink a *full pint* of *Guinness* on Friday after work as I tried to socialise on some level with the team who have been *so patient* in covering for me. I know who it was, it's the same guy I caught doing a line of cocaine in the toilets, rubbing off his nose with a buzz in his eyes as he came out of the cubicle in a world of his own; surprised to find me washing my hands. I never felt the urge to tell tales, why did he? Fortunately their Doctor is great and supportive, tells me that I have a legally recognised disability and that he can see I am doing everything I can to get better. He shakes my hand as I leave his office on Wimpole St and I wish he were my GP.

HR bring me in for *the talk*, they have read the Doctor's Report and he says *I'm fine*, so they can't understand why I have been off seeing my own Doctor again. Two minutes of debate defines what the Doctor has actually said, that he agrees with me entirely and not only am I clearly going through a tough time with my diabetes, a registered disability they cannot sack me for, but that I am also doing everything in my power to get well.

HR send me an email, they want a second opinion and arrange an appointment with a Company Nurse: pretty much now. Do you ever

287

get the feeling someone is trying to trip you up? The hired for bureaucratic, health insurance and staff morale purposes lady happens to be an ex Diabetes Specialist Nurse who takes one look at me and says, 'You need to go home.' I explain that I can't although I'm chalk white with sugar levels fluctuating between the twenties to the twos in the space of any afternoon, 'I have so much to do and under so much pressure to have it done. I do not have the time to be ill.' She is looking at me, like this is fucking awful.

The Director, stopping at my desk and giving me the patriotic speech with the *main man* smile, 'Hey Paul, we really need you here,' someone is clearly fresh from eighties yuppie fallout, reading *Sun Tzu's 'The Art of War,'* thinking it will give him the competitive advantage in superior Account Management skills. By this late stage I think he will need to be a bit more practiced. – So I pop out to inhale hard every ounce of comfort I can from this desperate deck of cigarettes.

HR bring me in for *the talk*, requesting that I give their Doctor full access to all previous medical health records and to sign the consent waiver form. The form is prepared in front of me with a pen on top; all I *need* do is sign. They also state that I may, should I choose to, list issues on the form that I do not want him to gain access to. This cheap bullying does nothing but make me want to run and I inform them that I'll talk it over with the good Doctor before I sign anything. The good Doctor informs me of this being, *"A common strong arm tactic implemented by HR Departments who do not know their boundaries,"* and that there is no reason why he would want or need to read, nor benefit in any way from gaining insight to my past medical records. He tells me to stand tall and that I am protected by law.

Seem to be getting better but every time I do I get worse. Touch of toothache one evening and a chunk falls off into my mouth. I pop to the Emergency Dentist and the root of the upset to my diabetes is revealed. Turns out to be none other, and no more than a hidden gum infection. Tooth extracted and it feels like someone has lifted a blanket from over my head. It's exactly as when I was diagnosed with diabetes in the first place. – Should have come as no surprise, I've been up almost every night needing sugar from the age of sixteen, going back to sleep without brushing.

I pass on the Medical Expert's explanation, that this is what was causing me to be ill for the past months on end: backed up by their Private Doctor. Every time I was getting better, the hidden infection would rear back up and set me off. My body trying to cope with the infection, the fever altering my temperature and this combined to cause massive fluctuations in my blood sugar levels. Compounded by the massive stress I've been put under to perform. I explain this as I put my extracted tooth down onto the desk of HR.

My sister calls to let me know my gran is passing away. I'm still recovering from being ill for so long and it's taking me everything I have to try and arrange to get back to Glasgow. I request that *Common Theory, Abbreviation and Dwiddle* stop calling; they have called four times today already with dumb questions about websites, all calls starting with, 'I'm sorry to hear about your gran, but...' 'You offer the same solution to all of your clientele, as a company you have not had an original idea in years. How can you possibly have to ask me questions at a time like this?' All email communication drops, my calls fielded and none returned. Night of the Wake and I explain to my mum that I am falling apart, that I'm falling to bits with the pressure and the stress of my failing health, work and family responsibility. Not managing any of them properly. Train back to London after the funeral and I receive a call from my Boss. I have been sacked. It seems Grandparents are not considered direct family members and as such I had no reason to be upset. HR want to bring me in for a *talk*.

I know from the silence that the woman was calling me from a meeting room, with no sign on the door but titled in earnest *The War Room*. What I was really feeling all along but never said, 'I'm crying out: I'm so SORRY. I'm trying so hard to get here and work hard. I am trying everything I can to get well. I'm doing everything I can to get here in the morning and stay a full day. No one feels as let down by me as I do for letting you down so badly and consistently. I've never been this ill before: it's going to fuck me up even more if I lose this job. Can't you get cover for me for a little bit longer?'

What catches in my throat, the refusal to return my favourite shirt; sent me a transcript of every Doctor's note, every correspondence building up their untidy little case, but not my favourite shirt. Broken the Cardinal rule of not being profitable in the first ninety days, what more should I expect? Tribunal? Unfair dismissal? I don't have it left in me; they know that, they are betting on that. Fucking tooth, bloody infection screwing over my diabetes for I don't know how long, at least two jobs of inconclusive obviousness.

# Career exhaustion

I seem to be working for one company after another where fluctuating health is considered to be a completely unforgivable pain in the arse: victim of an immature digital age perhaps? Hiding my health woes has always proved impossible, as it's always within the three-month induction period that I fall, and why should I pretend not to be who I am? Breaking the Cardinal Rule of ninety-day profitability is no longer a problem, I can't even manage that long. I bet '*The Godfather*' never put up with this shit.

I'm sick of being the elephant in the meeting room, sick of receiving the looks of, 'Why can't you just have better health like everyone else? Stop expecting to be mollycoddled.' I'm sick of always feeling like I'm camping it up, always feeling like I should just get over it: sick of going home too early to everyone's bemusement. I don't know if I'm any longer suitable for the kind of career where pressure is involved. I don't know if I'm ever going to be well enough to deal with stress in any satisfying manner, both to the employer and my own personal wellbeing.

Most of all, I'm scared of letting people down. When did diabetes become my full time occupation? It used to run in the background, now it's all I can think about. How do I get it back to how it was? Pressure mounting for a pound of flesh I don't have left to spare, it is time to find something a little more relaxing, and certainly something I believe in. The recession is biting though and even Recruitment Agents are no longer calling. I know, I'll attend the *Production Show* in *Earls Court* and find my own job.

Job number three: great, if short, period at *Adjective Binary*. The best move I could have made, even when my train caught on fire. Meant to attend the *BBC* talk but turned up at the wrong seating area or the right seating area on the wrong day; caught Many the Boss man giving a speech to four people on the nature and benefits of streaming media to agnostic devices; thought, I know a thing or two about a thing or two and introduced myself. Angel of Islington; clients in the Fashion Industry always amusing; never heard so many people putting on posh accents, never seen such disorganisation book afternoon meetings just so they can escape their Boss, breathe and maybe go home early once in a blue moon.

Nothing sorts your life out more than looking forward to going to work in the morning, 'Hachoo,' and another bloody bug from the disease zone caught between East Croydon to London Bridge; share Natasha's taxi and arrive in plenty of time for a bacon roll, latte in a *Styrofoam* cup and a banana, whilst standing outside having a puff and chatting to the team about all manner of common insignificance: seems the Boss man has fucked off to Turkey to get married to the Art Director, 'She clearly got to pick her own job title.' – Oh that's rude, who said that?

Nice to be able to support one of the Developers, when going through hesitation in ability caused by the duress of asthma. 'Don't worry about anything at all this end. Your health is more important than the client's website.' And having half a brain I have provisioned time for my team to have understandable personal moments. Also

292

confident that as a professional member of the team, his brain will spend far more personal time ticking away in the background problem solving on the project than any time spent in absenteeism.

All around us we hear rumblings of organisations laying off entire floors of employees via email or through text messaging. Haven't seen anything like this since *Enron* took down *Anderson Consulting* and it's proving to make me feel grateful for having a job, even at this reduced rate, in the first place. 'Hachoo,' and Natasha has brought back something special from a flight to Munich on a business trip. "19.0" how can my blood sugar be back up at nineteen, when all I've had this morning is a brew and a bacon roll? I didn't even have brown sauce! I can't think, I can't concentrate to take in the entirety of project strings and I can feel my sugar getting higher inside me, 'I'm sorry Richard/Ashley, I need to go home till this settles.' Thank God they treat this like adults and don't throw a hissy fit, while on a one time only agreement with a client my personal home landline is provisioned.

Giving up smoking through the use of *Zyban,* on the advice of my excellent Programme Manager Richard, worked for him; seems a great idea; continue smoking and have a tablet once a day for the first week; quickly realise I don't want a cigarette and when I do try to have one it makes me vomit from every fiber of my being. Seems a great idea till it amplifies every bad feeling I have all in one go; distress to the point of pulling out clumps of hair, and images in my head of rope over beams. *Zyban,* the drug with limited clinical feedback prescribed to smokers because anything is better than cancer. Still, nice to spend more time getting on with things and less time puffing in the rain. Not that the big Boss would notice, he is honeymooning week five with a core member of my team.

I'm leaving the company because they are running out of clients to the point where Ashley, my Finance Director presents a competition in the pipeline, "If they win the competition, we get the business!" Unsure of the company's ability to make wages at the end of the month; a bonus excuse for me to be honest, my body is in meltdown catching a new commuter flu every day on route from fresh countryside. Don't these plague carriers understand the concept of working from home when you're ill? Phone goes, 'Listen man, I don't even work there anymore. I can't answer your questions about why the wrong colours of dress are displaying.'

...

Job number four, Consultant in my title and a whole batch of new shirts to live up to it. Forty-five thousand pounds per annum basic and the same again in bonus, – WOOF! I have been applying and meeting with *Aspirational and Tuna* for two years now and finally my big break?

I can't believe I'm working from Romany's old desk, looking out onto a cabin by a fire escape once improvising as a secret Edit-Suite, sans planning permission. This is the floor where I could book a *local* English speaking camera crew for anywhere in the world; where Barry signed the backs of my Passport photographs to send me off to Zurich the following morning; where Danny decided he was going to give it all up to become a Stand-Up Comedian; where I had a short term Boss who was so terrible at paperwork, I got an extra week's holiday that year. This is where the Bookings Team dreamt of making movies and on a Friday afternoon this self-same fridge was filled to the brim with beer to see us all happily into the weekend, and under the helm of an ever approachable Managing Director, Mark, we mostly looked forward to coming into work again on

Monday. I grew up here.

New colleagues, fucking hell; Consultant one gives utterance in a series of poorly researched articles, 'Yoga; foodie; sharp knives, blue sky thinking on a greenfield plan.' Consultant two obsessing over *Sketchers* trainers, Consultant three is not worth mentioning, meanwhile Consultants X through Z are on secondment at a client installation, available only through conference calls they advise in acronyms deficient of substance and I don't know if it's the ingredients in this *Diet-Coke* but I want to scream.

What's happened to these people? When I met them two years ago it was within the walls of a major broadcaster and they were changing the face of modern media. – Now sealed off from a once ever too busy to help Dispatch Desk and the wisdom of Paul Beale, who taught me first thing, how to spot a bullshit client at twenty paces. I stand beside a rented kettle plant watching a hired in man, hired once a week to water the thing! At this exact same spot where my last memory is of going through menus with Runners late on weeknights and letting them order whatever they liked. Feeling as though I haunt the place, it's as watching the girl you love being unhappy with somebody else. This building will always be *Megalopolis-Transmission* to me, and for them it means nothing; they actually welcome the day when the new train link has her pulled down.

Week one and the Boss man's pregnant wife is diagnosed with *Swine Flu*; news and media coverage *spraffing* ape-shit about how serious this is. Last week it was *Avian-flu* we were all going to die of, today, piggy snuffles. Doesn't feel like a snuffle now he has transmitted it onto me, feels more as if someone is hammering nails through my ear canal and drying my hair with a paint stripper. Phone call to the Doctors in Uckfield because they don't want us anywhere near – yes

Natasha can't see green cheese – and diagnosed rather efficiently as one seriously endangered species. 'Diabetes man, you're pure fucked,' is what the good Doctor would have said had she grown up where I did. Taxi Drivers making a killing on prescription pickup and delivery through the letterbox: paint a black cross on my door as I call in on my second Monday to declare, 'I've been quarantined for five days,' perfect way to start a new job. Few days of suffering and back in action; then important interruption; part one of two stage vaccine that makes me feel worse than the flu I already had, but super important I have it none the less because the Government said so and me with my diabetes, well I'm simply counting the days if I don't heed warning.

Client meetings and none of this is adding up; how can a consortium of members not want to attend *any* meetings when expecting to be paid, and the project to run successfully? 'What do you mean as a registered charity you only put your name to the project to get it off the ground? What is this understanding, you can be too busy for further involvement? You do understand your target audience of this Video on Demand project are those least likely to be computer literate, have broadband or visit a Library to use the Internet as they struggle to control their children and cower from Social Services? Oh you do understand. Then... you have never actually met a poor person before have you?'

Pulling out my emergency blood sugar test monitor, one that's designed for old people with arthritic claws, sounds like '*Robocop*' has entered the room and beeps intermittently for the hard of hearing. Big screen, "12.0" readout in digital font, 'Brrreeeeppp, whinnnnneeeee, grrrrrind BEEP,' before eventual crunching halt. 'Why do you keep doing that?' asks the man up until recently I had been so impressed by. 'Well, if I test my sugar now it means I won't have to interrupt the meeting to have sugar later.' Why does it concern him? How selfish of me, that poor big Boss man.

Shuffle around the audience requirements? Certainly an interesting objective at this stage; having won the tender. Yes the client will hold rights to all educational videos they have commissioned through us, using the experts you supply. No you won't be able to license their own work back to them at a later date. The experts are doing this for free and you are charging how much? No, a VAT adjusted increase from fifteen to seventeen and a half percent cannot equate to that much.'

Being fired for, *'Political reasons,'* by a man ostensibly objecting to my testing blood sugar; questioning it every time. Sure sign of weakness in his eyes. What a hindrance I must have been for him. Sacked, at least this time not for diabetes, at least I can sleep at night.

...

Trebled my income throughout these times of ill health; not bad going, but of no use now I'm on the shelf. My blood is clogged with anguish and my heart heavy and still. Everything is difficult and working against me, but it's not worth getting angry about. I can only get better; and the fear and the panic then the calm. Not scared of the pain, not scared of dying, I've become afraid of being afraid. My blood is like acid dissolving me from the inside; feel it burning through my arteries and taste it in my spit. Anxiety runs through raw nerves, my heart palpitates, thoughts turn negative awaiting a childhood state-of-mind; and it's all just high sugar. All I need are a couple of day's good blood sugar and I know I'll be fine.

Worse still, when did I become a meek person and how do I make myself better? Quivering hollow bag of nerves, I'm nervous to pick up a pen. I'm nervous to go to the gym, I know if I go there I will feel human again and everything will slip back into place. My confidence weeping on the floor, the thought of travelling into work seems exhausting enough and memories to the point of expectantly waiting to become ill are not helping. I want to get over this so badly.

Go to see *Pearl Jam* play live at the *O2 Arena*. Tash grants my wish to take six weeks out from work and concentrate on doing my '*Moco*' comic book. I can see now that in addition to wanting to reach for a dream, I am also clamouring for rest. A real long rest that I can't see the end of; one whereby I know I'll be better on completion. Natasha secretly just wants me to give in for once and sleep.

# Promise

It seems having an *outstanding balance* isn't a good thing. Even my *Starbucks Card* is being rejected. Financial stress levels beyond all control and destroying my diabetes on a whole new level. I can generally gauge my Hba1c by how I conduct myself on phone calls with the Bank. They are all debt collectors at the end of the day. Still bemused by the girl at *Visa* who stated that I'd agreed to a *promise*, 'What *promise* is this?' I enquire. 'The *promise* to pay back all the money on time,' she divulges. 'I never promised any such thing, why would I accept emotional blackmail from a credit card company when you just shafted me for my PPI?'

I have, during a spate of high blood sugar managed to swear such abuse at a Debt Collection Manager that his company will no longer have me as a client, passing my details back to *EDF Energy*. Something along the lines of,

'You're through to the Manager of *Low Life Scum Debt Collection*, Mr Cathcart. How can I assist?' – In a pissy arrogant tone of voice.

'Well you can start by not calling me every twenty minutes.'

'What do you mean?'

'Well your automated calling system rings me on twenty minute intervals at least fifteen times a day, and when I pick up there is nobody there, this is harassment.'

'We do not call you more than once a day.'

'Yes you do, that's why I have asked to speak with yourself, and the call log on my mobile lists you as having called eight times today already, and you actually called me sixteen times yesterday.'

'That's not us.' – In the tone of voice of a liar reading from a sheet of pre-written responses.

'Yes it is. It's your company who answered when I called back just now, and you are on the phone.'

'We do not.' – Said without the decency to be ashamed, as my gran would say.

'You do. Stop it and take me off your system.'

'No Mr Cathcart, we will not take you off our system till your debt is cleared in full.'

'Look at your system; I have not missed a single payment so take me off your phone list.'

'Are you able to make final payment for the reminder of forty-seven pounds now?' – Officious twat voice.

'No, but I don't have to, take me off your phone system.'

'Breathy silence.' – From him.

'Listen you wanker, I have made my payment this month and the next is not due for another month, take me off your phone list.'

'Mr Cathcart you cannot speak to me like that, I'm warning you.'

'Listen, you're a wanker and you work in a call centre, so take me off your phone list.'

'Mr Cathcart, I will not remove you until the full amount is received and I remind you that this call is being recorded.'

'So even though I've paid each month you are going to keep calling.'

'Yes.'

'So you are a wanker?'

'Mr Cathcart you have an outstanding balance to *EDF Energy* of forty-seven pounds.'

'Wanker!'

'You cannot.'

'Why not? Wanker!'

'You cannot speak to me like this.'

'I can. Wanker. Take me off your phone list and don't be a wanker?'

'I will not.'

'Because you're a wanker.'

He hung up. – I think I've ruined his managerial stance by now, and it's his own fault for being a debt collection wanker. I wonder if they use that recorded call in their training. I'd love to see it on my *Experian Credit Report*.

Blood sugar of "18.0" and my cats have better Health Insurance than

I have; they are even covered for diabetes.

...

Now I look up on-line the place where I grew up; there is a posting from the guy whose hand-me-down clothes I used to wear: thank Christ my mother never let me get involved in his pink jumper phase; says he is in pieces to have heard his childhood best friend GT has died.

# Demons, and dawn sugars

Defeated myself, where do I go from here? Sit and lick my wounds? Hide? Stay indoors amongst a pile of sketches and childhood dreams? Pop out now and again, and stare up at the sun? Shivering in the night, awake and staring at the ceiling, waiting on glimmers of confidence. Health can only be around the corner, right? I just need more time to get better and an easier approach to a new position. I can't manage that train journey any more, the long hours, the hypos, the negative confused expressions waiting at the other end, the chilling panic as I face another day, the relief and presiding wave of calm as I brush through the office door; my own unapologetic look, "You say you are trying harder but you're ill again." Talking to myself, 'May as well turn tail back to your basket before you end up back in hospital, this world is not for you. I hope she sticks with me or I will be lost again. Lost without her, then who will understand? You can't be the only one going through this, not the only one. There has to be a way out of this and health is the key. You just need to get better, but when did health become such an issue?'

So I'm sitting here now, thirty-two years old and my spirit is prematurely exhausted. I'm so meek that I'm sure to inherit the earth, and I'm so fucking over. I can't imagine holding down a job never mind developing my career. The walls are literally closing in.

It's moved beyond guilt, it's altogether fear. I'm scared all day long, the world is passing me by and I feel as though everyone is having a go at me, then I react like an angry teenager. Mid-life crisis caused prematurely by my stolen fifteen-years so far, and fifteen more lost at the other end. I have truly lost my nerve. How will I ever get back on my path? Leaving this behind me, only to be looked back upon as a learning experience?

...

I'm back at the Diabetes Clinic, this time in East Sussex; filled with an air of hostility and even further and more difficult to get to than any clinic in my past. There is a middle-aged guy; I only witness him in a motion blur; just beyond exploded and stormed back out past me via the corridor leading to the waiting room. His blood sugar obviously through the roof and a fury far outreaching my own: chairs scattering, people still in them. Behind the glass fronted reception kiosk, all mutterings for once fallen quiet. Not their fault he has had enough of sitting there for hours on end, not their fault his appointment was changed six times over, and he doesn't feel too good. Perhaps he is a little grumpy and needs to have some more insulin? I suspect they expect he probably has a dry mouth, but can't see the wood for the trees, what's this fuss all about? Meanwhile in the waiting room, everyone now sitting in a more semi-circular formation is thinking to themselves, 'I know exactly how he feels, the poor bastard.' Finally I am called through to see the Diabetes Expert Consultant; only this time I have a Locum with larger ambition.

Before I can, 'Utter more words.' 'This I want you to look at. This is my new website, in development for diabetes.' 'Cool. That's what I do for a living. Well before I got so ill, now I'm having a break to get well. That's why I'm now struggling at the gym as I was saying because I'm so used to sitting down.' 'You build websites? For whom?' 'I was more a Project Manager in recent years, did a lot of Consultation work for *GSK*, worked on *Shell Oil's* sponsorship of *Ferrari F1*, that kind of thing.' 'So how would you...*request for information...?*' 'Can I ask first, my blood sugar is going totally off the rails all of the time. Peaks when I haven't eaten. Troughs when I go near the gym.' 'Ah this is because a short burst of exercise will force the body to produce sugar; prolonged activity will burn sugar.' 'I had no idea; so when I'm on the Cross-Trainer...?' Tell me, how do you get the people to look at them?' smile in his face, rubbing his hands together. 'Social Media and preferably building to word-of-mouth are the fashionable and certainly the most effective roots when possible. But with my sugar...?' 'Tell me this; how much can you make on doing advertising?' 'Banner advertising you mean?' 'Yes the adverts on the screen; I want to take my knowledge and put it on there for the world to see, and I see these people, do they pay to view the banners?' 'No, you would preferably sell media space on your site. And be paid on per-click advertising revenue but it can cheapen the quality of your content and put off your audience.' 'These people do not know what I know,' grin, 'They will pay to use this website.' 'Eh, shouldn't you as a Doctor be more... I don't know... forthcoming?' Odd look received, this man in on a mission to buy a mansion, paid for in reluctant knowledge. 'You mentioned about burning sugar, how do I look out for...?' 'Well thank you for coming in Mr Cathcart? Your blood sugar results are quite high; you should make an appointment to see our D.A.F.N.E group. They are very good for helping you.' 'Okay. Thanks for your time,' hope you get rich quick on our backs you gleeful bastard. Who the fuck is Daphne?

...

'Oh that's next week, we won't be talking about that until next week.'

305

– Dose Adjustment For Normal Eating (D.A.F.N.E) Induction Day, ten white people in a room and any information actually disclosed, through much prompting is given on a strictly need to know, rolling back of eyes, basis. 'Three mm vs. six mm needles?' 'Anyone?' Dietician Specialist Nurse tries to chime in when Diabetes Specialist Nurse interrupts, 'That's my bit, that's week five, and we can't possibly talk about that till week five.' Festering looks between the two dissuade further group questions, then another that just had to be spat out, 'Why is it that ah get cravings fir the worst kinds aye junk food when ah get a hypo?' asks one Scottish middle-aged father of two prepared to break uncomfortable silence. 'That's your body informing you it needs sugar,' informs Diabetes Specialist Nurse, as though winning the quick buzzer round. 'But does anyone else hiv the craving ah get in the middle aye the night?' 'For ice cream and pink shrimps?' I add. 'White mice and *Wham Bars* I get,' says another. 'Half a bag of sugar on my cereal or an entire packet of *Hobnobs*,' things are picking up. 'Those things are more addictive than smack!' continues a conversation outwith the scope of either Nurse's comprehension. 'How don't ah know when am hivin a hypo anymore?' asks that same guy with much concern, 'That's why a've come here.' 'We can go onto early warning signs when the course progresses,' lands swift rebuttal from Diabetes Specialist Nurse. 'Why are ma sugar levels higher when ah wake up thin afore a've even went tay bed, even if ah hivney eaten anything?' 'The same for me,' says a tubby lady. 'It knocks me completely off just when I think I'm getting on top of things,' I follow up, looking to the Nurses for answers but none follow. 'Did everyone else have that *Swine-flu* inoculation? That's been playing on my mind,' says one of us, could have been any of us. Four answer at once, 'Yes I was wondering that, made me feel terrible. When is the next?' 'Not any worse than the normal flu jab they give. I haven't heard back about my second injection. I don't think I want it.' 'I was worse with the Pneumonia vaccine.' 'They are tryin tay give thame tay ma kids.' Dietician Specialist Nurse tries to put a cap on this *discussion*, 'Second part inoculation was cancelled; the Government decided it wasn't worthwhile. It was only ever a response to panic,' sticking her ore in on behalf of her *employer*. 'You didn't have to have it in the first place if you didn't want to. You could have saved the *NHS* money,' comes her colleague – we're being tag-teamed. 'Did anyone have a choice?' ask all our expressions. Diabetes Specialist Nurse, 'If we could move on?' She has had enough but I ask anyway, 'While we're all here, bearing in mind we are never around this many diabetics, doesn't it makes sense to ask and share experience?' Pushing my luck says her candour; the other smiling to agree then looks down. 'That is one of the many benefits of the class,' swiftly interjects Diabetes Specialist Nurse and shut down, everyone home.

Jackets on and pensive looks, then an excited female voice from a previously silent chair, goes for it, 'Does anyone else get an itchy bum when their sugar is high or am I just lucky?' we all begin to chuckle. 'I get a right itchy rash around my groin,' comes another. 'I get sweaty feet.' 'I break sweat all down the one side of my body,' a room filled with love ever so briefly. 'I never get as ill as all of you make out,' says some prat completely unaware of his own condition: our own kind even putting us down, trying to suck up to the Nurses, makes me sad – more for him than us.

So basically an afternoon spent with two Middle Management Department Heads acting like disgruntled children, so overly protective of their position, behaving as more gatekeepers to the *fountain of knowledge* than people wanting to make a positive difference. Prophets of inadequate solution fathomed on the excuses of an inept audience marketing condition; a standard set, anything

307

has got to be better than nothing: too scared to be blunt because they will give up. But will we give up? Is what they are offering any better than holding our hands as we drown? Rather than requirements gathered and defined based on the principles of rightful understanding belays just responsibility. What they had to say was, 'I could tell you but then I would have to kill you,' quite apt with consideration to their entire course reduced to the principle, 'Have as much as you like; live on takeaways; drink *Cola*, eat fudge and bathe in custard. Just make sure you have enough insulin to cope with it, *as taught to us by the Pharmaceutical Industries*, and don't think to concern yourself about long term damage, blindness and amputation blab la bla. That's all part of the long term business model we aspire to.' And all for only fifty pounds return in a taxi times eight weeks; may be cheaper and more productive to just snuff it.

...

Picked this book up a couple of months ago when hardly paying attention, had the word *"Diabetes"* written on the cover and I'm a sucker for a get well quick scheme. I can capture my demons along with *dawn sugars*. It is the insulin making me fat and ill. Everything I am doing is wrong; everything I am doing is killing me slowly. The prescribed complicated carbohydrate diet knocking me for six, the combination, eating at me over the years; poisoning me; poisoning you; I was a kid who thought new trainers would make me run faster, but I can't let that happen to you.

I got my life back from this book I found in *Heath's Coffee Shop*, Uckfield, East Sussex. Hats off to *Dr Richard K. Bernstein, M.D.* The first Diabetes Expert I have found after seventeen years of searching, who actually knows what he is talking about. '*Diabetes Diet: Dr. Bernstein's Low Carbohydrate Solution*' has improved my life immensely (thanks Doc).

In truth; as bad as I thought it could get, and the dawning of a solution; at the drop of a hat and back down to four injections per day. It was all so simple. In the same relief, to be taking insulin and getting better when I had succumbed to this condition as a child: I now feel that exact same way about giving up carbohydrates entirely and reducing my insulin intake to a fraction. All the sweets and the no added sugar drinks I can do without. I'm better. I am finally getting better (tears everywhere).

I feel like me again, and back to the Doctors where the Receptionist instructs me to the waiting room downstairs. 'Where are the stairs to go down?' 'The waiting room on your left,' it barks. 'That's not downstairs then is it? That's the ground floor,' I nod exhaustedly at her, though nice to be able to stand up for myself again. In to see the GP, now reading a letter from her system, am I in trouble? 'How are you feeling Mr Cathcart?' 'Good, thanks, really, really good; I have lost over a stone since last week and need to up my blood sugar test sticks prescription as I'm now doing it right and testing eight times a day.' 'It says on here that you didn't attend the D.A.F.N.E course, and they have limited places.' 'Yes I got a copy of that rude letter too. If they passed on messages at their Reception Desk they would have known I was not coming. I called them on numerous occasions and never got through to speak with anyone proper, directly. Fifty pounds a week in taxis, there is no way I can make it when I'm not working because I'm off having a break due to poor health in the first place.' 'These test strips Mr Cathcart are expensive. And you are looking for how many a month?' 'When am I getting my second part of the *mandatory Swine-flu* inoculation you forced me to have?' 'Four hundred test sticks a month. Yes that is fine; we can have it set up to have them waiting for you at *Boots*.'

...

And finally I am developing a rightful understanding; now to attain a just responsibility.

# The three bears of blood

# sugar

How do I make myself better?

Fat bear: too much insulin. Skinny bear: sugar too high. Just right bear: healthy, happy diabetic.

Let's for a moment, forget the experts and let us concentrate on me the diabetic instead. Like the cave man my body does not expect to eat every day. My body by default, collects and stores energy till it seeps through my diabetic veins, peaking my sugar levels, disrupting my salt levels, polluting my blood into acidic syrup; and after fifteen years, making me cry out for help: all anyone could tell me was to have more insulin.

Insulin makes me fat; it's a foreign synthesised chemical hormone injected into my body to process sugar, storing the excess energy as fat. The more insulin I take the more my body resists. The more my body resists the more it blocks and backs up, creating insulin pockets. These pockets then randomly infuse with my system as a massively unexpected dose, leaving me in one hell of a hypo, and my body burning off fat and muscle producing sugar to fight it. And there I go, straight back up into the high blood sugar numbers tail spin again.

Carbohydrates make me fat; my body cannot digest them in a timely fashion with the insulin. They cause spikes in my blood sugar, which peak and trough out of phase from my five hours analogue insulin timeline. They don't really catch up and round off, Dose Adjustment For Normal Eating (D.A.F.N.E) style, but slowly degrade the quality of my blood, and clog my organs forcing my body to react in the early morning trying desperately to process them with dawn sugars; and there it is back up to "18.0" again when I went to bed with sugar of "7.2."

High sugar makes me skinny, unable to properly digest food, hold water or heal; my body melting into a puddle of acidic sugar as it did prior to first being diagnosed with diabetes. Easy to slip back in and out of when combining too much insulin, in meeting with the requirements of feeding off the wrong kinds of food for energy, topped up by too much sugar in chasing the tail of excessive insulin.

These very same ups and downs are what aggravate my temper, tire my soul and over time negate my character. Far simpler to digest protein and green leaf vegetables; easy, slow burning energy matching a, small quantity, five hours insulin timeline: synchronising my body while negating fluctuations. I'm far less likely to build up pockets of insulin under the skin, avoiding numerous side effects at later stages. It's metabolic meditation. We are all just flowers really; I can feel myself begin to wilt after only a few days of uneven blood sugar, then after only two of even levels I feel uplifted as though the sun has come up. It's really ninety percent diet, ten percent insulin, to be in control.

# Metabolic meditation

Your hand running out in front of you, nice and steady from left to right. That's your insulin; it's a little miracle doing its thing, five hours at a time. Now imagine a line running complementary and parallel; both of these lines synchronising the duration of; breakfast, lunch and dinner time. That is your protein and green leaves digesting over three consecutively matching periods of five hours, beginning to end. With one final thin line propping them up underneath for the full twenty-four hour long day, leading from your evening injection right through a tranquil night's sleep. The moonlight caressing you as your head lies snugly on a cool pillow. The sun rises and you open your eyelids, springing out of bed all sprightly like a rabbit, the whites of your eyes actually white for once, and no furry tongue. Turning off the alarm before it has even rung, you eagerly approach the day ahead. Eggs and a matching quantity of insulin for breakfast, ready to continue the cycle. People around you thinking, what a calm and collected individual.

Now imagine if you will one of those shock newspaper financial headline charts; a red line darting up and down like numerous lightning bolts strung together, and for good measure, picture this at random instances with insulin shots at various points between a twenty-four hour supportive timeline. That's your temperament on a

313

modern day socially acceptable diet. And imagine – you may not require much imagination – a psychotic character in a made for television movie holding a gun at a Gas Station; the Police screaming at the top of their lungs, 'Put down the FUCKING GUN. Drop your weapon!' and he is crying, angry, righteous indignation, no one treats him right; eventually being led away into a cage. Those are your emotions as a result of over fifteen years on a, *carb counting, eat what I like*, life balanced approach to your condition diet. Leading to your diabetic solstice; eyesight failing, feet numb, kidneys on a go slow, skin like a three packs a day smoker who works in a greasy spoon. GET BACK IN THAT KITCHEN AND COOK SOME EGGS! Tuna for lunch, chicken for tea; look at you bouncing back all tickety-boo like a little spring lamb. – I am so proud of you.

Before we reach the calm, we have a little storm of emotion, hunger and fatigue to weather. So if possible, take a week off work. That's right, treat yourself; extending yourself a week's courtesy at this vital stage will extended your quality of life immeasurably.

...

My piss smells like someone has pissed in it. The same hollow echo throughout my organs, flicking at my bones, draining my muscles as I try to sleep. The amount of salt coming up in my barren mouth, '*Throat noise,*' feels like flu, headache, lethargic and my shits are ungodly. Perfect sugar, and weight falling off me; there is only one way for it all to come out and it's pretty grim. You know when you're shitting green sludge-grease that your body probably didn't need it stored up all that much. Hypo, I'm having a hypo; test my sugar, "6.4," "4.8," over and over it's perfectly level though the sensation has me on tormented tenterhooks. Two hours now, three hours back up at "6.8", six hours, "5.4." Eight and it's "4.1" going on "3.8," but I now know my dawn sugars will lift that back in no time. "5.4" and time for insulin and eggs for breakfast. 'Let's pop to the cinema, I don't want to be stuck in all day.'

Emotional like listening to late night radio. Sick, like having twenty cups of coffee on an empty stomach, and the classic feeling, feeling as weak as a kitten. Under any other circumstance I would feel completely emasculated; waiting to be pushed over by some angry teenager on an underground platform. But today it stands for something.

Can't sleep but I'm focused, fuck me I am focused: this must be what it feels like to be an Oxbridge type, and the clarity; endless, I feel a completely different person. Sharp details I would never think to notice, and brilliant, brighter than ever. Calm, who is this calm? Maybe the Dali Lama but he has China knocking on his door; and this is when it hits me. I have nothing to worry about. I lead the most fortunate life.

That's all well and good until three in the a.m. still I can't fall off. Three fifteen and I've turned my pillow as many times. Got a full on erection. Come on Natasha, wake up, 'Snore,' right in my ear. Well at least that's put me out of the mood. I'll just get up and hang out with the kittens for a while. Funny how the hunger is not so bad when I'm up and around, just laying there was killing me, and I've got so much to do.

Walking around all tearful inside, head's all emotional and I don't want it to wash away; it's like being caught off guard by a touching scene in a film or when Lem died in 'The Shield.' November and I'm alright. This, this is what it's supposed to feel like to be human. I have missed this for seventeen years of desperately clutching at straws, trying to be happy. It feels as amazing as it does equally unfair. It's so fucking unfair. I can't even begin to recognise what I've been through and it's bottled up inside.

And that person in your life who does not think you should take the time out to recover; they never say it out loud just imply through change of subject when it does not suit them. You are not their main concern; they are of no real concern to you. No one who does not wish you health and support you one hundred percent can any longer be allowed to influence you.

...

Chicken, fish, red meat and a *hegg*, lots of eggs; green leaf salad and a selection of vegetables; *metabolic meditation*; ingredients destined and digesting in alignment with my insulin intake. Is it really this simple to completely change my life? – Yes, it makes diabetes seem natural.

Will I get my full health back? After only a single day I could feel the benefits; and much like when I was a kid on *Prozac*; it meant the world and more to me, knowing that someone else understood; this time it was Dr Bernstein. And that there was a solution, I jumped for joy. Two days in and my face is gleaming with smiles, and the thought of eating junk food, oh it's disgusting as people smoking around me at bus stops. I never want to poison myself again.

'Why is this food so cheap and mine stupidly expensive?' Chalkboard, my favourite food in the world is up there; spaghetti bolognese, tagliatelle with carbonara sauce, pepperoni pizza, sausage and mash, baguettes with everything on, desserts all so tasty in such huge servings. This bacon is lonely and needs a hug from a sandwich and a kiss from brown sauce. A Doner Kebab without the pitta bread, what's the point? Going to the cinema and I can't even have a foot long hot dog, where is the justice? The week loops around once more;

tired on a Thursday and I can't even call on *Pizza Hut*, Friday night and no Chinese Takeaway.

Saturday in town, still pining after the *Specials Menu* and it's eating away at me, *"Burger and chips with any pint for a fiver," "Lasagna and garlic bread for near fuck all."* Sitting in the pub and having the one beer I'm allowed; this would be nicer and last longer if I were having it with chips and even the marinated in lemon juice olives are off limits. I have to order something from the main menu, and shit a steak with fries is going to cost Natasha seventeen pounds and I can't even have the fries that come with it, 'Maybe they can swap them for mushrooms?' 'Silence,' and a look, 'It's starting to feel like the world is against me.' – This is where I have to be if I want to give up sugar, in the same way I had to want to give up smoking; it's an addiction I have no doubts about that, the way my body is climbing the walls.

...

*Tesco* Uckfield; I'd better ask someone so I approach an obviously polite and well-presented woman in her fifties, 'Excuse me, could you tell me the difference between salad and vegetables?' She doesn't know quite what to think. Clearly I'm a remarkable idiot; the glint in her eye, am I joking or not? Sharpening to a frown of, that's what the world has come to and how did you ever make it this far. 'This aisle is salad, over there are the vegetables.' 'Thank you,' I beam, ah mushrooms I recognise you from pizza; cheeky tomatoes over there pretending not to be fruit, so long my little friends. Now walking hypnotised past muted veggies into the brightly coloured crisps and the juice spectacular, *Toblerone* and packs of *Hobnobs*, man how much did I used to enjoy them? Can't I even have the one? No. No, no. Hold on, who are the people eating this food I can't have? As I look around, ninety-nine percent of all the edibles in this store will make me sad,

317

like these people. – Oh, I don't want to end up looking like that, they all must feel like shit.

There is only one way to do this diet, it's by sticking to it one hundred percent and enjoying looking into the mirror every couple of days (minutes) watching as my body develops muscles I never even thought I had. I can get severely good looking on this diet. My thirty-six inch waist jeans no longer fit and my t-shirts hang off me like tents. There is a hidden expense in having to buy new clothes.

It's all back to giving up the things you thought you loved to get better, and putting up with a few things you don't want, to feel great. The trade off, I have to give up on the sensation of sweet taste, the very sense – or sensory deprivation; well that's the *dis-ease* part covered. Oh, and controlling of hypos does not depend on how many *Chocolate Buttons* I think I should have; the general rule of thumb, as soon as I start enjoying them, I've had enough. I learnt that lesson the boring way.

Then the saving grace, it turns out, when you ask, when you simply mention you have a *small dietary requirement* and I get over being concerned, 'They will think I am being a difficult freak,' that Chefs from the smallest of cafes and coffee shops, from high street chain Italian eateries right through to the finest hotels and restaurants, will take enormous pleasure in bending over backwards to assist us. It's like you have given them something interesting to do. Their passion is food, they want to create, they want to innovate and satisfy and you are the perfect excuse. Imagine if you will, a Chef is cooking burgers and pasta for idiots with no taste all day, then we come along and they have a chance to do something mutually beneficial. Even the unhappy woman who throws my change at me swapped my toast and tomato for some extra slices of bacon.

Decreased to three injections per day and there are other ways to experience sweetness.

# Wish you the health to use

# it (maybe too late)

Do I want a beer? Yeah I want a beer; I want to drink cold beer all day, every day. I want half a dozen pints of *Guinness* in the evening. I want to smoke two packets of *Marlboro Reds* and I want to get rid of this fucking smoking ban. I want to knock back shots of *Sambuca* with my hand rested on some pretty girl's thigh, I want to do fucking cocaine like the *Rolling Stones*, but I'm going to have black coffee instead. Thank God my fiancée has great legs.

It heightens all of your other senses to compensate; they used to say that in primary school; does that include your sense of not being able to cope and wanting to throw yourself out of the window to an equally sorrowful death. If only you could figure out how to unclasp the lock because you can't find the key? I'd better go look at as many pictures of Tera Patrick as possible; I imagine a blinds man's wank bank is invaluable.

...

They would then ask, 'Would you rather have been able to see first and then go blind? Or would you be better off, being born blind, not knowing what you are missing?' Well, what they actually said was, 'See goin blind in aww that? Ah pure couldn'y handle that man. Fuckin so freaky scary man. Ad be shittin maself big time. Am pure shittin it right noo jist thinkin aboot it. All yer other senses get better when ye go blind. You can hear better and smell stronger.'

'I, smell yer maw.'

'You shouldn'y laugh at blind people cos you might get hit ower the heed way a scafoldin pole nd go blind yerself. Happened to ma mates Uncle.'

'No it didn'y.'

'I it fuckin did.'

'You're pure fulla shite.'

'I an you've really goat the new *Celtic* strip at yer granny's'?'

'I a hiv.'

'No yeeve no ya wee fanny.'

'All boot you in the fanny.'

'Will ye fuck. But would ye think ye would rather be blind or be born blind?'

'A'd rather see colours first.'

'I, me anow.'

...

Perfect sugar balance and the loss of three stones in weight; I feel

321

like '*Spider-Man.*' Get this letter from the Diabetes Eye Screening Clinic, informing me I am in the first stages of going blind. An appointment made for a second opinion, Private Diabetes Specialist Eye Doctor.

I'm so scared she leaves me because she can't cope and I can't blame her. Anyway, my gran used to say, "Wish you the health to use it." Man I'm so scared of going blind. I'm going to sign out for a while now.


Paul

# Short break, waiting room

Maybe best to get the drinking over with in one go; where I got myself into trouble mixing insulin with alcohol, it's a bit of a recurring theme and I wouldn't want you getting the wrong idea. I am from Glasgow none-the-less and it was one of the only things I was always supposed to be good at.

# Take one – JD and Pepsi

# Max

Life's yellow in the Virginia Galleries just off George Square, wrinkled jeans splashed in ink and red plaid shirts; Mo with his ginger goatee is advising, while laughing at me, on how best to shave, 'Go way the grain. No bother at aww.' I'm still amazed at how a spot of shaving gel foams up massively when touched by droplets of water.

Somehow I've managed still to have my full thirty-six pounds wages in my pocket, somehow having gotten out of paying my ten pounds dig money and triple somehow having had a bit of extra cash left from somewhere to cover my Travel Card. So Greg's gran has Alzheimer's and she is off to some special old people's social housing with red string and a triangle to pull on when she needs attention for the rest of her life, and Greg all sympathetic is planning a party in her *empty*. All we need now is some booze and they serve me just fine in the Queen St *Haddows*, so a bottle of *Jack Daniel's Old Number Seven* for me; tastes just like liquorice. I tried a sip of Nolan's last week when we sneaked into *Nice N Sleazy* and it was lovely. I'll mix it with *Pepsi Max* so I don't need to worry about the sugar content. Plenty of planning and preparation there then, now I just have to pour out some of the three litres of *Pepsi* bottle to make room for the *JD* and there you go. Voila, the perfect brew for swigging in the street and no one will ever know. 'Are you sure if I have this now, and I have about eight pounds left to buy beers later, that'll be enough to see me through the night?' I'd already discounted for fags and chips, see, careful planning. 'That should be loads man,' replies Greg in his painted vinyl heavy metal jacket, brandishing that iconic lyric, *"Death to the apocalyptic napalm city."* WTF? 'Geeze a swig aye that. Ahh. That's fucking good man,' lays in Greg.

So we gulp away and pass the time of day, chatting to our hippy mates on the balconies of tie-dye t-shirt shops, alternative record stores and *Mr Ben's* second hand leather jacket shop; always cycling back onto critical subject material, which bands are the best, '*Nirvana* and *Alice in Chains*,' and whose hair is going to be the longest; only stopping to smile at the pretty girls walking by, as they keep on walking by.

'I have an idea! Let's chip in and buy Grungy Flora a new pair of baseball boots. Here Flora, we're all gonna chip in and buy you a new pair of shoes! They're knackered man, look at the state of your shoes, they're terrible. How can your mum let you wear those shoes?' – Friends are laughing in shock. I think I'm harmlessly funny with a reasonable point to make. 'Look at them though they are in terrible condition. No point in getting stroppy, it's not my fault your shoes are falling apart and Kurt Cobain's dead and your shoes look unhappy. I know it's the Grungy look but you have gone too far. Is it true you save time in the morning by just not getting washed? Awwe fuck it then we won't get you new shoes if you're going to be like that. I only wanted to help your feet. A nice new pair of shoes makes you feel

325

nice.'

Things take on a bit of a blue tone from there; I remember being in the back of Liam the Joiners car heading over to the South Side, and asking repeatedly, 'So are you a *Vajoiner?* I remember feeling quite sick; Liam pulling over to the crossing of the Clyde on Bridge St and Greg going off to find me a poly bag to throw up in. Rice and tinned pineapple chunks leaking all out through a hole in the bottom, bacon risotto everywhere all over the back seats, just before I got loaded into the back of an ambulance.

It's all black from here, and I'm glad I missed the worst bit when they pumped my stomach. Someone must have told them I was diabetic or they saw it on my dog tags, as the Doctor is screaming at me to wake up, 'ARE YOU STUPID? DO YOU KNOW YOU COULD HAVE KILLED YOURSELF? DO YOU KNOW HOW A FULL BOTTLE OF *JACK DANIEL'S* COULD KILL ANYONE? AND YOU ARE DIABETIC; YOU COULD HAVE BEEN DEAD IF THEY NEVER GOT YOU INTO THAT AMBULANCE ON TIME.' Oh, I'm in the Royal Infirmary, I'm in the same corridor where I seem to have spent my entire childhood with cuts and blows; James Black's chin going through my head when playing races in the playground; my eyebrow split open by a pebble after going off the little rainbow wall on my BMX; arm fractured from falling off a wooden frame and Mum thinking I was only moaning for attention so ignored me till the following day; waking up on my way here one frosted evening having slipped on black ice, then becoming diabetic and finally being knocked down. It's like home from home, but with my mum waiting on Social Services to interject. But no one is talking to me now so I'm off to Nolan's house for a nice cup of tea.

Up I get playing human pin ball with the rest of Glasgow's finest,

'Oww, Sorry, oww oww sorry, Are you all right there pal do you need a light?' guided by touch and bruised shins, making it out under moonlit sky, somehow eventually making it to Steven's parent's home. 'Whit's happened to you son? Are you alright? Is he alright? Is Steven with you? Are you drunk? Is he drunk?' where they sit me down on the sofa and get me to test my sugar, "*High*," then ask, 'How ye feelin?' 'I'm a bit drunk but my body's telling me to do push ups to burn off the sugar (well at least those are the words I think are coming out my mouth),' before they kindly pour me back into an ambulance. A combined twenty-five minutes later the screamie Doctor says, 'We were wondering where he went,' before having me sit around for seven hours under observation, then sending me home.

I get home, get a bollocking, get suspicious of foul play as my jacket lining is all ripped open, my money and *Walkman* missing: post experience has proven this to be just me. Vomit, reach, vomit; yellow stomach bile blistering the roof of my mouth; sugar test results of "17.0" it's coming down. Have some insulin and fall asleep face first on the living room carpet. – Sorry for wasting the time of the *Glasgow Royal Infirmary*. Sorry Steven's parents. Flora never spoke to me again. Liam the Vajoiner sold his car. Greg still only ever calls me *Paul Daniels*, and I'll never drink *JD* again.

# Take two – Single Malt

# ghosts of Pitlochry

Pitlochry with the sun dimming toward the end of a pale yellow day; July touched by November, we duck into a confined den. A local band is playing traditional songs, singing insular vernacular plucking accustomed instruments; gives pause to ask the eight strong crowd of regulars, 'Before we go on. Do we have any English in here tonight?' I'm laughing now; Natasha is so in for it. 'Go on, tell them.' How bad can it be? She is thinking, bravely raising an arm, 'SILENCE,' from every corner. Silence thrown on the floor, 'This wan is called *Tartan Warrior King*, it's aboot how Robert the Bruce took own an killed eleven thousand English, single handily in the Battle of Bannockburn afore ultimate defeat at the haunds ay they filthy cheating scum.' I'm almost on the floor, and Tasha thought they were taking requests, 'Are they kidding?' 'No, but they think William Wallace is Australian. Let's go.'

Next stop hotel bar has a massive range of Single Malt Whiskies' on offer, for the tourists, the connoisseur and amber gantry decoration. I fancy some of that! Barman recommends their house label, 'Distilled, just up the hill *ken*, to the highest standards, rate it to stand tall amongst all Islay competitors like,' and it would be rude to decline. Down the hatch and a question forms on my lips, 'How come you still sell *Bells*? My grandad and his mates won't even drink that anymore because they suspect it's distilled in England.' Question ignored, and maybe he isn't a mad racist; quite nice and I leave him to think he has a chance chatting up my fiancée as I go mingle.

'Ahh they have *Deacon Blue* on the Juke Box, I've not heard them in years,' prodding Natasha from polite conversation with the Bartender banging on about how he manages the place and where he hung out in London, 'I love them; this is going to be a brilliant night!'

Tash is keeping a gentle eye over me as I'm knocking back large doubles like there is no tomorrow; savouring the bite; maybe a bit too quickly even for the bar crud, coining it in. And I'm singing away to myself back and forth to the Juke Box with handfuls of silver coins before going into full conversation mode, 'Do you not like *Deacon Blue?*' with the equally inebriated and couldn't be less interested, only popped out for a small libation, who the fuck is this guy?

'Let's go back to the room,' Tash tentatively suggests; I sense hidden cringes, so arm in arm we venture forth back and forth then forth once more to our own hotel. Half dozen or so family measures have taken their toll and just about managing to keep my arse off the ground, slurring along the lines of, 'Whaa, whaaa whaaa, yes whaa,' just have to make it up these four flights of tartan carpeted staircases, past paintings of suspected-pretend old people and empty suits of armour, 'Is that bear moving?' and home free. 'Oooops. Owww, laughter giggles, whaaa whaaa whaa,' the key does finally make it into the lock, give or take, 'Whaaa, I'm having a tremendous time,' minutes. Tasha makes an instant bee-line for the bathroom

329

and starts throwing up, 'Whaaa'ts wrong? Shouldn't that be me? Did you even drink much?' Poor girl pausing between hurls to explain, 'I think it might have been the steak from earlier. HAAUUGGGAAA,' head back in the toilet, just an echo pronouncing, 'Sorry I dragged you home, I was feeling really sick.' 'You should have said.' 'But you were having such a lovely time and I've not seen you, HURL, this happy in ages. SPEW.'

Laid back on the bed, finding my shoe laces and keeping an eye on the bathroom door trying to keep her chatting, 'I thought it was me being a pain in the arse,' when all of a sudden and make no room for error, I so desperately need to pee. There is no option for waiting here and no chance of getting in there, so off to the balcony; peeing into the wind, singing to myself and the void, *'DIGNITY,'* and back to me she blows.

'OK I need to get into the bath now to wash my legs. Natasha, there's been a technical issue,' as I shuffle past gaunt face and paler arms to figure out a shower attachment that plugs into taps. Back onto the bed wrapped in a towel, 'Natasha, who are all these people in the room?' 'What?' bemused, washing her face. 'I can see the shadows of people in the walls; they keep coming into and out of focus from the pattern.' Chalky back of forehand placed on my forehead and neck; I'm neither too hot nor cold, maybe a bit warm then she has me test my blood sugar, "22.0" 'SHIT.' Attention drawn, looking up into the corner by the window frame into tourist tartan, 'They keep coming in and out. Is this place haunted?' I'm not really panicking but I'm not sure if I'm seeing ghosts or I am hallucinating due to the combination of high blood sugar and drinking spirits, but this has never happened to me before and I am far from enjoying it. 'Maybe they hate the wallpaper?' her comment appealing to my drunken side and pulling me back from possible fear.

Tash comforts till I settle; all hugs and cups of locally bottled Scottish water sourced from Tweedledee Springs just up the Glen, and explains that many people can hallucinate from drinking too much Whisky. Seems reasonable, with my sugar knocking my system's ability to digest and deal with the poison, it's clearly not helping any. Insulin and a kiss on the head then off to sleep with a packet of '*Traditional Scottish Shortbread*' under my pillow and all is well when I awaken to the clatter of breakfast trays and '*The Scotsman*' newspaper being shoved under our door, but still ashamed of not being there for Natasha when she needed me, when she had sat up on her own throwing up for the next three or so hours. I'll never drink Single Malt again.

# Take three – Pink Sambuca

# at the Sherlock Holmes

A trip into London, I've not been here for months and I've not seen my old mates Les and Neil for even longer. Natasha is working over in Swindon today and to commute there and back from Uckfield in a single day seems pretty painfully pointless when we can stop over in a *laterooms.com* for a cozy stay of room service. So *The Sherlock Holmes* on Baker St it is and tomorrow I'm popping to the *Production Show* to see if I can land myself a job; the *BBC* have a slot about the *iPlayer* and I plan on passing around a few CV's. But today, today is for me; I'll catch up for lunchtime drinks with my old chums while she's at work then she'll come join us after. Perfect!

The *Low Life Bar*, very friendly little hub not getting the crowd it deserves, so the drinks are on special and it's a tenner for four bottles of *Peroni*. A joyous impromptu occasion by the best of standards and we have one or two or three, then *Paul's* eyes are dazzled, caught by the glimmer of the gantry: Pink Sambuca! I've not had it in ages, used to drink it like crazy down in the Spanish Bar with a lesbian photographer and I never stopped with the stuff when living it up in

West Hampstead, so let's have a few on the go. Lovely doing a shot with a beer, and close friendships that will last forever; seems so complete, then having to pop outside every fifteen minutes for a cigarette, to stand under scaffolding acclimatising to ice-cold. Back into warmth, raise my glass; I could do this forever.

Well it was great to see everyone and we're back to the hotel room, it's gorgeous in here like its own little apartment and I'm ready for our *KFC Family Bargain Bucket* with *Rolo Ice Cream*; ignoring the complimentary bottled spring water in favour of *Pepsi Max* and eying complimentary shortbread for later. 'This head cold is horrible,' I say, when the shadows draw in around me; in an instant I am back to where I was in Pitlochry, only this time it's a whole lot worse.

'YOU'RE GOING TO KILL ME.' 'Paul, Paul, look at me. No, listen, listen to me. It's me, breathe,' kneeling beside me, holding gentle eye contact, stroking my hand, trying desperately to calm. 'I'm too scared even to think.' Forcing me to test my sugar takes more than some convincing, "28.0" 'SHIT.' The place is spinning. Part of my brain knows high sugar and alcohol is responsible. 'Just leave me alone. Just leave me alone, I want to go home. I just want to go home. Let me go,' convinced Tash is out for murder. She tries again desperate to comfort but each arm around me is more terrifying, drawing me into death. I can see her face, the woman I love, I can see in her gestures only compassion but somewhere in my head is very mixed up and everything is wrong. Some self-preservation instinct has me take my night-time insulin but now I'm sure there are other people in this room and I want so badly to go home to Glasgow.

'There are ghosts in here. This is way worse than it was before,' speaking in one sentence, fearful of what I think she is in my next; she could be the Devil. Breathing has become erratic and not taking

333

any chances, so while I'm busy slipping in and out of consciousness a shaking hand dials zero through to Hotel Reception arranging for an ambulance. Two knocks to the door and two very burly Security men are waiting outside, only reassuring us, 'An ambulance is on the way,' and one of them is nearly in tears at the state of me. 'She is trying to kill me.'

Paramedics come in and kneel beside me, we go through what I have had to eat and to drink, 'Keep her away from me. I'm sure she is who she says she is but I know she is trying to kill me.' They ask if I have had anything else other than alcohol and I've not. They ask if anything like this has ever happened before, I muster explanation over hyperventilation that only a matter of months ago I was taken into an ambulance as I found myself on Great Portland St not knowing where or who I was with blood sugar of "19.0." 'It's the same scenario here only... Can I have a hug?' The Paramedic declines for a cuddle and a tearful Natasha walks nervously behind us and into the back of the ambulance.

Things are starting to become a bit clearer now with the insulin making its path through my system and my breathing now less heavy and more controlled, 'The usual concussive chat.' Sugar is "16.0" by the time we get to the Royal Free Casualty Department and again I'm laid out on my back with a line of fluids in my arm, holding onto Natasha's hand, 'How long can this go on?'

'ROAST BEEF. POTATOES. GRAVY. YORKSHIRE PUDDING. CUSTARD. SAUSAGES,' comes calling out from behind the white curtain two beds down. 'What the fuck? Anyway...,' trying to mind our own business, 'Things have clearly gotten even worse and I'm completely losing control. Why should something like a few drinks push me over when it never has before? Why didn't the UCH with their Diabetes Ward fix me before rather than sending me home and writing me off as, "You'll be fine, you just need more insulin." At this rate I will be scared to go outside soon and I'm so sorry.' 'APPLE PIE AND ICE CREAM, SOME TOFFEE...' It's hard, we're both of us trying not to roar with laughter and hold onto a smirk instead, and 'I feel like I'm dragging you down with me.' 'It's okay; you need to just not have spirits again that's all.' 'I can't believe I asked that Ambulance Driver for a hug because I'm frightened. I'm so embarrassed.' Squeezes my hand and smiles a little tearful. Tash and I, hushed giggling to ourselves at the neighbour's menu requests when a ten year old boy who pulls the curtain closed behind him, and has come into stick a *routine* thick needle directly into the artery of my right wrist, explains about the man calling through, 'His sugar is so high, his body thinks its low and he is craving everything his brain can think of. He is on Sunday Roasts now, been at it for hours.' 'Fucking hell!' 'It never stops,' as he pulls back the curtain on his way out. 'Aw shit Natasha, I can't let that happen to me.' 'The first thing we need to do is give up alcohol. That never seems to agree with you anymore, even when you only had a few beers you have started having the most terrible hypos, maybe stick to just having a glass of wine?' 'Deal,' and I pull off the Mary blue knit blanket when we're both kicked out of the hospital after the results come in: that it was just high blood sugar and there are no signs of ketoacidosis in my *Blood Gas* so I'm in no immediate danger. Taxi back to Baker St; walk of shame past Hotel Reception, I'll never drink Pink Sambuca again.

Thanks to the staff at *The Sherlock Holmes Hotel* for your concern, I'm sure I'm the last thing you need on a quiet Wednesday night. Shame though that the next time I stay over your bed falls apart and the headboard skelps me on the noggin.

# Take four – Big orange

# Glucose Syringe

Heading back the way home from the gym; third time this week and it's only Thursday; haven't had a drink since whenever or a smoke in forever, don't know how many more holes the cobblers will manage into this belt. Had enough; time for a treat, a packet of cigarettes, a one off, probably not even smoke more than a couple? *Diet-Coke* o'clock to stay out of the house for a while longer and this little bar round the back of the shopping centre seems friendly enough to pass an hour with notepad in hand watching the world go on by. 'A *Diet-Coke* please?' and I pop out the side door for my second, 'Puff,' delicious, and back at the bar reading the paper.

A local gives it the, *I've arrived,* pulling his barfly pew; sparks up a conversation with the waitress, 'God, I'm a writer, why do I struggle so hard to write a text message?' he protests too much in Geordie accent and his dime store poet routine is lost on me before it began. More a *wafter* blogger than a Writer: innocuous chat over a cigarette, 'What brings you to Royal Tunbridge Wells?' Something about an *Hons* in Literature at a prestigious University he lives off the memory of, near where I used to live up in Scotland; humour and, 'I think I'll join you on that next *Guinness*. Not had a beer in a long time.'

'My round,' he proclaims; I check the bank and there is enough in there. 'Check my sugar,' and its "13.0" so have another shot as he makes a meal of downing a vodka to amass the courage to press send on the now two hours' long deliberated text. 'Just ask her if she wants to meet you for a coffee after work.' 'Ah can't man, ah don't know why I just canna manage.' He clearly gets off on this lonely guy at the bar crap; too intelligent to conform to society, doesn't own a TV and that kind of thing, another round comes by. Bar nuts the food of the early evening, 'They stopped serving meals months ago because they have no customers,' another pint of the black stuff and onto loves lost. 'Everyone I know has got married and I'm alone. I was with a girl...' 'Surely you can't be that bad at meeting girls, even with all the *anything for the lady* conversation?' Sugar of "13.4" it's time for another shot of insulin; onto another pack of cigarettes; pretty wankered by now, 'Has she still not replied?' 'She never does.'

Glaswegian takes his seat at the bar to the left of gloomy writer boy, picks up on my accent and let the customary gruelling trip down memory lane commence, where he grumbles so strongly I have to lurch forward to understand a word, 'Hey, it's a different world doon here.' I hate this shit, the face of a *heavy* that's been spanked a few times, absent of any good memories and heritage presumed diseased as his liver, but that cheeky *M&S* jacket is dead giveaway and he will be back to middle class and good times when the door swings shut behind me. One more shot of insulin, I think I'll need it; needle half way in my tummy with t-shirt held up and a cotton bud fallen out of my pocket: denying that's mine; everyone who is anyone can see my belly. 'Prrp,' text messages received, "*At station*" "*In taxi*" "*Outside*" and I look up through the door to see Tasha in a white cab waiting on me.

337

Delighted; tuck myself back in and out the door; old pestilence can go back to being Champagne Boab.

Back of the taxi I broker the deal to have Pizza for supper, as I'm *all out enjoying myself* and have made a friend; skirting by a row of green traffic lights and cozy on the sofa telling her about my day before I even know it. 'Hold on, I'm going to be sick,' make my eventual return, 'That was at least three pints of *Guinness*. Aw no, my sugar has climbed to "19.0" but I'm long overdue my night-time insulin and it should catch up and come down soon.' – Nothing like drunken diabetic math. 'Should you have more insulin with this garlic bread?' 'Eh, not so sure, I lost track of how much I had earlier trying to keep up with the beer to be honest. Test again in twenty minutes; see how I am getting on?' 'Yeah, I'll help you keep an eye on it.' '*Pooh Bear*, I love you.' 'I love you too puppy. Glad you had a wonderful time.' 'Oh I'm going to be sick again.'

'How much did you have?' 'Not that much I don't think,' cats all over me, seems strange but a sure sign of a hypo; test my sugar for the forever time and "6.2" that was fast, better get eating. 'Pass me the *Chocolate Fudge Brownie* please? Plenty of room for it now. – Can't eat any more of that, need to bathroom. BARF.' There goes all the pizza and ice cream, now for a poo. How much did I drink? Aw hold on, I'm getting all shaky, 'NATASHA.' 'WHAT?' 'CAN YOU PASS ME IN MY BLOOD SUGAR TEST?' 'COMING.' 'Sorry, thank you.' 'That's okay, what is it?' 'Fuck, it's "3.8." 'I'll pour you some *Cola*.' – You know love when your partner passes in your blood sugar test when you are having a poo! I'm out of there as fast as I can and sitting on the sofa swigging back an *Eeyore* mug full of bubbles. 'Maybe better have some glucose powder with syrup in, this feels like a bad one.'

Have about as much *Starbucks Caramel* and *Dextrose Powder* dissolved in water as I can handle, 'Feel sick now; that should be plenty.' 'What is it now?' 'Fuck, "2.8" fuck!' How much more of this syrup mix I can stomach I don't know but I'm worried, I keep pouring it back and testing over and over again. Every time I reach the safety of "4.0" it bombs back down and I vomit everything back up. 'This is bad.' 'Should I call a Doctor?' 'I can't, I'm drunk; it's my own fault. The fuck, I've had loads more – *hiccup!* – too much insulin.' All I can remember now is having more and more with each pint. 'Shit, I'm going to go into a coma.' 'You won't it will be fine. Drink more. You have *Glucogel*.' 'Get it.' A tube of that in my mouth all at once and I feel even worse, 'Going to be sick, HURL, that's got to be it now?' 'Test again?' 'Fuck, its "2.4," I can't hold anything down to keep it up.' 'I'm calling an ambulance.' 'No don't, they are only going to inject me with the *Gluco Syringe*. Pass it to me.' 'Are you sure?' 'I don't have a choice.' 'Let me read the instructions first.'

'The size of that needle!' FEAR, 'That's going to touch bone.' 'It says you should be unconscious first,' shaking up the contents and removing the cap as I stare at the bloody thing. 'Well I'm going to be if I don't have it now. I'm vomiting everything I eat and all the insulin has nothing left to feed on but me.' 'Do you want me to do it?' she says knowing she can't. One last look at the long thick, longer and thicker needle, 'How the hell is that going to pierce the skin, needle, what? I'm too drunk I can't do this.' 'I don't know if you could, sober.' Pinching, pressing, pressing, still pressing, press again and finally break the skin. I can feel every inch of the thing and just want it over with, reaching my thumb up and over the plunger and pushing for the longest time. Retracting the needle for ages in shock, run to the bathroom, 'VOMIT. SPEW. I'M GONNA DIE.' 'No you're not. Test again.' 'Give it another minute to kick in... "4.2" it's working. I'm gonna barf,' knees on wet floor, rinsing with mouthwash and praying at the porcelain altar for a good long hour, 'God I'll never drink again. REACH,' all the way till the final bar nut lifts out and finally I lay down. 'Are you okay?' 'That was fucking horrific.'

# 41

Holding myself together.

A shot of insulin, a shot of Sambuca, a breath for fresh air.

A shot of insulin, a shot of Tequila; drinks at the Spanish Bar late after work.

A shot of insulin and more friendships that would last forever?

That smell when moisture from raindrops falls upon the summer's dust.

Sad as a Sunday, and my grandad is sitting at home alone drinking himself to death while I'm down here unable to help like a complete cunt.

Is this all I ever was, binge drink and complain, binge fuck and chain-smoke and swear like a Sailor? Taking health for granted, now begging for a sporting chance at redemption.

Back to the fear of God, it is the same God and the same fear but you never get used to it. Perhaps if I did, it would become mortal fear.

It's as though living in the moment when I glance at my watch; the second hand is stuck, nothing changes, all value and intention removed. '*Tock,*' and relief, everything is fine, but I never get to leave that moment ever again. Hands over my face, fingers kneading against bone of sockets, eyes clasped so tightly black has become red; heat emanating through deep tissue and sinew muscle: I can't stay here forever, I can't find comfort anywhere.

Could do with some manly advice round about now; think I'll have to man-up instead.

Cynicism as a coping mechanism: fucking Diabetes Expert Dwarfs.

It's weird, but going to the gym is like praying to myself to get better.

I believe in me.

So am I the product of what I came from derived in poor health, or can I live free?

Why did he leave me with this wound that won't heal?

My father was in a mental institution, and I'm terrified to end up in one. I wonder if anyone has ever ended up in a mental institution because of acting out from high blood sugar?

And on a good day I am happy, and I am lucky to have lived all those days.

A better person when my sugar is level.

I'm nicer to be around.

Content not frustrated.

I do this because there is no other way.

Hold it together Paul.

Hold it together man.

Maybe I'm just Glasgow enough to get through this; maybe I've been physically and emotionally toughened up enough to break the preordained pish. This Cathcart boy born in Duke St, hear it for Glasgow, GLASGOW, GLASGOW!

# Fight or flight: Fight

"Do you suffer from, low sex drive, flaccid penis, tightened skin around the penis, bad skin, bad penis, bad breathe and no one wants to see your penis? Etc. when your sugar is high?" – Thanks for reminding me.

Much like a diamond appraisal, Professor Chung looks into my eyes for signs of diabetes using a magnifying lens and intensive torchlight. I force my eye to remain open, unflinching glaring into light. 'Look up. Look over to my left. Look at my right ear,' well this is make or break right now and I've given in, all will past over, whatever he says is how it is and I'll move on or stand still from here. Little roll back on his wheeled stool and an understanding nod, then comes an explanation; I do have the first signs of diabetes in my eyes, and being made up of the smallest blood vessels in the body, my eyes shall deteriorate if I do not get on top of my diabetes. – But not yet, God he is talking in future tense, saying not yet, he means not yet. Please mean not yet. 'This should be seen however, more as a sign of future danger, such as when a person suffers Angina and this being the body's warning of future heart failure.' – It's an early warning sign; my eyes too have early warning signs, 'A shot across the bow,' God I am going to be okay. I am not at this moment further into blindness, it can be avoided and with good control it needn't get any worse. Feels as though the sun has come up and I never thought it would rise again; this is chance at life, new born baby joy; tingles from head to toe and I say nothing; relief, I sit as confused as the sparrows. Hold eye contact, paying respectful service to moving lips while the voice in my head is the only voice I'm listening to, 'I'm going to be okay. I'm going to be okay,' squeeze coming from Natasha's ever present hand, 'I'm so lucky to have you.'

Professor Chung pushes back and away a little on his matchbox stool and you can tell he loves wheeling around on that thing with a sense of play nearly as much as his chosen vocation. 'Thank you for your time.' very restrained, I want to hug the man and kiss his head, I want to allow the build-up of tears to pour but I'm savouring that for when we get outside together and home free before someone changes their mind, and I can hold onto her and relish in the end of this. We exit to the street, make it about as far as the expensive café and I hold onto her for a moment that means a lifetime. I could explode, fall apart, cry this out, have a nervous breakdown, 'I'm sorry about how much that cost.' 'Don't be so silly,' pulling in to face me and see if I'm okay because nothing else matters, 'Peace of mind is priceless. I just wish we had come here sooner, when you started getting more ill, when we lived around the corner.' 'How much is the follow up appointment?' 'With Dr Abraham? About three hundred. Don't think about it. It's fine. You're fine.' Home and relax with a headache and sleep for a week; catch up on that other stuff later.

...

All very civilised, no children kicking their mothers in the face, whilst drinking from bottles of bright pink chemicals, but steadily stream a supply of glowing and calm individuals, many as old as they are very well heeled. The value of wealth over health easily

345

established, it in no doubt helps, and the classical definition of disease as an equaliser amongst men failing in context within this condition. Life well and truly in perspective, I don't know if I'll ever worry about general things again.

I see a little African boy with his mum, he has the entire glow of the world in his cheeks, and I know just by looking at him he will never suffer the diabetic ups and downs as I have. A smiling Receptionist points me out to a Nurse, who approaches to collect me, shaking my hand, a natural smile as though every day is a worthwhile day. She weighs me and converses, ready to discuss every question and topic variable I can muster, from panic and frustration to sugar fluctuations caused by ground coffee and losing weight; she sees it all every day. Before pointing out my blood sugar test monitor is way off the mark giving wholly inaccurate readings. Job title of Nurse, she clearly understands more than any *NHS* Diabetes Expert Consultants I have encountered and more importantly in some respects, she declares an environment I want to be in when I am ill. I'm still taken aback the Receptionist hasn't brought her personal life into work with her, having failed completely to suck air through her teeth, raise her hand to inform she is on the phone or tutted at my inconvenience. Not used to this I almost feel cheated.

Dr Abraham's understanding of the diabetic is a revelation. I always knew I was not the only one going through this, but he and his team know *me* well. I talk him through my situation and he actually listens, sneezes, and then congratulates me on making myself better. Explaining that in taking this relatively short time out to get better, I have extended my lifespan by years. As relieved as I am to hear his professional understanding remove perceived objection from time to get better; am I simply asking for justification and permission, again, not just to be ill but also to get better? 'Counselling is an option,' he offers after my enquiry, 'It is perfectly natural with the build-up of guilt you feel from being ill, and anxiety, that you may wish to see a Counsellor. Though in time with your health improved, I'm sure you will find the layers of upset and stress breaking down like layers of an onion, and you may no longer feel this need,' knowing from experience nod of his head, 'We do have Counsellors available across the hall, if you do wish to make an appointment.' – Thoughts interrupting again, that awful metal sculpture of an onion to represent different layers of society when I was a kid.

We further discuss; ninety percent him ten percent me; how diabetes is affecting all aspects of my personal life, social life and career, before he delves effortlessly into a couple of horror stories; people still conversing, with sugar of one point six; people rushing for work and running up the escalator, collapsing into comas at the top; people nodding off into a high blood sugar daze at the wheel of a car and crashing into a family saloon. All right captain morbid, Shit! Now I'm thinking, I don't really need to know this, and he turns things around by advising that I have an insulin pump. Not an *NHS* pump; a high-grade pump that tests for sugar levels and takes care of the technicalities for four thousand five hundred pounds. Four thousand five hundred pounds for the initial base unit only and then on top of that the cost of cartridges to keep it operational. Or if that figure proves unreachable at this juncture, then there is the possibility of a lease. Has this whole thing been a sales pitch? No, it's just that I don't come from the same world of wealth as *they* do, and my cats have better health cover than I do, but this time it's a good *they* and seeing how the ageing gentry are performing in the waiting room dictates to me the path of my own future. Hold on though; four thousand five hundred pounds for an artificial pancreas solution, didn't I come up with that idea seventeen years ago? I can't afford to buy one, I don't think I'd even want to have one attached to me; the

347

very idea is creeping me out. I do feel more confident though that he recognises in me I have made myself better and he recognises in my prior advisors, '*A backwater in diabetes knowledge.*' He is equally confident that all things in the body, eyes included, will heal.

Fight.

# Getting better, state of

# mind

"It's like having my son back." – Mother

Tearful yet unwilling to rollover, remorseful, am I mourning my lost seventeen years? Why did I have to hold in all the stress as a child? Why couldn't I just have peed the bed and let it all out? So much to think about, Dr Abraham explained to me, the times when I was on my way home to collect late insulin, vomiting yellow stomach bile and half asleep: that I was actually incredibly close to falling into a diabetic coma with ketoacidosis. When I think about the circumstance of how this happened, how my friend's sister decided she didn't like me, and hid my insulin, how I decided on so many occasions to stay out over night when I never had insulin with me; it shakes me to think how close I came. And that's the easy stuff, that's just the physical cause and effect. It's the emotional head trauma of realising what this disease has done to me, how it has warped my behaviour throughout the years that's going to take its toll to recover from.

When my sugar is high, I get this feeling; I am waiting for something

349

bad to happen. When it stays high I have nightmares about being bitten by dogs and people coming into my house. The worst is when I awaken and the fear stays with me; mix this with strong coffee and it's a recipe for panic attacks and wanting to curl up on the sofa to hide from the world. The only way to remedy this; eat properly, drink lots of water to flush out the simply imperfect blood sugar and watching a good comedy often helps.

...

Release of anguish, well enough for long enough to begin to look back, and look forward.

*Before*

*At present I am lost, my character thin, my confidence gone, expectations extinguished, soaked through with doubt, nurtured in worry, close to giving up entirely. I used to be better than this, I used to look the world dead in the eye and I thought I could stare down the sun, now the world's gotten the better of me. Responsibility for everything and it's all too hard but I'm going to make myself better. Maybe it's the time I find on my hands, or my current health status. This book just seems right.*

*After*

*Seventeen years of feeling like that fly, banging its head off the bar window.*

*I'm a better person when my sugar is level. I'm nicer to be around. Content not frustrated. I do this because there is no other way. Please stay with me.*

*Now*

*Week four of being human and I have no intention of leaving this island. I crave new challenges, I want to be involved. So this is what it feels like to be young?*

*I don't feel uncomfortable all the time anymore, I feel fresh and capable. I can't remember feeling like this since I was a kid.*

*Clearing out the cobwebs and now to come to terms with having been ill for seventeen years.*

*Writing this book has made me realise how I see the world. Made me realise how high sugar has changed me. I'm actually quite a nice person.*

*I hope I'm nicer to be around and for me it's great to see how lovely the people around me are. I don't feel like everyone around me is having a go at me anymore. I don't take everything to heart and no longer feel everything is a poor reflection on me.*

*Six months on*

*Every day is lovely, the trees show me how young I am, cool breeze refreshes me, water reflecting sky and I am privileged to walk around here in the company of all you beautiful souls. The smiles of others light me up and I know tears can be recovered from. It's time to create some little ones, a George Victor, a Jack Nolan.*

*We should never and I will never again allow myself to feel guilty over being ill. I know I am doing everything I can to be healthy and that's way beyond what most non-diabetics do.*

*Thanks for letting me get this off my chest. It's true, it's not good to keep it all bottled up inside.*

*Thank you, Paul*

# Sugar levels ill, sugar levels

# well

Taken some time out to write through fluctuating emotions caused by ever-changing blood sugar levels, as defined in my situation and specified by my blood sugar test monitor results.

*Sugar levels ill*

"0.0" Call my mum, the boy's pan bread. – Fortunately this hasn't happened, yet. "1.0" Call an ambulance, the boy's in a coma (and "1.5" I expect). "1.8" Inject me in the leg with that big orange *Gluco Syringe* please! Don't worry I'm totally unconscious, I won't feel a thing as that thick needle pierces my skin and if I do then maybe the intent is for the pain to bring me back. "2.6" *Dextrose, Coca-Cola, Snickers bar* and ice cream, everything to feed the hunger: oh now my sugar is "21.0!" "3.0" *Dextrose* please, for that balanced hypo approach. Although I'd rather have a bag full of all those cheap 'n' nasty sweets we ate as kids, pink shrimps, white chocolate mice, *Wham Bars* and a big bowl of ice cream. In fact just parachute me into '*Willy Wonka's Chocolate Factory.*' "4.5" 'Now is not the time for discussion. I know my sugar is bottoming out so pass me the sugar; all of it.' "5.0" Come on the diabetes! – Keep this up for a couple of days and I'll be feeling lovely, and the world's a better place. "6.0" 'I knew it was you; your period is due.' "7.0" 'Let's actually go outside.' "10.0" Taking everything personally, taking everything to heart and taking it all the wrong way. "11.0" 'I'm not in a huff, I'll test my sugar and if it's above nine then it's me. I'd better have some insulin.' "12.0" Feeling a bit pish, back aches and acid indigestion, 'I'm sorry for acting like a complete shit earlier when my sugar was high. I know you understand but you shouldn't have to put up with me acting like this and I feel like I am destroying your life.' "13.0" Unlucky, 'Don't even fucking look at me, AHHHHHHH. You have no idea how horrible this is, or what I am going through.' "16.0" Check I haven't left any plugs in. "19.0 +" Panic and confusion preside, I stand lost in my own street and the love of my life is a near stranger. An ambulance is en route to take me to A&E where they will drain a *Blood Gas* directly from an artery in my wrist to test for ketoacidosis then look at me like I'm wasting their special time.

*Sugar levels well*

"0.0" Am I still dead? "1.0" Big orange *Gluco Syringe* time, although I don't expect this will ever happen (again). "2.2" *Gluco Gel* on my gums please, and best I inform the people I work with that there is only a one in a million chance this could lead to me being on the floor and them having to get off their arse and do something. "3.0" *Dextrose Powder* in water please, but only three teaspoons to bring me up sufficiently then some eggs or something to keep me balanced. – I try not to panic and it's easier now that I know what has caused the hypo. Because I now take such small doses of insulin, I avoid having to chase blood sugar levels spiralling down then bouncing back up. "3.9" Double check I have not levelled out here, if so my body will soon work its way back up to "6.0." "4.0 – 7.0" One week of this and I

353

feel like '*Spider-Man*,' but best I try and stay closer to "5.0." "10.0" Check which mystery item in the shopping list is packed with secret sugar? The last one was an apple *lip-balm*. "11.0" I bet I have some kind of fever, thermometer, water and *Paracetamol* please. "13.0" This still happens sometimes; an awkward cup of coffee can be enough for me to convince myself that the Waiter has short changed me, so I request a receipt. But at least now I know why I'm being all over the top and things aren't all so personal. I'm still not giving him a tip though.

# Lifelines

*"I am the lord who heals you,"* *'Exodus 15:26.'* Quote taken from my local Doctor's surgery, carved on a plank pulled from a singing fish, positioned above a receptionist bearing more than a slight resemblance to *Dame Edna Everedge*, – I was really looking for someone with a more formal qualification.

When joining a new *NHS* Doctor, it is customary to meet with the resident Diabetes Nurse. It seems less customary for her to know anything about diabetes. She seems helpful enough though and based on written summation from my Private Specialist, has in hand the results from an additional thyroid test added to my standard blood work.

Borderline defensive because I don't trust these clowns, 'I expect my sugar levels to be high as they have been all over the place with my now three week long cold.' She seems to understand that having a cold affects diabetes and enquires as to my fluctuating levels, which I explain to be between low and twenty-two averaging on ten for the most part, 'Certainly the most common number on my blood sugar test monitor.'

Asking how my cold is now, I explain that it feels like I'm at the end of it, but I'm still quite feverish. She then informs my Hba1c was alright, reading at "7.8" from the results and she wants me to see the Doctor for antibiotics as my cold has gone on for far too long, especially *if* it was affecting my blood sugar. – Keeping it to myself for now, but quietly impressed by her interest. 'Fair enough,' I say and comment, 'It has reached the point where I'm getting jittery and nervous as my sugar has been all over the place for so long.' Now she looks at me as though I were an alien and replies, only because she feels she has to say something, 'You're probably just ill,' complete refusal to acknowledge a connection between the two. – That's what I get for showing faith.

'Oh before we go any further and before I forget, these blood sugar monitors are driving me nuts. This one is my third and was sent to me directly by *Accu-Chek* because others were faulty, and even this gives me constant "E number" error messages. Can you recommend another one, as I'm wasting so many blood sugar test sticks and so much blood?'

'Oh we usually have loads in from the *Reps*,' – troubled, her thoughtful mouth and jaw reaction is to chew from either side in pause, 'But I don't have any at the moment. What kind is it? Oh you don't like *Accu-Chek*?'

'I'm platform agnostic, as long as it works, and I got this one because the last was out by over one unit when compared to the equipment at the Private Hospital.'

'Oh that's quite a lot.'

'Well yes, based on four to eight, that's a quarter of my blood sugar tolerance. It's a lot!'

'Well you can get tests now which read ketones from your blood.'

'Excellent, I'd like one of them.'

'I can't remember what they're called or who makes them, but I'll look into it for you and get you one in. I'll make a note to call you on Thursday. I only work here Thursdays. I cover half of the County.' – All very impressed at her own single-handed contribution to the diabetic landscape.

'Thanks that would be great, but can you prescribe me one from *Boots* in the meantime?'

'No. We don't prescribe them, we are dependent on the *Pharmaceutical Reps* to supply them as demonstration units, and then we can only prescribe test strips. They are very expensive!'

'Yes, but they give them away because they make their profit not from the machines but from the repeat prescriptions on test sticks. Like cheap printers and ink.'

Looking at me again like I'm an alien.

'Now your cholesterol, this really is high.'

'What is it?'

'Six-point-nine'

'What should it be?'

'Four'

'Oh that sounds serious, I was expecting it to peak though with the change in diet and having lost well over three stones in such a short period.'

'I will need to put you onto a course of *Statins*, to bring it down.'

'I'm sure it's just my body breaking down excess fat, it should clear up in no time.'

'Well, we will test it again in another three months to see *if* it has come down. That should have given enough time to adjust to your *diet*. Then we will need to put you on a course of Statins to bring it down.'

'What are Statins exactly?'

'They are *just heart tablets* which you have each day to help with cholesterol.'

'For how long?'

'Forever.'

'I'll go on with my new diet and exercise. I don't want to be on more medication forever. What are the side effects?'

'They can make you feel sick and your muscles hurt, head-aches and the usual side effects expected with strong medication.' – And she says this without even flinching, without acknowledging for a second what this would mean to me.

'I'll see if better diet can fix it. Even the indents from scars on my legs, caused by the boils I contracted on becoming diabetic, and first injecting, have started to finally heal-up like they should have, on this diet.'

'OK, well I'll book you in for another three months, if it's not down by then,' nod of, you will do what you're told, 'We are very strict about *persons with diabetes* taking them.'

I just look at her and laugh to myself, I mean for fucks sake I'm thirty-two years old, any intention for better or worse of playing strict is going to have to include a corset, stilettos and her holding a whip. And that's not even a rubber Nurse's uniform. What really gets me though is the qualified intention to help. But qualified by whom? No questioning of their own methods or practice, just a pride in being able to hand out doses of strong drugs and intolerable side effects with zero thought given to any alternative or the impact this will cause to the patient's life. Paying no attention to my notes stating I've lost weight already and I'm clearly on the mend. Don't get me wrong, if in the long term I do have an issue with cholesterol, which I don't, I shall be appreciative and accepting of long term discomfort in return for watching my kids grow up. But even so, I would want that handed down to me by a Heart Expert. Not a Diabetes Nurse who clearly does not understand diabetes and has yet to get back to me with a functioning blood sugar test monitor.

...

Far from the only one; advice presented in afterthought, divulged, though often with such confusion and lack of context, never mind incompetence and danger, it was never properly administered. The friendly nudges in the right direction going so against the grain of everything I had been taught, there was no room for comprehension only dismissal.

'This appointment was made for me by your Diabetes Nurse Practitioner, over concerns she has over my prolonged cold with respect to diabetes, and you have prescribed to me Vitamin C tablets filled with so much sugar, it reads on the leaflet, "*Not suitable for people having trouble digesting sugar.*" – Awesome work.'

Diabetes Clinic appointments, changing date in a flurry till I lose track: resulting in nasty letters saying I have been signed out from their care. And this seems reasonable?

Diabetes Friendly Turkish Delight; got the skids and high sugar. Yay!

Flu jabs, from now on, get the hell away from me.

Pneumonia vaccine? Only poor health care put a healthy young man in the path of such an old-farts alert.

Social Science mandatory injections enlisted and cancelled by the Government on the whim of poor advice and Public Relations debacle, deciding with no further notice that it was not so important after all. So what exactly have you filled me with?

'You need to give yourself a good shake,' said the spinster I worked with behind the bar; thirty going on dead with three cats. How dare I be tired in her presence? – A good shake, shall I mix that with elderflower?

'All that natural sugar in milk can't be doing you any good Paul,' says Bill, in his unconscionable tight fitting t-shirt; biceps bursting out the workplace kitchen; as I fill up my bowl of *Weetabix* to the brim, counting them out as two carb units each. I take heed with a pinch of salt, as milk being firstly natural sugar and secondly low in sugar content, before topping up to the brim with more milk my half-filled pint mug of digital filter coffee; knocking sugar levels through the roof, unable to put two and two together.

Personal Trainer at the gym, 'Yeah we have been learning on and taught to instruct diabetes patients. You need to stop eating carbs and potatoes. Not to have any sugar when you work out.' – Five foot of ginger freckled Australian nodding to the *Twix* bar in my hand. 'Amanda, if I gave up eating complicated carbs and never had this sugar to top me up, I'd fall into a coma mid workout. You can't just tell people to stop eating, when they are on prescribed doses of medication.' 'Oh, I've been doing it all week. Is it really bad?'

Contact lens appointment; the lady advises with a straight face, 'Do not take these out and clean them with your tongue, no matter how dry and uncomfortable they feel.' 'You're kidding: people actually do that?' 'Yes it's very dangerous; the best thing you can do instead is place a warm damp tea towel over your eyelids at night, this will help to keep open the glands.'

Speaking with my GP's stand in, 'He sent me to see a Specialist, who told me I was a *matter of urgency*. He then called in his Boss who further instructed I was *top priority* for fear of *imminent blindness!* He then took two weeks to even send out the request to the Eye Specialists to get me onto their waiting list. I've been left worried sick in fear that my eye sight could deteriorate to blindness at any moment.' And she replies, 'People do have varying definitions of urgency.'

Went for a hearing examination; diabetes check box on the *form to fill out*. Friendly Expert Hearing Aid Dispenser man (that was his job title), advises with an air of authority on how type two diabetics don't have any issues with hearing loss, as, 'They only get low sugar, though type one's often have an excess of sugar built up in their ear canals.' Next he is going to tell me this is where sugar cubes come from. – In actual fact it concurs that Natasha only starts conversations when on a different floor of the house with a hair dryer in her hand. – 'What?'

Went for a massage day at the spa, again with ticking the diabetes box; this lady will only give me a gentle rub down as, 'A proper massage will hurt diabetic patients.' 'It's okay; I'll just have a full back massage. You don't have to worry about my diabetes.' 'Oh well, I

361

know this to be true, I have been a masseur for four years now.' I give up. – You fucking rub backs for a living, but I'm not saying that out loud.

Damp proofing specialist having surgery in his eyes every six to eight months, caused by poor diabetes control, and the telephone engineer who visited; half his stomach removed and a bag inserted to help reduce excess weight and take the strain off of his type two diabetes. But he put it all back on in no time and now has type one diabetes: though both of them still completely unwilling to give up eating bread! – Some people just don't want help.

Living in denial of the detrimental effects of our condition; over and over pushing near escape to the backs of our minds through want of being normal. To some extent we are all guilty, but in truth, only with a rightful understanding can we accept a just responsibility. – Please don't just have some more insulin.

Then again, this is coming from a guy who sat at the window in *Starbucks* and watched a teenage boy drink carton after carton of cranberry juice; obviously trying to quench an undiagnosed thirst, and moments away from collapsing on his way home. You know how in a film when you see a horse fall, and you know it's a stunt horse and you know it's going to be fine, but it still makes you feel sad? It was a lot like that; I really should have stood up and done something to help.

It's not about guilt, but there has got to be a point when saying, "*Its not my fault.*" is not enough.

And finally, "*Cautious optimism is how we choose to approach this condition.*" – Wonderful Australian man at *London Medical*.

# My Yin is all over the place

A nine-hour flight and only up a couple of times; cool in the cabin, it never occurred to us to bring shorts for the landing. Thirty-four degrees and a layer of moisture bleeding through the shirt I was hoping would get me a free upgrade. Double check insulin stored in the '*Spider-Man*' lunch box with ice packs (makeshift *cool-box*) is doing fine and climb aboard a little red whippersnapper seaplane to our Maldivian Paradise.

'Breathe in for the body, out for the mind.' he speaks meaningfully; breeze circulates as we transition into the next pose, turquoise waves wash gently onto a perimeter of island sand. Every muscle in my body awakening in harmony with my new diet, discovering an inner calm further illuminated by its effects on my diabetes. A heightened awareness acquired I never thought possible.

Balancing your mind, your spirit, your Chi, however you come to define inner self-equilibrium. My blood sugar will not falter with this heightened sense of being; one's complete removal from the Western World and its many abstract accomplishments. I can see clearly now that insulin is a little miracle not to be abused. When mixed with the right balance of diet and exercise, it allows my body and mind a level of health unfettered.

Eggs, sunny side up, got to be. Bacon strips, 'Mmm,' for breakfast and its another glorious day. White sands meeting aqua going on forever, more beautiful than maybe I thought the Earth could be. Open-air shower, straw hat and shorts: sandy walkways through lush vegetation, 'AHH. BIG LIZARD MIGHT EAT ME!' wooden decking leading to our table, and pouring black filter coffee, 'Yawn. Aww so relaxed I could fall over,' the gist of things.

'Two weeks more of this to go, I don't know how I'll handle it.' – Almost me.

'Was I right to book in for the fortnight instead of only ten days?' – What's left of Tash.

'Absolutely. I had no idea the world would be this good,' feet caressing sand, 'This paradise is exactly as living in a *Bounty* commercial. So glad we came; my brain can hardly take in that this is the same planet.'

'You made it here.' 'I think I did. You brought me here. Thank you... Look a baby shark. I can't believe how far in they swim.'

'And the Sea Turtles are enormous; we need to find some without going too deep in the water.'

'Can you tell we're not from around here?'

'Ha. Because they think I'm a giant...Do Stingrays sting?'

'I don't know but Rab Crowlin's Goldfish lived till it was eleven.'

'How?'

'His dad replaced it every time he had to flush it and he couldn't tell the difference. Sorry, my head is so relaxed for once it's full of gibberish.'

'Please don't be sorry. I brought you here because you deserve to relax.'

Shoreline stroll holding hands, mustn't get any closer, feet in the water we paddle our first few steps into warm sea, little angel fish dancing all around my ankles, 'Ahhh, whit's that? Fish are freakin me out.' Huge smile, 'You're an idiot!' Jump up and down, take some photographs, say, 'Hi,' to a few now familiar faces. Passing near our abode, 'Those birds get so close. They are so cute, what are they?' 'Little Maldivian Pigeons?' Walk on by the Fish Grill Bar, 'Come back here tonight?' 'Sounds a perfect plan, we can look up at the stars.'

Standing on our head following sunrise and an attempt at running along the beach, splashing, giggles and falling over each other most of the way; stop to hold hands, looking out over the ocean is total all-encompassing calm.

*Indian Ayurvedic Body Type* following omelettes for breakfast, the man looks at my tongue and tells me I have diabetes; course of massage focused on my shins to engage the pancreas as prescribed in an ancient diagram and I am floating all the way. Red powdered bark, 'For diabetes,' handed over in a jar. Our Yoga teacher comes over to wish us well and explanation that in its original setting, the contents of this jar would be a cup carved from the trunk of red husk filled with rain each evening. The water turning red by morning and a remedy created to deal with diabetes. I've to drink it as tea, have far less insulin.

Bottled water by the hour and a dunk to cool down; pasty Germans chain-smoking by the bar submerged within the infinity pool, backs to the horizon. 'Bit of a budgie smuggling contest on this island Tash, are you loving it?' 'Why is it always fat bald men who insist on wearing bright orange trunks?' 'Perverts!' looking away as I whisper because they look almost as hard as their fluorescent wrinkly wives.

Missed Yoga this morning, were sound asleep.

Half past ten in the morning at a push and flashing wrist bands as *golden keys* cutting circulation from the wrist, the English contingent drowning in off-brand spirits they wouldn't even consider purchasing back home, determined to get their money's worth. Medieval diets and deep red sun burnt tattoos look in agony but nice as pie, 'We come here every year...Is that to test sugar? All my family have diabetes.' – I'm counting down from five in my head. Tash prods, 'You need more sun cream,' twisting me about and lifting my arms to apply then spinning me round to get at my nose like a three year old as I continue conversation. 'You got here a week late because of the volcano? That's heart breaking. We're hoping it kicks off so we can stay forever and ever.' Someone spots the Fruit Bats flapping from branch to tree overhead, 'AHH I'm frightened of bats,' Tash splashes everyone in the face and into their drinks to get past and hide. 'We're more city dwellers you and I Natasha, do you think? Are you ever coming back out?' Still cowering behind me, 'But they are huge orange furry things.' We climb out of the pool together, 'Ah ah ah oooh owww hot hot hot oww oww,' over tiles to reach our flip-flops left over by empty sun beds. At least we made the Germans raise a smile.

...

'I can barely lift my head from the table. I'm so rested,' exhales Natasha. 'You need to get up and pick your own food. I waved over to Chef on my way in; I'll be eating something special soon... AHH ANTS!' a little crowd of them gathered over a piece of dropped fruit by my ankle, 'Do they eat you?' 'I don't think so, they are eating fruit.'

'Think I saw it happen once in a film. Are we going for a massage after this?' 'Yeah.' 'How is your book?' 'I don't know, I've been reading the same chapter for four days.'

Over lunch the following day, 'What if it rains and the tide comes in and the wind makes a big wave take over the island and we get eaten by fish?' 'It's not going to happen. This island has been here for a thousand years.' 'I hope not, I hate getting wet feet.' 'You are such a *'Muppet'.*'

Another day another lunch, 'I never want to go home,' someone is contemplating becoming a refuge. 'Still can't believe we're here,' she starts squeezing and shaking my hand over the table, playful like a toddler, 'I can't even believe this place exists. I love you.' 'I love you too puppy. Just try to relax, you made it.' 'On a different note, can you believe she tells me her eyes are fine? How many years have I worried sick about her eyes, getting Nuns to pray on flights and everything? *"Odd shaped nerve ending. Gets a bit dry. Got eye-drops for them."* Unbelievable, and she's known for years; waits until I bring it up to tell her I'm fine, to tell me her eyes are fine. I just said all that without swearing, I must be calm.'

Fish for lunch, Chef is delighted to assist in personally preparing all three meals a day in meeting with *all-inclusive* dietary requirements, then he pushes a step further, 'You are having *Bitter Gourd* yes? *Indonesian Bitter Gourd?*' 'Oh this sounds fancy, what is that?' I'm getting excited, then onto an explanation. 'This is what we use and people on the surrounding islands when no insulin.' 'So to resolve diabetes?' I'm thinking to myself, I don't believe in homeopathic remedies, but around here they *have to be* nothing short of wise decision and functioning solution. 'I will prepare for you with dinner.' 'Cool. Thank you Sir.' 'Less insulin,' big smile of instruction. 'Okay.'

It's grey-green, everyone else is having chicken curry and I'm handed a cup of something the same colour as my eyes but the mucky texture of muck, sludge extract and plant things; appropriately mixed together but not really mixing together at the same time. 'You want me to drink this?' respectful but please no. 'Yes, this is good for reducing sugar,' all knowing nod. Wink, and down the hatch in one; wasn't so bad; face of smelling someone else's fart in a lift. Smile then he toddles off, not even bothering to ask how it tasted. 'So what happens now?' I ponder to Tash. 'What do you think was in it?' 'I have no idea, assuming it's a local plant, which reduces blood sugar. Is that all I'm having? Am I not getting fed now?' concerned smirk. 'How much less insulin did you have?' 'Eh, a little bit...' and a couple of sad minutes pass before I spot Chef winding his way back through tables returning with a plate. 'Can I ask, what was in it?' Chef smiles even brighter, 'It does not taste so good, it is from the root of bitter melon,' then disappears back into the kitchen because he can see in the background someone is doing something he isn't happy with. 'Oh spicy meat, glad I'm not having cheapo curry,' sticking my tongue out, 'You can still have pudding Natasha, I won't cry. You are on holiday.' 'Did you see all the cakes?' grin. 'HA.' 'I nearly ate all the cakes! If I wasn't diabetic, I'd be a fat bastard... Ohhh I need to go to the toilet NOW!'

Hell for leather for three hours, reading comic books on the pan.

...

Night-fishing on calm surface; wooden construction, thin, red paint and a little lawnmower engine on the back: pretty to look at provided you take your mind off, 'There are sharks beneath us.' Sun is settling pink through cobalt and the darker blue water is where it's gotten deep, right where we are. 'Shut up Paul you are freaking yourself

368

out.' Bucket of fish bits handed out and skewered onto hooks held over rocking edge, 'I've caught something. No, I'm stuck on a stone. I've caught something. No, I'm stuck on a stone. I've caught something.' Girl behind us also shrieking, her boyfriend has caught something. 'No, I've caught your boyfriend. I've caught something. No way, I've caught a Puffer Fish! I can't eat it? No don't put it in the bucket, put it back in the ocean.' Basking in my own glory, 'Hey Natasha, I caught a Pufferfish; I'm going to go on about this forever.'

Two minutes pass, 'I'm hungry. I need the toilet.' 'Hold it in.' 'Thanks for your support.' Clasped hands and no sign of land, 'Seriously, I need to go to the toilet, that stuff is cleansing my insides, I can feel it scraping a layer every time I go and I need to go now.' 'Tough.' Taking my mind off the toilet, 'This thing sinks and not a whitey on board is making it to shore; fish with heart attacks from feeding on us. Look at us though, Western tourists, who would out-swim the sharks if this sunk? Not us. Look at the locals, pure health. How lean and muscular not being able to afford living on crisps and *Cola* all day, faith forbidding alcohol; you can see the point, it's got to be for the best. Although to be fair, there are people up and down Glasgow with darker tans than that.' 'Shut up.' 'I still need to pee and poop.'

Barbecued prawns and a cheeky Piña colada under silken maroon drapes, feet back combing sand and looking off into lightning bolts in the distance, 'Rainy season starts tomorrow,' sighs Tash. 'Still praying that Icelandic volcano kicks off and we need to stay here for another month?' 'Do you think it will? They would need to keep us here and feed us!' 'I could work here for free, it would be worth it.' 'Me too; how are you getting on with those cocktails?' 'These are the only time I've had to take more than a quarter of my insulin dose with all that Arrivederci medicine in me. And I'm only on two injections a day in the first place.' 'Do you think it's working then?' 'Yeah, I do. Do you

369

think it's all Hocus Pocus medicine? It seems to be working more than a little bit. A lot more than a little bit. How else can people out here without access to modern medicine survive with diabetes? Although I don't think I'd ever have gotten ill if I'd been born out here.' But I'm damned if I'm going to risk taking it through customs.

I never want to go home…It's nice, just for a while, not forever but for a while to turn off and not think about other people's problems.

…

I've got the skids, and coming home to *twenty-four* hour news is like having a guy with a, "*The end of the world is nigh*," placard sitting on my sofa. Done pestering single mothers, the Government are moving toward the impact *diabetes* is causing on society, unable to distinguish our condition from the sufferer. "*Zombie apocalypse… thirty-five percent of all National Health Service budget to be spent on diabetes by two thousand and thirty five…MP twoddle requests that all obese type two diabetics pay for their own medication.*" 'Boo!' "*…National figures published today show diabetes numbers are booming.*" Cut to unimaginative imagery of sugar cubes, syringes, fat people with faces covered by black squares walking down the street but you can still tell who they are and graphs without numbers on. "*Are they coming up out of the floorboards to steal food from your plate? You won't be able to put shoes on your children's feet because diabetes will either eat your kids or the elderly will claim all your benefits,*" up the tempo, "*Chances of seeing a Health Practitioner in times-of-crisis are slim; diabetes is overburdening the state; the elderly refusing to keel over.*" – State? We live in the United Kingdom. Times-of-crisis? Are we descending into Armageddon? Are we heeding, "*Death to the apocalyptic napalm city.*" – Have I missed something or do these people just really not want me to turn the channel? "*Prime Time Zombies in the day time?*"

'Diabetics and Pensioners, what a bunch of bastards,' I tell myself. A profoundly negative media reminding us who we are; never more than six feet away from a rat, a sex slave, a diabetic about to take everything you have, a Pensioner who just won't kark it and a *Coca-Cola* in this country. Enough of this!

Open the paper, *"Johnnie's mum's coming to terms with her teenage sons diabetes,"* image of his blood sugar monitor is reading "301" so can only presume he is dead as I'm reading this, or some journalist has identified a new buzz word to target an *as a mother* article around. Get some shows on the go to keep me occupied, and here we go; *Sherlock Holmes* has managed to dismiss a suspect based on the culprits type two diabetic inability to open a jar; hence he couldn't possibly have hurled the murder weapon? Clearly they never interviewed him with high sugar. And now some melodrama has a kidnapped diabetic child standing in for a time bomb; if she doesn't have her insulin in time... what she will probably piss herself? Right, put down my *iPhone*, get off the pan; we are moving house again tomorrow.

Perks of living back in a fairly large town; alternative therapies; Yoga classes; Chinese Herbal Medicine – distilled through a millennia of knowledge, only tarnished by a love of Karaoke and a pong-shong for Shark-Fin-soup; Chanting; Detox Meal-Deals, you name it we got it. But I'd rather, now my head is clear, detox from those people who only ever call when they want to make themselves feel better by bringing me down with them. 'Why aren't you drinking?' 'Not coming to the pub?' 'That's not cool man.' 'Yoga?' 'I'm not meeting up for breakfast. I'll be drinking till three. I'll be in bed hung-over.' 'What's wrong with you?' followed by a Friday night text, *"At the Spanish Bar, friends down from Glasgow but never invited you because you wouldn't like it."* Because I'm an adult and I'm happy and I don't need to escape from life; quick change of mobile number and my world is a clown free zone.

Chances of duplicating Maldivian alternative therapies back home? *Wii Fit Yoga* takes the edge off and it's nice to see my avatar slimming down to perfect Body Mass Index from the fat little tosser he was before. The scales have even stopped groaning when I step on them, giving me further confidence to join the local sports-centre. Downward Facing Dog and Sun Salutation three mornings a week helps cleanse my system; core strength invaluable, helping with what had become for me a *hypo shame* in having to ask for help. And the positive roll over effects to diabetes has reached a plateau of living on a single injection per day, night-time insulin only. Pop out to the fashionable Herbal Therapy store, over the road from, *"Each as much as you possibly can for £5 Cantonese cuisine."* When enquiring for *Indonesian Bitter Gourd* a man is called out from the back room to assist and convince, 'The essence of *Bitter Gourd*,' as he so uncomfortably puts it. 'Does it contain the root of *Bitter Gourd*?' 'Not so much, it is more the essence of.' 'But what is actually in it?' Smiles instead of answering, dressed in all whites, in the essence of a medical man. 'That white plastic tub in your hand; what are the ingredients? What is the chemical composition?' 'As I said, it's not so much the substance; it's more the essence of.' 'So seventeen pounds for nothing I want then. Can I make payment by essence of money?' What a cock, I'll try the local Chinese store for acupuncture and wacky pills next. *Bupa* aren't interested.

# Living with a machine

On one of my many trips as a lad to see Sister Shepherd I asked, "Don't we just need a machine that measures your blood sugar and gives you the correct dosage of insulin throughout the day?" That seemed the obvious solution. They looked at me as if I was talking about space ships. Seventeen years on and two billion pounds later, we now have the artificial pancreas.

...

Have placed my claim on Payment Protection Insurance (PPI), those bastards at the Bank have been proven thieves in their excessive desire and governance has pushed them to refund the aggrieved, plus I want my thirty-two pounds back for that packet of couscous they gave me a charge for. Foreseeing a potential payback, and although they are staying shtum on the amount, I calculate a sum in total equal to the potential purchase of said artificial pancreas; pondering what I would be giving away in return.

The very purpose of an always attached, always switched on, twenty-four/seven artificial pancreas is not functionality meets necessity, but the perfect marriage of product development and marketing. Finding a problem three hundred and fifty million people should not have, then *leasing* a solution, further keeping them off balance. An oversold amenity for every child; I mean, what is the point if you are feeding them the wrong types of food and over compensating with insulin in the first place? – Though I understand this to be a very personal judgment call. Giving in, giving up on self-knowledge; handing over power; human nature rendered redundant, passed over for a processor to the behest and profitability of majority shareholders. Maybe it's not the same for you, I'm sure it's different for us all, but for me it's a convenience gone too far. At which point does a machine instil a confidence in independence? It never will: acting instead as another man made barrier between rightful understanding and just responsibility.

Pancreatic transplant; dead persons bits revitalising us sounds a wonderful plan but *immunosuppressant's* to stop the body rejecting the organ are more harmful than diabetes in itself, and prohibitive up-front costs moving our *stock* from black into the red, plus there would be a huge increase in *assisted* donors. Stem cell implants, beta cell transplantation to *cure* diabetes? Early doors in dangerous clinical trials stages: always another fifteen years or so to get it right? – Clinical trials for *once-a-week* insulin injections, hopefully not to be sidelined. The future of diabetic medicine is not a peripheral induced hypo when the microwave turns on, but I can see it happening.

...

Anything has got to be better than syncing my blood sugar monitor test readings to a mobile phone, and expecting it to upload wirelessly and successfully via *cloud services* to an I.T illiterate General Practitioner; further expecting the poor bastard to articulate a solution based on these, meta data, time stamps and statistics. Hasn't he got enough on his plate with near two-thousand patients at a rate of around forty per day? The Government is already turning our GP's into Accountants and now Pharmaceutical Industries wish to bestow upon them externally, promoting from *direct point-of-sale* to setting them up as boffins. When have I ever seen my Doctor not struggle to print off a prescription? I'm already preparing for those immortal words, 'Balance your sugars and have some more insulin. I will arrange for you to visit the Diabetes Specialist Nurse in a few weeks' time.' – Better off using my blood sugar test monitor results to predict *Lottery* numbers.

It is *again* diabetes intervention going in the wrong direction, offering no significant benefit to the sufferer. How many blood sugar test products have I been through, by how many brands? How many more competing products have I seen on store shelves? And taking into account the nature of software with its countless updates; it's complicated enough to keep track of my shit as it is. Now the option for the future, all this information, stored and uploaded to *cloud services* or downloaded directly to USB keys before access is granted at various levels to my Doctor, my next of kin, diabetic friends on Social Media and medical insurers (alarm bells). Like they are going to know what to do with it?

No way. It's back to keeping a diary of every time you masturbate and handing this over with your urine sample; the Doctor's not going to get you laid; only you are fucking yourself. – Of course you could go private. The only ones to benefit from us going bionic is the *Diabetes Industry*, sell, sell, and sell again; a new product every fifteen years, we are subject to a drip feeding of help whilst indirectly chasing our tails: never truly educated, no rightful understanding, we are divided and fall an additional step from *just (read: non profitable) responsibility*. Insurance industries will love these though, when determining through much filtered glasses; *removing real world fluctuations*; that on assessing health data based over a timeline and defined objective curve, that we did not control our sugar levels sufficiently. We might only be in for a sprained ankle: payment declined.

...

Dr Joseph Lister meets a modern world of Nanotechnology; I foresee a mouthwash secreting insulin based on digesting sugar analysis; perfect measures to rinse and repeat every twenty-four hours.

# When we rule the world

Think I'm doing well not hankering after junk food till another *Domino's* leaflet falls through my letterbox. I put the *Papa Johns* leaflet straight in the bin. I find myself going on-line and ordering from the full menu selection; half Hawaiian, half Pepperoni, chicken wings, coleslaw, *Ben & Jerry's Chocolate Fudge Brownie* and *Caramel Chew Chew* ice cream, *Diet-Coke* for now, normal *Cola* in case I have a hypo during the week, by the time this wears off. Insert voucher code to get my twenty-five percent discount, all the way down to pressing the order button. Then I stop, close the browser window and head downstairs to make myself an omelette, patting myself on the back for preventing myself going blind.

*Starbucks* are the worst though, those limited edition *Christmas, Gingerbread Lattes* are almost worth losing a toe for. Maybe a small one? Venti is only forty pence more, 'Venti Black Americano please?' 'Space for milk?' You are making me sick with marketing tripe, – you want my name and email for a cup of personalised coffee, 'Seriously?'

Better diabetic social conditions: how about a blood sugar test monitor that takes into consideration the lifestyle requirements of the *everyday diabetic*; including our sleeping partners. Soft glow display, so as not to wake up the house, and reading to two decimal places: resting inside a cradle to charge, with pot for used test strips for my convenience. – Analogue insulin results delivered in digital quantities, I just want it to shut the fuck up! Most important of all: use of standard (read: cheap) test strips, which will not be superseded periodically on the day I run out. In fact, make the whole thing truly backwards compatible by using off the shelf components, and have the *NHS* order them in their millions as a patent free standard solution. Don't worry about complicated ketones; I'm more than happy to piss on a stick for now.

Fifty-three million diabetics in Europe alone and all we are offered in public is *Diet-Coke*. They will know when the diabetic uprising occurs, when the cake shops burn and *Fanta Zero* pours from every tap. Speaking of which, three hundred and fifty million diabetics world-wide, times what we spend each year on self-help solutions in all their guises, let's just *chip-in* twenty pounds each and buy our own Diabetic Pharma Inc. – Feel that? That was the quake of *the man* shitting himself.

# You thought the plague was bad; wait till you try the tiramisu

Three million diabetics in England alone, there must be five people in this bar thinking, 'Will I have the *Diet-Coke*, the *Diet-Coke* or the *Diet-Coke*?' shortly before giving in to thoughts of, 'Sod it. I'll have a beer and a burger, and while I'm at it may as well have the tiramisu.' But how did we get here, why do we make the jump so easily from being careful to being moderate, through to, 'Oh I'll just have anything and jack myself up full of insulin. It'll do me no harm?'

Why is it that all other medicines are prescribed in minimal quantity to maximum effect ratios whereas insulin is prescribed, 'Here help yourself?' You wouldn't encourage a chain-smoker to carry on and just have more chemo. Again, we are back to this common misconception of insulin as a harmless hormone overcome by simply having more sugar, leaving the diabetic to get on with the sugar fluctuations.

...

Post nineteen eighties, we are the first generation of diabetics with a proficient opportunity to keep our blood sugars level, through a combination of both long and fast acting *analogue* insulin injections supported by clear dietary requirement. – Those Scientists knew exactly what they were doing. But things needed to be more profitable. – No one really knows in what condition our collective bodies will form, following on from the dreaded fifteen years insulin dependency time bomb, never mind beyond the age of sixty; rendering conventional wisdom based primarily on previous generational National Census (read: almost unavoidable death) completely invalid.

Yet each and all of our influencers still manage to define unique conclusions; those self-same gratifying Mentors, Celebrity Chefs, Consultants, Dieticians, HR hacks and low grade smart phone programmers offering up varying propositions of treatment, whilst feeding from the very same pool of inaccurate information not derived from any real time – human being analysis. They can only be giving half the picture (unenviable solutions).

So derailed is this *Diabetes Industry* in decision making, as to be unable to agree on even the most basic of fundamentals dictating the paths of our lives, such as: Which are the best injection sites? When is it appropriate to have additional insulin? What are level blood sugars, 4 -8? 5.3 - 6.9? Are 9s OK? Can we get away with 9? What should and what shouldn't we eat? Can you really fire me for having attended the Diabetes Clinic?

This is where the tell-tale signs are blown out of the water and we realise from an intimate perspective, that the vast majority of people, of whom this *Diabetes Industry* comprise, do not actually have diabetes let alone understand life as a diabetic on any real level, yet come to define the crux of our lives; enabled only by a complete lack of governance.

The ones we hope for when dreaming of a better future; the '*Dr House M.D's*,' highly skilled at *making the world a better place*; ingenious medical minds always on the cusp of a cure. We don't have them. Those great minds are few and far between, and busy elsewhere, swatting malaria, while we're stuck here in the doldrums with our *Diabetes Experts*. You know the ones you meet in every Diabetes Ward, the Head Consultant Expert, the one at the forefront in a field, somewhere, of diabetes medicine, 'The finest mind in research and development,' well that's what he tells the Nurses. We've simply got the numpties' who think they know about diabetes in the same way that all big sisters think they know how to cut their little brother's hair.

For members of the medical profession, the study of diabetes is very rarely a calling. In general medical circles diabetes is treated merely as a development opportunity, a fashion, a new department in which to get involved with its rapidly expanding patient list and inevitable allocation of funding. For everyone else this *Diabetes Industry* has grown to become an *everyman for himself* boon to the global economy and in the worst cases it's a cash cow. – Ghost-writers of sugar free kid's books, if my kids speak like you I'll be sending them off to boarding school at '*Dawson's Creek*'. – Just for my thoughts, if I was a bastard and I had money (hopefully not too long now) I'd invest it all in fast food and pharmaceuticals.

Medical Politics and Global Corporate Finance further intrude to undermine a true, valued solution, as Governmental and Private Institutions decline to share resource or take leadership from one another. The result, insurmountable time and energy; those tens of thousands of years combined medical knowledge wasted as competing factions diagnose busily in circles, purporting to train and sell each other *Diabetes Solutions*, whilst drawing ever more opportunistic profit growth forecasts on boardroom walls or pessimistic declining red lines in health care reform plans. Depending on which side you're on.

A Diabetes Industries' self-fulfilling prophecy does not wish us well; a position easily deniable through global governmental refusal of funding for research and development grants into new medicine. Sellers of shovels in times of a gold rush, *Avandia*, heart attacks? *Rezulin*, liver failure? Purveyors of poison and snake oil oddly thrive in times of desperation. Has the hard sell of insulin really got something to do with reduced patent exclusivity; surmounting pressure to claw back development funding? Hasn't the patent on insulin and blood sugar test monitors run out already? Then why still so expensive when surely attractive as white label service to anybody with a lab coat and license to replicate medicine? And we are back to marketing and a lack of true governance, given in to unhealthy reliance and building upon the informative black hole. Diabetics pimped out in there millions: the best interests of over a third of a billion people swept under the carpet.

We speak now of being the financial ninety-nine percent and history tells us diseases past were considered great equalisers amongst men; forsaking any right of status or means of wealth. In this respect, diabetes is unique; a disease brewing in the genetics of the unqualified, waiting on the everyday people's diet; junk and snacks combined with stress to tip it over; left to the ignorant to treat, hand in hand with the greedy. That tiramisu, social conformity has led us to become our own worst enemies.

We are a sensitive market, being devoured by vultures, a commodity more lucrative than the illegal drugs trade of heroin or cocaine. A resource being mined for all our worth, and we're worthless when we get well. Eventually, as proven through tobacco and alcohol, trust will crumble as the number of diabetics' increases to critical mass and tax gains from sales of what got us there over cheap-solutions no longer top the cost to society in terms of health care and lost man-hours. The question is whether a taxation and condemnation of harmful foods will follow or precede the diabetic having to pay the unrealistic cost of medical expense.

Financially viable but where are the educated decision makers?

# Type three diabetes

It's easy to point and laugh, point at the fat family walking past, 'Fat bastards way fat wains, – and giggle. No wonder their children are fat, look at the parents eatin massive *Grab Bags* a crisps and drinkin full fat *Cola*. Fat fucks; it's no fair on the children but is it? They're the ones going to be diabetic by the time the dah dies aye a heart attack. Fat fudge eating bastards; how do they even shag each other? It must be disgusting. Probably stop haulf way through licking *Sprite* oaf each other for a *Mars Bar*, "I canny help it. It's ma glands, it's ma glands," as they shove it in. Fried breakfast and no exercise, *KFC* eating chubby-chasers, they mustn'y give a shit aboot their children.'

...

*Get the shopping in then pick up my boy. "KFC Nacho Stackers, Walkers Deep Ridged Crisps, McCain Drive Through Oven Chips," these signposts everywhere drivin me nuts. Quick, duck into the shop before I end up in McDonalds again. Ninety-nine pence Arctic Roll, three hundred percent extra free bright pink Cherry Aid; these family size packs of chocolate bars, that's my second month's supply this week. These multi-buy crisps work out cheaper than three individual bags. Chicken Tikka Lasagna; oh that's getting me wet just lookin at it. – Fed up eating at home all of the time by myself though and freezing ma baws aff standing beside these fridge-freezers. Local café or restaurant instead?*

*Sounds a bit cheeky. Push the boat out a bit? Gee that a go.*

*Walk up the road, "Buffet, as much as you can eat for £6. As many trips to the pasta bar as you can manage with your XXXXL cheese pizza and garlic cheese bread. Remember kids eat for free." Remember? I a remember; Brittany loved this place. I still expect to see her in the kitchen every time, putting out the plates, waiting own the delivery boy on his scooter. Always calling him oot when it's pissing doon way rain; funny as fuck. Ah pure miss her so much. Right, pull my pish together, get the menu on the go. Fancy something different, the steak or a fish; eating pizzas every night, it's no good. 'How much is that?' Fuck me; I canny even afford to look at that page own the menu on a single parent's income. I'll stick to the Specials Board offerings for normal people. Pizza it is.*

*It's not happening; back to the Shopping Centre instead, football own the telly so a case aye beer is cheaper than four bottles and I'll get the barbecue burgers and sausages in, plus a dozen types aye breed rolls in case the neighbours come over and make friends like they do own the adverts. Pair of cheeseburgers, Jaffa Cakes, and Quality Street; pure quality man; they cherries look crackin, aww deep and red, the kids would love thame but who can afford four pounds fir a punnet? Cherry tarts, how slutty. Ahh Cherry Bakewells, six for a pound: dirty and slutty. Same way these cheap ice creams; ice cream, like blow-jobs, there's no such thing as a bad one. Those double loyalty points will come in handy with Barack growing out of his tracksuit bottoms faster than he is being bullied out of class. Jeans no longer come in his size, till he turns twelve. Puppy fat av'e telt him; like his dah. I.*

*Take my boy to the Doctors on his teacher's advice, but he's just big for his age like me and we thought it was good he is eating up all his school dinners? Tripping over five year olds still in prams and fifty year olds parking mobility scooters; bloody methadone addicts outnumbering the "don't smoke" stickers, till wee Tracy finally waves us on through tay the stuck up bitch, 'Come in and take a seat.' as if she has never seen us before. 'Blood sugar has come back "7.2"* that is borderline type two diabetes in a child; better start him on these tablets to rein him in before it's too late, and a course of Statins to keep his heart big and strong like his father's. Don't want young Barack being taken by the Colonel like his dear mother or being whisked away by Ronald for that matter now do we?' – Speaking in code awe aye the time, the boy is overweight not stupid. 'Is he staying active?' 'I, he is own that phone aww aye the time, its pure crackin.' 'And how is Michelle?' 'Aw Michelle is doin great thanks, they goat her own that Social Networking at school, great for her to be speaking with kids her own weight. And next week they are doin that Guitar Hero; well after the school sold oaff they playing fields to the Property Developers; it's good fir thame to hiv something else tay day, and tay be honest the kids much prefer it. Hiv you seen thame go at it? Aww they get all caught up, singing along like mental, it's great fir their asthma.' 'And how about you? Anti-depressants going okay? How are your varicose veins? Blood pressure running high? Anxiety? Your ulcers? I will write you up another sick note for the Welfare people? Two months may not be enough; I'll put you down for six: gives you plenty of time. Could do with buttons on this keyboard just for anti-depressants and insulin, would save me lots of time.' – Always struggling to fill out and print auf a repeat prescription. Someone should teach her how tay use that thing. 'And how is your diet may I enquire?' 'I, been workin hard tay follow they celebrity cook books you recommended me. Piyin the extra fir they microwave diet foods way the logos own. I even goat a pair aye they trainers that firm up yer bum when yeh walk. An av'e been lookin intay that D.A.F.T.E.Y course own the Internet at the Library.' – Looking up to see the Good Doctor has lost all interest, ushered us back out of the door with a glance up. Was just aboot tay tell her aboot the evening walks way the pedometers we goat free in they giant chocolate honey caramel coated cereal packets; we've all three of us goat wan each; it's pure magic. Trust the Good Doctor must have urgent business to attend to, and tay be fair she might be a bit jealous because she is nearly the same size as me now. Just relieved my children are in good hands. Certainly no made tay feel am just a number they collect a monthly income fir, fir jist for hivin us own their books.

...

Believe it or not, it used to be hard to get diabetes.

# Evolve

Heartburn like no other in the middle of the night, with the accompanying blood sugar of fifteen; have insulin, try to sleep it off. Assure Natasha in the morning, 'I'm alright,' and she descends to work. Sugar is still hovering between fifteen and sixteen, now vomiting up stomach bile and getting dizzy, telling myself not to panic. Ketoacidosis it has to be. Can't find a Doctor to see me, nor receive a call back to arrange confirmation of my suspicion. Certainly don't want to waste the time of an ambulance, but now I'm hazardously stepping around, guts on fire and *NHS Direct* have just instructed me they can't help: it's the same with the nine-nine-nine. Emergency Services Operator making clear she can't be wasting their time on me. Now following I don't know how much convincing, certainly she went quiet on her end at least twice, 'When will the ambulance get here?' 'Within an hour with no blue lights.' Thank God the Paramedics dismiss her instruction and are at the door quicker than I can call a taxi.

Ketoacidosis, Appendicitis, generally the other way around the Paramedic tells me. 'Anti- depressants; no they won't be affecting you.' His dad also died recently; these ambulance people so understanding. When I was a kid I used to pray to God to remove all the bad parts of me and keep the good. Absolved!

Two days sitting around just to make sure, fair enough.

Prepping me for surgery, they hook me up to a *Sliding Scale*, a drip of insulin still dependent on them to come in to test my sugar on the hour, still requires me to have my own bottle of *Coke* as their instruction sheet doesn't instil any sense of urgency in getting the patient some sugar when they do need it, 'No a yoghurt is not suitable. Yes I did have *Cola*. I couldn't wait on your forty minute round trip; I'd be in a coma by now. I know I'm not allowed to eat before surgery, you just offered me a yoghurt?' She has fallen out with me now and comes back in an hour. 'So tell me about this sliding scale, it's Antrapid insulin and I won't need my night-time insulin with it? But I don't take Antrapid insulin; my body will take weeks to adjust to it. Your colleague just explained, it's going to push my sugar through the roof.' 'This is what it says on the sheet.' 'Well that sheet is no good to me. You know all about diabetes from that chart? Do you know what it's like to have your fiancée bring your sugar and test sticks into the bathroom when you're caught having a hypo during a poo? Trust me, you don't know a thing about diabetes and I'm going to make you listen to every word I have to say.'

'Not worth the paperwork,' arrogant Anaesthetist forceful and disdainful that he knows more than I, but if it's all wrong then what's the use? I engage him to ensure I won't fall into a diabetic coma, 'Test my sugar throughout, this drip doesn't take into account I'm not due any insulin and I've not eaten for two days,' and when he resigns himself to my insistence, I pass him my eyeglasses, 'Good, that's all I wanted to hear, take those for me.'

I awaken with blood sugar sky high, could have been easily avoided, could have negated blood loss and muscle tension further adding to my recovery discomfort, but no one wants to listen. 'Have you done a course?' the Recovery Nurse asks as I scream for pain meds. 'It will hurt, you have undergone surgery,' informs the self-important scrotum, 'The pain meds may take as long as twenty minutes to *normalise* you.' 'Did you know you can take sugar readings from your ear lobe?' adds a second Nurse standing around with her thumb up her arse. When did saving lives become a blinkered occupation? I'm unable to ask myself in white poker hot seething pain.

Excruciation over, I awake to my room: insulin within reach of *Beef Hoola Hoops*. D.A.F.N.E it is. Well I haven't eaten in thirty-six hours, throw a dog a bone and pass the morphine. Eighteen hours later I'm assisted scream-stumbling and faint into a taxi home.

...

Sitting outside *Starbucks*, mid to late November, chain-smoking, late forties, looks sixty, rollups and breathing for Methadone. No traditional signs of war on his form, though all the classical hallmarks of family well established within society, very much the modern tramp. On first name terms with the Police, I sit on the chair beside him, a thousand reasons why I should be in his place and he mine. He sees my discomfort and is nurturing as though I am his own kin; incredibly well spoken, tells me about having his appendix removed when he was a child, how he fell through the railing on his bed during recovery and tore it back open. He tells me of how in Darwin's eyes the appendix was, 'Remnants of the tail through an act of evolution. Would you like a couple of Valleys to help with the pain? On gratis of course, I don't want anything for them.' 'You're good thanks.'

Two weeks into recovery, I'm up and about hobbling from room to room desperate for fresh air. No signs of diabetes taking me longer to heal, the very thought of it taking fifty times longer is ridiculous, and if anything my good diet and healthy lifestyle has me healing faster than regular people. Ready to begin biting my feet with cabin fever, 'Natasha, take me out for a coffee?' 'You can't go out yet. You nearly keeled over on Monday.' 'I insist you accompany me out for a coffee, or I'm sneaking out on my own when you're at work.' 'Okay, you're an idiot.' Savouring a Black Americano, she a *Red Cup Venti Christmas Gingerbread Latte*, ventures out of thought, 'I have an idea, you know your mum is coming down for Christmas, and my parents are over, shall we get married on Christmas Eve?'

# Out of step

How will it happen? Waking up during the night, blind in one eye, too frightened to go to sleep from then on, until eventual loss of sight in the other? Vision gone blurry near useless, unable to see my children before switching off completely? Stupidly looked it up on-line; the usual diabetes foray, one hundred and one ways I'm going to die, scaremongering equals book sales. I'm taking this all in and shitting myself. A clear repeat of the *NHS* Specialist's, "As soon as the newly developed vessels leak, they will haemorrhage blood into the path of the retina, un-mapping the pathways of nerve endings to the brain resulting in blindness. Laser surgery treatment, resultant scarring, loss of night vision and peripheral vision; blurred down the middle unable to read expressions a best case scenario."

I'm going to be half dead. I'm thirty-five, directed in the continued *hangover story* from the seventeen years or so poor diabetes control of my youth.

'Am I going to be blind in the coming weeks? Will I make it till I'm forty? What is the worst-case scenario?'

'Well I wouldn't be so pessimistic.'

'Fucking hell, after what you've just said.' – Inner voice.

'Well, what is the best case?'

'That we keep your eyesight exactly how it is. That's my job.' – All smarmy because he can afford to be. All that's missing is his slippers and smoking jacket, and any sense of him knowing what he is doing. 'But first we have to get you seen by a Specialist, who can tell us exactly what it is and then they can do laser if it's required.'

I thought he was the Specialist? I'm being jammed into his definition of a *diabetic story*, which he is using to identify himself as a *Diabetes Expert*. A panic merchant repeating out loud, *the story*, with seemingly no reasonable world experience backing it up; sitting back half eagerly to have found something, half terrified at what he has found. 'You're very young to have this.' Turns out to be a fucking Optician, sitting in an *NHS* Hospital Consultancy. I can't believe I fell for it again.

*NHS* Specialist appointment received in three weeks' time to take place in six weeks' time. *NHS* Specialist appointment received in four weeks' time delayed to take place in twelve weeks' time; should have sent it in braille.

...

Thirty-two degrees of random hot summer's day this year in England, 'I'll have *Diet-Coke*,' half the glass filled with ice. God please, don't let this be the summer I go blind. Ten pounds and twelve pence for two *Diet-Cokes* as we sit, my wife holding onto both my hands outside the restaurant next door to *London Medical*. Still haven't paid for my last visit to this Private Medical Centre. Now in a Waiting Room waiting for someone to come on over and tap me on the shoulder.

...

I awaken during the night, head on the pillow, duvet tucked about my person by Natasha in my sleep. I peek open my eyes, I can see down the hall to the ensuite bathroom. I can see. I smile; I rush with emotion. I don't care what there is tomorrow because just now I manage to hold onto you. Close my eyes, remembering his words of, 'We practice a professional cautious optimism. There is no reason in this day for any diabetic to go blind.' – Prof Victor Chung (Hero). Out of step, eyes and diabetes, deterioration of sight, two years to catch up and lagging behind rejuvenated health.

...

A week today I had laser surgery to remove *abnormal* blood vessels from my eyes, and a pioneering injection of unlicensed *Lucentis*, both controlling Macular Edema and preventing further growths in legacy of poor diabetes control. All I want to say is that should this happen to you; do not be afraid.

# Dis-ease

This dis-ease, it loops and it never ends. *Starbucks, "Nine days till Christmas,"* cakes for a pound; Carrot Cake coated in icing in the fridge, *Venti Vanilla Latte.* Fucking cunting bastarding coffee and cake. Could cut out my tongue, which would be as committing suicide because I'm tired. If I eat this, I risk losing everything. I'm not a child but I act like one. Always an excuse, always an opportunity for too much insulin and a hypo outside a cake shop; always a push for permission, 'Just this once,' it never ends. Just responsibility down to me: I eat this shit and I'm dead. It never ends.

# Conclusion: my problem is

Trying so damn hard, that's what we do. If the events of dis-ease could be described by the methods of its victims, then diabetes is all about trying just so damn hard. For us, everything is in the property of the struggle and we push on.

Strange writing this conclusion, in a good way; so far removed from how my head worked such a relatively short time ago, dis-ease: the very idea of being ill has become alien to me. Skin glowing in the mirror and bouncing out of bed in the mornings, horny as a rabbit: switched on and calm, calmer than I've ever been. Allowing for time to think things through, the importance to me clearly relative to what I observe as the difference it has made for those around me. Never have I been stronger or more capable. In control, though acutely aware I'm only a single bottle of *Cherry Cola* away from it all crashing back down; I'm not scared anymore. I have great confidence sprung from health and stand evermore humoured in the notion, no one could tell from looking at me that I am *persona non grata with diabetes*.

When I started work on the project, it was all personal hurt and resentment. How can this be happening to me? How could I have been let down so badly by the people whose job it is to protect *the likes of me*, to the point where I would go blind! How could they let this happen? My biggest fear coming true, being left to rot between the cracks, I was a, *"Very angry young man,"* indeed; retribution and redemption required in equal measure; the better part of me wanting to support others. – Still I felt lonesome.

Following on from my first six months of scribbling, I reached out to the *Diabetic Community* for thoughts and opinion – would this mean anything to anyone else? Where I was fortunate to make friends with Amber, age twenty-four from Tallahassee; a bubbly girl whom had contracted diabetes only as a secondary complication to the removal of a cyst from her pancreas: in itself a secondary sacrifice to already suffering far more severe Cystic Fibrosis. I received an email from another lady, aged fifty-six from somewhere in America; reeling from the emotional toll of having been diagnosed diabetic one week prior to her sister's death due to complications from this illness. More recently I heard from a furious girl who fell to diabetes mere weeks after reading a book about a diabetic ballerina; she now spends her life trying to find the book that will make her better. And Eddie, no one told Eddie he had to eat when taking insulin, so he was hypo-ing all over the place for six months. No one I heard from felt his or her diabetes was an anonymous statistic or a randomly generated genetic conclusion; all of us acknowledge this in our *state-of-being*.

For us diabetes amplifies everything; if you feel just-not-right then broken blood sugar will make it wrong, as alcohol does an alcoholic; every bone of contention, every pulse of ill will, slight upset or lull, every wave of exhaustion and misunderstanding all amplified. Deformation of sadness, doubt, and dependency; symptoms lost in a bigger world, it leaves us wilting. We push on.

Living with a *profitable* disease is a double-edged sword, sure *they* are going to make us new medicines every fifteen years once patents for the last have run out, and these on some level will spell vast improvement over previous. But it's for us to direct and decide upon, which of these medicines is suitable *again* in meeting with our *state-of-being*, not solely encapture the requirements of a mass *Diabetes Industry's* profiteering. – It's not such a bad situation to be in; on a good day *it's not such a bad disease to have.* Our health is readily manageable with the right communication: no miracle medicine in the world is going to work without precise communication. My problem is the same as yours: my solution the same as yours.

*Before*

*At present I am lost, my character thin, my confidence gone, expectations extinguished, soaked through with doubt, nurtured in worry, close to giving up entirely. I used to be better than this, I used to look the world dead in the eye and I thought I could stare down the sun, now the world's gotten the better of me. Responsibility for everything and it's all too hard but I'm going to make myself better. Maybe it's the time I find on my hands, or my current health status. This book just seems right.*

*After*

*Seventeen years of feeling like that fly, banging its head off the bar window.*

*I'm a better person when my sugar is level. I'm nicer to be around. Content not frustrated. I do this because there is no other way. Please stay with me.*

*Now*

*Week four of being human and I have no intention of leaving this island. I crave new challenges, I want to be involved. So this is what it feels like to be young?*

*I don't feel uncomfortable all the time anymore, I feel fresh and capable. I can't remember feeling like this since I was a kid.*

*Clearing out the cobwebs and now to come to terms with having been ill for seventeen years.*

*Writing this book has made me realise how I see the world. Made me realise how high sugar has changed me. I'm actually quite a nice person.*

*I hope I'm nicer to be around and for me it's great to see how lovely the people around me are. I don't feel like everyone around me is having a go at me anymore. I don't take everything to heart and no longer feel everything is a poor reflection on me.*

*Six months on*

*Every day is lovely, the trees show me how young I am, cool breeze refreshes me, water reflecting sky and I am privileged to walk around here in the company of all you beautiful souls. The smiles of others light me up and I know tears can be recovered from. It's time to create some little ones, a George Victor, a Jack Stephen.*

*We should never and I will never again allow myself to feel guilty over being ill. I know I am doing everything I can to be healthy and that's way beyond what most non-diabetics do.*

*Thanks for letting me get this off my chest. It's true, it's not good to keep it all bottled up inside.*

*Thank you, Paul*

*Taken from 'Getting better, state of mind (original notes).'*

This new lease of life has cost me, and I'm never going to stop being upset that it may have been entirely avoidable in the first place, but again I'm more fortunate because I'm not the one watching a loved one crumble under the weight of misinformation; I haven't even lost friendship with a single person I couldn't get over. My life past this stumbling block plays out as I had wished for.

As for Stuart Cathcart, well the way I have been thinking on it; for all he took away, what he never gave me was anyone to live up to, so I have always been free, always been my own person. Whatever it was he found at the bottom of a bottle, which he couldn't find in his family; it's not important, it doesn't change anything in my life ahead. And should my son behave as my father had, would I be able to forgive him? Not for all of it, not for much of it. I'd have to work hard with him to move past and be proud of him where I could for the sins he has made as a human. The way I have treated people and I still look myself in the eye; I couldn't just walk away. They say you can't learn from other people's mistakes, but my father taught me a lot and my mother is worth a thousand of him.

My victory will be in living a prosperous life: not sink or be caught in grief, not to become defensive and stop caring and not deny. No giving up or running away. I choose to make life my own and let the past be the past; guiding me as it should.

Still, lessons learnt; I won't ever feel guilty again for being ill, not when I'm supported by you and we are trying harder than most. I will continue to go against the grain of the *Diabetes Industries'* propaganda, which has convinced so many of us for so long that we should be grateful for the drip-feeding of care and attention, leaving us eternally grateful to be chasing our own tails. – It will forever be in our hands to teach the *"honeymoon period."*

I have also learned to appreciate that most people do try to help us, and do try to understand; they just aren't professional care workers or mind readers and we have never properly informed them how to do so. Though common decency does not require a Psychotherapist and many should be ashamed. It is left to us as diabetics to lookout and offer support to our diabetic Brothers and Sisters. The opportunity to perpetuate rightful understanding for just responsibility is ours.

It does stick in my throat that on the day I started researching *'Persona non grata with diabetes,'* there were an estimated two hundred and fifty million diabetics in the world. Forty-eight months on and the same pharmaceutical company are claiming three hundred and seventy-one (million). A combined population larger than the USA! How accurate can this be? I ask how much of this is to bolster shareholder confidence. I wonder if it will help sell this book. With numbers like that though, there is certainly no room to feel lonesome.

Old scars have heeled and again I look the world straight in the eye, convinced I can stare down the sun. How I love the smell when moisture from raindrops falls upon the summer's dust.

I hope you read this and it helped you figure things out a little more. It helped me feel more human just writing it and knowing you are there.

We eat well; we train, this does not kill us.


Paul - April 2013

# On-line component: 'our

# D'

Sharing hindsight for the benefit of each other. www.pngwd.com (our D).

'Building on the foundations of the written publication, 'our D' works in conjunction with the typescript, encouraging you the reader to open up and share diabetic experience through *key life defining moments* designated under chapter headings taken from, *'Persona non grata with diabetes.'*

> *"Borne of the realisation that in writing, 'Persona non grata with diabetes,' I overcame many of the emotional quandaries cycling with the physical burden of this disease, and as such the motion of writing through the diabetic journey; especially through key life defining moments: has been of equal importance to me as any benefit gained from changed lifestyle, medication or diet."*

Taken from 'our D'

This live compendium of shared experience, working to inform social consciousness; I'm dealing with what I'm going through; just. I'm scared of what you are going through. Let's use this to give each other a heads up.

Statistics gathered; priceless data, real time disclosure of true lifetime diabetic experience, the benefits of medication, side effects and ailments. Analysis available to meticulously cross reference with unlimited numbers of clinical trial outcomes benefiting the diabetic community as a true on-going voluntary census to better inform the development of our medicine.

...

Note to reader

I will build this when the book has generated enough sales to afford me to do so.

# Coming soon: 'Persona non grata: life without insulin?'

Introduction to the next step in, 'Persona non grata: *life without insulin.*' How do diabetics in poorer, less developed countries survive? I test their combined meditative and dietary solutions on myself, while assessing, is the West responsible for the development of man-made diabetes? Should this not bear fruit, I intend to undergo beta cell transplantation to *cure* my diabetes.

ETA: January 2016

3695935R00255